THERAPEUTIC PHYSICAL MODALITIES

Therapeutic Physical Modalities

Kamala Shankar, MD
Physical Medicine and Rehabilitation Physician
Veterans Affairs Palo Alto Health Care System
Palo Alto, California

Clinical Assistant Professor (VCF)
Functional Restoration Department
Stanford University Medical Center
Stanford, California

Associate Clinical Professor
Department of Physical Medicine and Rehabilitation
University of California, Davis, School of Medicine
Davis, California

Kenneth David Randall, MPT, GCS, ATC
Lead Physical Therapist, Livermore Division
Veterans Affairs Palo Alto Health Care System
Livermore, California

HANLEY & BELFUS, INC. / Philadelphia

Publisher: HANLEY & BELFUS, INC.
Medical Publishers
210 South 13th Street
Philadelphia, PA 19107
(215) 546-7293; 800-962-1892
FAX (215) 790-9330
Web site: http://www.hanleyandbelfus.com

Note to the reader: Although the information in this book has been carefully reviewed for correctness of dosage and indications, neither the authors nor the editor nor the publisher can accept any legal responsibility for any errors or omissions that may be made. Neither the publisher nor the editor makes any warranty, expressed or implied, with respect to the material contained herein. Before prescribing any drug, the reader must review the manufacturer's current product information (package inserts) for accepted indications, absolute dosage recommendations, and other information pertinent to the safe and effective use of the product described.

Therapeutic Physical Modalities   ISBN 1-56053-434-6

© 2002 by Hanley & Belfus, Inc. All rights reserved. No part of this book may be reproduced, reused, republished, or transmitted in any form, or stored in a data base or retrieval system, without written permission of the publisher.

Last digit is the print number: 9   8   7   6   5   4   3   2   1

CONTENTS

1. History of Therapeutic Physical Modalities 1
   Tanja L. Kujac, MD, and Kamala Shankar, MD
2. Superficial Heating Modalities 7
   Doug T. Ota, MD
3. Deep-Heating Modalities 18
   Kevin Ochs, MPT, Upinder Pal Singh, MD, and Kamala Shankar, MD
4. Iontophoresis and Phonophoresis 37
   Nirmala Nayak, MD, and Kenneth D. Randall, MPT, GCS, ATC
5. Cryotherapy 47
   Kirstin Young, MD, MPH, and Eugenie Atherton, MSPT
6. Aquatic and Hydrotherapy in Rehabilitation 55
   Sandra L. Symons, PTA, and Maynard M. Tabachnick, MSPT
7. Ultraviolet Light and Laser Therapy 77
   Kevin M. Means, MD
8. Magnet Therapy 87
   Sonia Williams, MD, and Butchaiah Garlapati, MD, MPH
9. Electrical Modalities in Musculoskeletal and Pain Medicine 98
   Viviane Ugalde, MD
10. Therapeutic Exercise 121
    Rajeswari Kumar, MD, and Michelle Voss, DPT
11. Massage Therapy 143
    Sanjiv Jain, MD
12. Spinal Traction 161
    Ernest H. Winkenwerder, MPT, and Kamala Shankar, MD
13. Joint Mobilization 177
    Ida Hirst, PT
14. Taping Techniques as an Adjunct to Rehabilitation 194
    Wendy S. Burke, DPT, OCS, and Cindy Bailey, DPT, OCS, SCS, ATC
15. A Practical Guide to Biofeedback 209
    Daren Drysdale, BCIA, BSC, and Kazuko Shem, MD
16. Acupuncture in the Management of Neuromusculoskeletal Disorders 227
    *Alice M.K. Wong, MD, Simon F.T. Tang, MD,
    and Henry L. Lew, MD, PhD*
17. Basic Principles of Injection Techniques 239
    Jeffrey L. Woodward, MD, MS, and Ted A. Lennard, MD
18. Promoting Functional Independence through the Use of
    Assistive Devices and Durable Medical Equipment 261
    Sarah Eggen-Thornhill, OTR, and Jennifer Fouché, OTR
19. Mobility Aids 284
    Kenneth D. Randall, MPT, GCS, ATC

INDEX 301

CONTRIBUTORS

Eugenie Atherton, MSPT
Physical Therapist, New Orleans, Louisiana

Daren Drysdale, BCIA, BSC
Clinical Psychophysiologist, San Jose, California

Wendy S. Burke, DPT, OCS
Assistant Professor of Clinical Physical Therapy, Fellow, Medical Education, Department of Biokinesiology and Physical Therapy, University of Southern California; Supervisor of Outpatient Rehabilitation, USC University Hospital, Los Angeles, California

Cindy Bailey, DPT, OCS, SCS, ATC
Assistant Professor of Clinical Physical Therapy, Fellow, Medical Education, Department of Biokinesiology and Physical Therapy, University of Southern California; Director of Physical Therapy, Los Angeles Orthopaedic Hospital, Los Angeles, California

Sarah Eggen-Thornhill, OTR
Staff Occupational Therapist, Occupational Therapy/Physical Medicine and Rehabilitation, Veterans Affairs Palo Alto Health Care System, Palo Alto, California

Jennifer Fouché, OTR
Staff, Occupational Therapy, Occupational Therapy/Physical Therapy and Medicine, Veterans Affairs Palo Alto Health Care System, Palo Alto, California

Butchaiah Garlapati, MD, MPH
Resident, Physical Medicine and Rehabilitation, University of Arkansas for Medical Sciences, Little Rock, Arkansas

Ida Hirst, PT
Practice Owner of Physical Therapy Specialties, Pleasanton, California

Sanjiv Jain, MD
Medical Director, Inpatient Rehabilitation, Carle Foundation Hospital; Medical Director, Wound Healing Center, Carle Foundation Hospital; Staff Physiatrist, Carle Clinic Association; Director, Rehabilitation Medicine Services, McKinley Health Center, University of Illinois, Urbana, Illinois

Tanja L. Kujac, MD
Staff Physician, Department of Occupational Medicine, Kaiser Permanente Santa Clara Medical Center, Santa Clara, California; Attending Physician in Electromyography, Valley Medical Center, San Jose, California

Rajeswari Kumar, MD
Clinical Professor, Department of Medicine, UCLA School of Medicine, Los Angeles, California; Veterans Affairs Greater Los Angeles Health Care System, West Los Angeles, California

Ted A. Lennard, MD
Clinical Assistant Professor, Department of Physical Medicine and Rehabilitation, University of Arkansas for Medical Sciences, Little Rock, Arkansas; Private Practice, Springfield, Missouri

Henry L. Lew, MD, PhD
Clinical Assistant Professor, Department of Functional Restoration, Division of Physical Medicine and Rehabilitation, Stanford University School of Medicine, Palo Alto, California; Veterans Affairs Palo Alto Health Care System, Palo Alto, California

Kevin M. Means, MD
Associate Professor and Chairman, Department of Physical Medicine and Rehabilitation, University of Arkansas for Medical Sciences; Medical Director, Falls and Mobility Disorders Program, Central Arkansas Veterans Healthcare System, Little Rock, Arkansas

Nirmala Nayak, MD
Physical Medicine and Rehabilitation Staff, Veterans Affairs Northern System of Clinics, Martinez, California; Associate Clinical Professor, Department of Physical Medicine and Rehabilitation, University of California, Davis, Medical Center, Davis, California

Kevin M. Ochs, MPT, STS
Physical Therapist, Veterans Affairs Palo Alto Health Care System, Livermore, California

Doug T. Ota, MD
Staff Physician, Spinal Cord Injury Service, Veterans Affairs Palo Alto Health Care System, Palo Alto, California

Kenneth David Randall, MPT, GCS, ATC
Lead Physical Therapist, Livermore Division, Veterans Affairs Palo Alto Health Care System, Livermore, California

Kamala Shankar, MD
Physical Medicine and Rehabilitation Physician, Veterans Affairs Palo Alto Health Care System, Palo Alto, California; Clinical Assistant Professor (VCF), Functional Restoration Department, Stanford University Medical Center, Stanford, California; Associate Clinical Professor, Department of Physical Medicine and Rehabilitation, University of California, Davis, School of Medicine, Davis, California

Upinder Pal Singh, MD
Professor and Head of Department of Physical Medicine, All India Institute of Medical Sciences, New Delhi, India

Kazuko L. Shem, MD
Physical Medicine and Rehabilitation, Santa Clara Valley Medical Center, San Jose, California

Sandra L. Symons, PTA
Board Member, Northwest Aquatic Therapy Association; Seattle Veterans Affairs Hospital, Puget Sound Healthcare System (Spinal Cord Injury), Seattle, Washington

Maynard M. Tabachnick, MSPT
Vice Chairperson, Northwest Aquatic Therapy Association; Program Director, Outpatient Aquatic Physical Therapy, Veterans Affairs Puget Sound Health Care System, Seattle Division, Seattle, Washington

Simon F. T. Tang, MD
Associate Professor and Chair, Department of Physical Medicine and Rehabilitation, Chang Gung University, Chang Gung Memorial Hospital, Tao Yuan County, Taiwan

Viviane Ugalde, MD
Associate Professor, Physical Medicine and Rehabilitation, University of California, Davis; University of California, Davis, Medical Center, Sacramento, California

Michelle A. Voss, PT, DPT
Physical Therapist, Veterans Affairs Greater Los Angeles Healthcare Center, West Los Angeles, California

Sonia Williams, MD
Assistant Professor, Physical Medicine and Rehabilitation, University of Arkansas for Medical Sciences; Staff Physician, Baptist Health Rehabilitation, Little Rock, Arkansas

Ernest H. Winkenwerder, MPT
Outpatient Physical Therapist, San Jose Clinic, Palo Alto Health Care System, San Jose, California

Alice M.K. Wong, MD
Professor, Department of Physical Medicine and Rehabilitation, Chang Gung University Medical College; Chang Gung Memorial Hospital, Tao Yuan County, Taiwan

Jeffrey L. Woodward, MD, MS
Private Practitioner, Springfield, Missouri

Kirstin Young, MD, MPH
Private Practice, Redwood City, California

PREFACE

Modality—a method of application of any therapeutic agent; limited usually to physical agents.

Agent—any power, principle, or substance capable of producing an effect, whether physical, chemical, or biological.

Intervention—the act of interfering so as to modify.

Therapeutic—pertaining to the art of healing.

In this book, a variety of authors have contributed their clinical knowledge, practical experience, and the latest review of literature in the application of therapeutic modalities. The primary reason for compiling this information was to address the needs of physical therapists, occupational therapists, and physical medicine and rehabilitation physicians. In the case of the physicians and residents, we believe that this information is particularly valuable. Most of the emphasis in medical school is on the medical aspects of healing, and we believe that information on therapeutic modalities requires more careful consideration and attention. All elements of a prescription, such as reason, indication, contraindications, treatment site, intensity, frequency, and duration, should be assessed and well thought out. Additionally, the benefits of multiple modalities and their interactions should be understood by those prescribing them.

This book closely examines most of the therapeutic modalities and interventions in use today. In addition, we have included information on some of the less common modalities. In each chapter of this book, we have attempted to capitalize on the experience and insight of both physician and therapist. We believed that this was important given the traditional team approach that has been so instrumental in the success of physical medicine and rehabilitation. The chapter authors have attempted to condense the most useful information in their respective sections with emphasis on efficacy and practicality.

We would like to acknowledge all of the authors who have contributed to this text. The chapter authors and their staff have put much effort and time into this text, and we are grateful for their work.

Kamala Shankar, MD
Kenneth D. Randall, MPT, GCS, ATC

FOREWORD

This text follows in the spirit of the classic texts of Sidney Licht, MD, *Therapeutic Heat and Cold, Therapeutic Exercises, Therapeutic Electricity and Ultraviolet Radiation, Massage, Manipulation and Traction, Medical Hydrology, Medical Climatology, Orthotics, Rehabilitation and Medicine.* However, it differs by covering a large number of modalities in one volume.

Information on these various modalities is important, as there have been many recent additions and developments in this field. This book is especially valuable in reviewing and updating this information, and it nicely covers the indications and other considerations that provide the scientific bases for the use of a specific modality.

The value of this text is its thoughtful coverage of a wide array of modalities and its inclusion of the latest information on the rationales for their use.

Rene Cailliet, MD
Professor Emeritus
Department of Physical Medicine and Rehabilitation
USC School of Medicine
Professor, Department of Medicine
UCLA School of Medicine

DEDICATION

This book is dedicated to all those wonderful people who have influenced our lives and for those folks who encourage us to march forward.

Chapter 1
History of Therapeutic Physical Modalities

Tanja L. Kujac, MD, and Kamala Shankar, MD

Much of the history behind the various modalities discussed in this book has been thoroughly reported by Dr. Sidney Licht of New Haven, Connecticut. Dr. Licht was an honorary member of the British Association of Physical Medicine, the Danish Society of Physical Medicine, and the French National Society of Physical Medicine. Licht published a series of books in the late 1950s that have served as a foundation for physical medicine and rehabilitation, including *Therapeutic Exercise, Therapeutic Heat, Therapeutic Electricity and Ultraviolet Radiation*, and *Massage, Manipulation, and Traction*. This chapter will briefly revisit the history behind some therapeutic modalities that have been popular for many centuries.

SUPERFICIAL THERAPEUTIC HEAT

Superficial heat can be supplied in the form of conduction or convection. Conduction is the contact transfer of heat between two bodies of different temperatures, and convection is the flow of different temperature objects past one another. Ancient forms of heat included heated water, sand, oils, and grains as well as sun and sweat therapy. Wounded soldiers in ancient Rome were routinely sent to warm mineral springs to abate aches and pains. Other Romans used public baths as a form of relaxation and socializing. Licht noted that at one time there were over 800 public baths in Rome with water at varying temperatures so bathers could alternate exposures to both heat and cold, a precursor to today's contrast baths.[1] Today, contrast baths are most commonly applied to the hands and feet to treat rheumatoid arthritis and neuropathic conditions such as reflex sympathetic dystrophy (RSD). Soaking typically begins in warm water (43°C) for about 4–10 minutes alternating with 1–2 minutes of cooler water.

Hot water in containers made of animals skins and gourds once served as hot packs. Hippocrates recommended use of bladders filled with hot water for treating sciatica and rectal inflammation and wrote in *De affectionibus*, "When the ears become painful, bathe them and foment them abundantly with hot water."[1] Today, hot packs are widely used at temperatures of 70–80°C for 20–30 minutes. Common uses for these packs include analgesia, muscle spasm, hyperemia, and increasing collagen extensibility.[2] Other forms of conductive heat were very popular in the early 1800s through the turn of the century in France. Public hot houses used fire under a vaulted furnace that served as early convective saunas to open pores and produce sweat. Hot water baths were used to alleviate all sorts of pain. Around 1900, Gaspard Torella advocated sweating in an oven as the best way to cure small pox in 15 days. Licht noted that von Leyden and Goldscheider recommended warm water exercise in 1898. Whirled water baths were used in World War I, and the Hubbard tank was developed for aquatic exercise in 1928. Although Hubbard tanks are large and expensive to operate, they are still used today, primarily for cleansing large wounds.[3]

Barthte de Sandfort was first to describe a paraffin bath in the medical literature in 1913,[1] but melted wax was a common way to treat styes and ecchymosis of the eye in ancient times. In addition, the Romans immersed their bodies in hot oil for massage preparation. Today, paraffin baths are used primarily for treating contractures in patients with rheumatoid arthritis and tight skin and joints in patients with scleroderma. These baths consist of mineral oil and wax in a 1:7 mixture at around 52°C. Dipping is the most common method and consists of 10 cycles.[2]

DEEP HEAT

Ultrasound, a type of conversion heating (also known as a diathermy), had a number of uses in the early 1900s. The term *diathermy* was introduced in 1907 by Nagelschmidt referring to "heating through" of current.[5] As was noted by Licht, in 1912, British engineers used ultrasound to avert subsequent *Titanic*-like iceberg disasters using echoes from pulsed waves, and during World War I, ultrasound was used to detect submarines. In the late 1920s, ultrasound was shown to have more biological and physical uses. Harvey used ultrasound to destroy bacteria. Medical application of ultrasound essentially began in the late '30s with reports of ultrasound effects on various tissues. Licht noted that the first reported medical use of ultrasound was in 1938 in which Pohlmsan in Zurich used ultrasound to treat a woman with sciatica. An 800-kc generator with mineral oil as the acoustic coupling medium was used. World War II prevented further experimentation of the medical application of ultrasound until the late 1940s when Deniéré used ultrasound to treat various ailments including arthritis, asthma, scleroderma, and ankylosis.[1] Today, ultrasound is routinely used to treat RSD, tendinitis, degenerative arthritis, and contractures, as well as assisting with wound healing.[2]

The prefix *ultra-* is used in the word *ultrasound* because it uses sound waves above the human hearing range (18–20,000 Hz). The best tissue penetration occurs at 0.8–1.0 MHz, which in general causes temperature elevations of 4–5° at depths up to 8 cm. The depth of heating is dependent on the frequency used, tissue type, and the beam direction.[2] Fat is poorly absorbed compared to muscle, and the greatest absorption occurs at bone–soft tissue interfaces.[3] Penetration is much deeper when the beam is parallel instead of perpendicular to muscle fiber.[2]

Biologic effects of ultrasound are broken down into heating or nonheating. Nonthermal effects include streaming, cavitation, and standing waves. *Streaming* refers to tissue cellular movement, whereas *cavitation* is the formation of gas bubbles produced in tissue by turbulence. *Standing waves* are simply resonating sound waves within tissue.[3] Licht noted a number of studies assessing changes in blood flow caused by ultrasound. It was concluded that small ultrasound intensities cause vasodilation, and large intensities cause vasoconstriction.[1]

The application of ultrasound may be direct or indirect. Direct treatment involves placing the applicator on the skin and stroking or gliding a large flat surface (1–2 cm/sec). Indirect ultrasound treatment refers to the use of degassed water as the absorption media placed around the treated surface.[3]

Other forms of diathermy include short wave and microwave. Original shortwave treatment, also known as conventional diathermy, was administered using a spark gap generator. However, the development of the thermionic vacuum tube allowed for much higher frequencies, ranging from 10 to 40 MHz.[5] The most frequently used frequency is 27.12 MHz. Short-wave therapy is usually administered by way of capacitive coupling in which the body part being treated acts as an insulator between two plates. With the invention of the magnetron tube, extremely high frequencies called microwaves could be obtained. The two microwave diathermy frequencies used are 915 and 2456 MHz, although microwave therapy is rarely used today.[2]

MASSAGE AND TRACTION

Ancient mentions of massage describe different forms depending on the culture. Licht wrote a wonderful historical survey beginning with what may be the earliest mention of massage in the *Kong-Fou* that was written around 2700 B.C.[4] Later, massage was considered one of four main types of medical practice during the T'ang Dynasty (A.D. 600–900) in China.[4] In India, the earliest mention of massage was in the *Ayur-Veda*, in which massage was referred to as "shampooing and rubbing." The laws of Manoo that were collected in the 14th century described friction rubbing as a religious duty.[4] The term *samvahana* is a long-standing Indian term for massage. In Greece, Herodicus, a teacher of Hippocrates, referred to massage as a form of medicine that prolonged the lives of the enfeebled.[4] Hippocrates was reported to be the first to mention benefits and contraindications of massage. In his book *On Articulations*, he stated, "Friction can bind a joint that is too loose and loosen joint that is too rigid" and that friction "can cause parts to waste; moderate rubbing makes them grow."[4] Hippocrates was also quoted as saying, "Vigorous frictions harden the fiber, light frictions loosen it. When pursued a long time, weight is lost; applied in moderation they increase weight." Areraeus advised massage of the limbs for treating epilepsy and also recommended rubbing the legs for headaches and vertigo. Following Hippocrates, the renowned Greek physician Galen discussed specific massage techniques such as rubbing obliquely or transversely. He also classified massage into three quantities and qualities.[4]

Today, massage terminology and techniques are attributed to Per Henrik Link who, in the early 19th century, adopted French terms that arose from ancient writings. These include *effleurage, petrissage, friction massage*, and *tapotement*. Effleurage consists of stroking and gliding movements, petrissage consists of kneading, and tapotement consists of percussion.[2] The common uses of massage include general relaxation, decreasing muscle spasms and edema, loosening fascia, breaking up adhesions, and stretching skin scars. Average duration of massage is 5–15 minutes, depending on the therapeutic intent.[2] Massage is contraindicated over malignancy, infected tissue, and open wounds. Myofascial release is a form of massage that involves the application of prolonged pressure with simultaneous passive range of motion (ROM) to stretch focal areas of tightness.[2]

Although forms of traction date back as far as massage, the word *traction* was not used historically. Instead, traction was described in terms of ropes and pulleys. Licht noted that in Hippocrates' book *Mochlichus*, traction was applied to reduce "gibbosity."[4] Also, drawings dating from A.D. 900 by the Byzantine physician Niketas portrayed traction for reducing dislocations. In 1542, Guido Guidi, founder of the first medical school in Paris, translated Niketas' works into French, including over 100 diagrams of various forms of traction.[4] There was a revival of spinal traction in the third and fourth decades of this century, and Cyriax popularized lumbar traction in the 1950s. Today, traction is most commonly used for cervical disease, especially radiculopathy. Although lumbar traction trials are often used by physical therapists, lumbar traction has not proven to be as beneficial as cervical traction.[11]

THERAPEUTIC EXERCISE

According to Licht, the ancient Chinese form of exercise known as Cong Fou is the oldest example of therapeutic exercise. Developed around 1000 B.C., the Cong Fou were motions and positions prescribed by Taoist priests to relieve pain and other hindering symptoms.[9] Exercises consisted of breathing routines with little motions. Licht also noted that Hippocrates categorized three types of medical practitioners, one of which is a gymnast, one who studies diet and exercise.

Historically, exercise was recommended for a number of different reasons including weight reduction, mental relaxation, strengthening weak muscles, and treating incurable illnesses. Today, therapeutic exercise has been redefined to mean a specific treatment to a specific part of the body. This includes stretching techniques, range of motion exercises, strengthening, aerobic, and proprioception therapy.[10] Often these exercises are administered by physical and occupational therapists with specific prescriptions from the treating physician.

BIOFEEDBACK

Biofeedback is a form of operant conditioning in which one learns to take over his or her physiologic parameters (i.e., a highly specific response could be learned). The goal of biofeedback is eventually to remove the measure instrumentation (e.g., skin temperature, electromyography [EMG]) to control the desired response without monitoring.[6] For biofeedback to be successful the parameters must be measurable, the patient must receive continuous information, and the patient must be highly motivated.[6] Historically, biofeedback has been used to treat tension headaches through muscle relaxation, to control heart rate and blood pressure through voluntary visceral control, and to treat migraines through control of peripheral temperature regulation.[7] This type of autogenic therapy shifts the treatment responsibility to the patient. In the 1950s, Whatmore and Kohli experimented with EMG biofeedback, and in the mid 1970s electromyographic feedback was added to treat tension headaches. The Biofeedback Research Society was formed by a group of researchers in 1969.[8]

Other disorders treated with various forms of biofeedback include Raynaud's phenomenon, spastic hands, low back pain, overuse injuries, and excessive anxiety and arousal in athletes.[7] In the authors' experience, biofeedback is also beneficial for patients with chronic myofascial disorders and may be used as an alternative and adjunct treatment in refractory industrial-related injuries.

MAGNETS

In the early 16th century, a Swiss physician alchemist, Paracelsus, used magnets to treat epilepsy, diarrhea, and hemorrhage. In the 18th century, Franz Mermer, an Australian physician, had a popular magnetic healing salon in Paris. The purpose of the salon was to treat untoward effects of innate animal magnetism. Dr. Perkins used a metal magnetic wedge to cure injuries in Connecticut in 1799. In the late 1800s, Sears catalogue advertised magnetic boot inserts. In the late 20th century with the increasing interest in complementary and alternative medicine, magnet therapy for pain management has become a multi-million dollar business. In the 19th and 20th century, electromagnetic gadgets were popularized by many groups. Currently, magnetic necklaces, bracelets, mattresses, wrist supports, knee and ankle supports, low back elastic supports, magnetic gloves, and insoles are available, and with internet advertisement, use of these are all the more popular.

The use of magnets varies widely. Therapies can be divided into two categories: stationary and alternating. Stationary fields are generated by magnets whereas alternating fields are generated by electrical devices. Stationary magnets can be applied closely to acupuncture points of specific organs. Magnets have been used to treat muscle spasms, strains, tendinitis, arthritis, and chest pain. There is some literature on experimental benefits with epileptic seizures, anxiety, and depression. It is too early to determine if these anecdotal benefits reported have any long-standing therapeutic effect or side effects.

ACUPUNCTURE

The oldest records of acupuncture are found on bone etchings from 1600 B.C. The first book of acupuncture, which contains a wealth of details, is the *Huang Di Nei Jing* (The Yellow Emperors' Classic) written around the 2nd century B.C.[12] Between the Han Dynasty (206 B.C.–A.D. 200) and the Ming Dynasty (A.D. 1368–1644), acupuncture practice underwent refinement. The *Zhen Jiu Da Cheng* (Great Compendium of Acupuncture and Moxibustion) of Yang Ji-Zhou was published in 1601, which influenced acupuncture practice in Asia and Europe in the 17th century. In the early 19th century, French, English, German, Italian, and Swedish physicians experimented with this technique. Especially noteworthy are the teachings and publications of George Soulié de Morant during this period.

In Western medicine, we have an intricate knowledge of anatomy, microscopic anatomy, and the chemistry and biochemistry of the body but little knowledge of what actually makes it "tick." It was this energy at the root of all life that was the primary interest of the ancient Chinese. Thus, the ancient Chinese concentrated on the elaborate system of forces whose interplay regulated all the functions of the body. *Qi* ("life energy"), one of the fundamental concepts of Chinese thought, is the manifestation of any invisible force. In classical acupuncture, many energy channels traverse the body. In all diseases, whether physical or mental, there are tender areas at certain points on the surface of the body, which disappear when the illness is cured. These are the so-called acupuncture points.

All the acupuncture points belonging to any one of these groups are joined by a line; the Chinese word for this, *Jing*, means "a passage," or today forms part of the Chinese word for *nerve*. In the West, these lines are called *meridians*. There are 12 paired meridians and two in the midline. The twelve main meridians are lung, large intestine, stomach, spleen, heart, small intestine, bladder, kidney, pericardium, triple warmer, gall bladder, and liver. The number of acupuncture points along each of these meridians varies. The heart meridian, for example, has nine points on each side, whereas the bladder meridian has sixty-seven. All the acupuncture points on a meridian affect the organ after which they are named. The classification of the many acupuncture points to well-defined meridians is very helpful in practice, e.g. which organ patient has the disease, the acupuncture points in that meridian could be treated.

In certain medical schools in China, Chinese medicine and Western medicine are taught in different departments of the same university. In some hospitals, the two groups of medical practitioners work together in the management of some patients.

SUMMARY

Many therapeutic modalities and interventions have been in use for several hundred centuries for treatment of many ailments. Some continue to be used, such as superficial heat, while others, such as microwave diathermy, were once popular but have gone out of fashion. Yet others, such as acupuncture and massage, have regained popularity with the recent trend of complementary medicine techniques.

REFERENCES

1. Licht S: Therapeutic Heat. New Haven, CT, Elizabeth Licht, 1958, p 466.
2. O'Young B, Young MA, Stiens S (eds): PM&R Secrets. Philadelphia, Hanley & Belfus, 1997, p 602.
3. DeLisa JA, Gans B (eds): Rehabilitation Medicine, 2nd ed. Philadelphia, J.B. Lippincott, 1993, p 1238.
4. Licht S: Massage, Manipulation, and Traction. New Haven, CT, Elizabeth Licht, 1960, p 275.
5. Osborne S: Diathermy: The Use of High Frequency Currents. Springfield, IL, Charles C. Thomas, 1950.
6. Fadem B: Behavioral Science, 2nd ed. Philadelphia, Harwal, 1994, p 237.
7. Sinaki M: Basic Clinical Rehabilitation Medicine, 2nd ed. St. Louis, Mosby, 1993, p 554.
8. Winer LR: Biofeedback: A guide to the clinical literature. Am J Orthopsychiatry 47:626–638, 1977.
9. Licht S: Therapeutic Exercise, 3rd ed. New Haven, CT, Elizabeth Licht, 1961, p 959.
10. Shankar K (ed): Exercise Prescription. Philadelphia, Hanley & Belfus, 1998, p 498.
11. Braddom R (ed): Physical Medicine and Rehabilitation. Philadelphia, W.B. Saunders, 1996, p 1301.
12. Mann F: Acupuncture: The Ancient Chinese Art of Healing and How It Works Scientifically. New York, Random House, 1971.

Chapter 2
Superficial Heating Modalities

Doug T. Ota, MD

The use of superficial heat for therapeutic effects has a long history. It has been used in the form of dry heat such as the sun, heating pads, or water bottles, and wet heat, such as hot baths and saunas. Conditions for which heat has been used include pain relief, general relaxation, decreasing spasms, and improving range of motion (ROM). Superficial heat modalities, which are a form of thermotherapy, include hot packs, heating pads, paraffin baths, fluidotherapy, hydrotherapy, and infrared lamps. Hydrotherapy is covered in Chapter 6.

Regardless of the type of superficial heat modality, certain characteristics are common to all forms. Superficial heat modalities have maximum temperature elevations at depths of approximately 1 cm. This is a result of the limitation of penetration only to the skin and subcutaneous tissue. If deeper heat penetration is desired, for example, into muscles or deep joint capsules, then an alternative modality must be considered such as ultrasound.

Superficial heat modalities are considered to be an adjunctive treatment to be used in conjunction with other treatments including ROM, stretching, and exercise in order to achieve an appropriate beneficial response. For example, if the treating physician provides only analgesics and therapeutic modalities to treat an athlete's symptoms (e.g., pain, swelling, or stiffness), the athlete will not be able to return to activity safely or effectively.[1]

The determination in selecting and administering superficial heat modalities is multifactorial and requires an understanding of the patient, the condition being treated, and the characteristics and limitations of the modality. For example, the effect of superficial heating is a result of a direct influence on local tissues as well as an indirect effect on deeper and distal tissues. An understanding of direct and indirect effects of heat is necessary to choose the appropriate modality for treatment. Another factor to consider is that body habitus influences the modality selected in that subcutaneous adipose tissue affects the depth of penetration of many modalities.[2] Adipose tissue has a lower conductivity, which limits the ability of heat to penetrate through the subcutaneous layer. Also, in selecting a modality, one must realize that there are a few well-designed clinical trials demonstrating the efficacy of specific modalities to specific conditions.[2]

METHODS OF HEAT TRANSFER

Heat is transferred from one source to another source from one of three methods: conduction, convection, or conversion.

Conduction is the transfer of thermal energy between two bodies in direct contact. The transfer of heat occurs when there is a difference in temperature between the two objects. As the temperature increases in the colder object, the energy and, subsequently, the heat decreases in the warmer object unless there is a constant input of energy into the warmer object such as an electrical heating pad. Examples of conduction include heating pads, hot packs, and paraffin baths.

Convection is the transfer of heat between two objects of different temperature that are in direct contact with one another but one of the objects is flowing relative to the other object. The temperature gradient is maximized in this condition, which produces a higher intensity of heating. Examples of convection include whirlpools and fluidotherapy.

Conversion is the transfer of heat by the conversion of energy such as sound waves and infrared rays to heat and is dependent on the resistive properties of the material. An example of conversion is infrared lamps.

INDICATIONS

Analgesia

Analgesia is a frequent indication for the use of superficial heat modalities (Table 1). Although the direct effect of heat from a superficial modality is limited to the skin and subcutaneous tissue, the indirect effect of heat on pain modulation may relate to more complex mechanisms of impairment to nerve impulses from reaching the higher central pain centers. Inhibition of the pain impulses as described by the gate theory is one possible mechanism. Large alpha-beta fibers, carrying afferent impulses to the substantia gelatinosa in the dorsal horn of the spinal cord, inhibit the ability of A-delta and C fibers from fully conducting to synapses. The pain-generated impulses are blocked from reaching higher level sensory pain centers, thereby providing an analgesic effect.[3]

On et al. investigated the analgesic effect of local superficial heating following a painful electrical stimulus. Sympathetic skin response amplitudes decreased significantly following local heating and did not return to their initial levels within 15 minutes after the heat application was stopped. The analgesic effect may have been due to suppression of cortical pain sensation from increased levels of endorphins, as well as local inhibition of afferent C fibers.[4]

Additional studies have postulated a more direct effect of superficial heat on pain modulation. The application of infrared radiation over the ulnar nerve at the elbow in human subjects demonstrated an analgesic effect of the distal arm in the area supplied by the nerve. Also, when the modality was applied to the skin, demonstrated an increase in pain threshold was demonstrated. These effects were thought to be due to temporary conduction block.[5]

Spasticity

Spasticity can occur from various causes. Spasticity as a result of direct injury to muscles or tendons can occur from overuse injuries or direct trauma. Muscle spasms may also occur as a result of a guarding mechanism to protect associated structures. For example, a lumbar disk herniation may produce spasms in the

TABLE 1. GENERAL INDICATIONS FOR SUPERFICIAL HEAT MODALITIES

Analgesia
Muscle spasm
Hyperemia
Accelerating metabolic process
Improve joint range of motion

lumbar paravertebral musculature to restrict back motion and prevent further injury. The sustained contractions of the muscles produce pain, inducing further muscle spasms. This results in a spasm–pain–spasm cycle. Superficial modalities are used as an adjunct treatment to disrupt the cycle, allow resolution of the muscle spasm, and improve pain control. The mechanisms by which this may occur are not clearly understood. However, many patients find that heat has an overall relaxing quality that contributes to the decrease in spasticity.

One study showed that the application of heat decreased frequency of impulses along the gamma motor neurons.[6] The efferent gamma motor neurons innervate the muscle spindles, which are involved with the stretch reflex arc. Decreasing gamma efferent impulses diminishes the stretch reflex and subsequently decreases alpha motor activity. The result is muscle relaxation.

Fountain and associates evaluated the effect of ultrasound, hot packs, and infrared radiation on static forces of the neck in patients with poliomyelitis. They found that a decrease of resistance in passive lateral flexion of the neck musculature and, therefore, a decrease in spasticity, with each of the three modalities. The effect of the modalities remained 15 minutes after the application of the modalities had ceased.[7]

Hyperemia

Superficial heating has been demonstrated to produce hemodynamic changes. Heat produces a local vasodilator response in the superficial blood vessels that dissipates the heat away from the area. It has been demonstrated that forearm blood flow may increase threefold following treatment with hydrotherapy at a temperature of 45°C.[8] Correlating with the increased blood flow is an increase in metabolism. In the acute inflammatory stage, this may have deleterious effects because it can lead to increased edema and hemorrhage. However, in the chronic inflammatory stage, heat can assist with the resolution of inflammation from the vasodilatation effects by increasing nutrients, antibodies, and leukocytes and clearing metabolic elements.

Range of Motion and Stretching

Although superficial heat modalities have a limited depth of penetration into tissue, in areas where there is little adipose tissue or soft tissue covering, such as the hands and feet, application of heat is beneficial for ROM and stretching exercises owing to the effect on soft tissue. Several studies have evaluated the effect of heat on soft tissues.

An evaluation of the extensibility of a rat tail tendon under conditions of stretching, heat, and combination of heat and stretching simultaneously showed that extensibility was maximized with heat and stretching combination.[9] Additional studies have demonstrated that the extensibility of tendons can be maintained after elongation with the combination of heat and stretching simultaneously when the stretching is continued during the cool-down period. The experimental findings suggest that the use of heating modalities in conjunction with physical therapy increases extensibility of collagen tissues including tendons and joint capsules[10,11] and reinforces the notion that superficial heating modalities should be used in conjunction with other therapies to improve therapeutic response.

Wright and colleagues demonstrated the effect of superficial heat applied to the metacarpophalangeal joint. They showed that heating the surface temperature to 45°C by an infrared lamp produced a 20 percent decrease in stiffness in the joint compared with the stiffness at 33°C.[12]

CONTRAINDICATIONS

There are several conditions in which the treating provider must not use heat thermotherapy as a form of treatment (Table 2). Acute injuries, hemorrhage, and acute inflammation are contraindicated due to the vasodynamic effects of heat. In the initial stages of an acute injury, heat will exacerbate the condition by increasing edema and hematoma formation from the increase in blood flow and increased endothelial lining permeability. This ultimately will impair the healing process.

Processes in which hemorrhage is of concern should not be treated with heat due to the increase in blood flow with heat therapy. This includes persons who have bleeding disorders, such as hemophilia, or whom have chronic atrophic skin changes associated with prolonged steroid use that may result in increased friability of the capillary system.

The application of heat in an area of ischemia is contraindicated because metabolic demands are increased as a result of the application of heat and may exceed the supply that can be provided through the impaired vasculature system. This can lead to infarction of tissue. Also, burning of tissue can occur more readily in ischemic areas as the rate of destruction exceeds the ability of the body to supply the necessary elements to repair the tissue. The risk of burn formation also increases, because heat will accumulate when the arterial inefficiency prevents adequate shunting of heat away from the heated area.

Areas that are insensate should not be treated with the application of heat, because the ability to receive pain feedback is impaired. The patient's ability to report excessive heat depends on intact receptors and pain pathways. Heat and pain fibers begin firing at approximately 43–45°C,[13] and tissue damage can begin at 45°C.[14] The inability to sense heat and pain prevents the treating provider and the patient from knowing when the safe levels of pain threshold have been exceeded. This factor increases the risk of burns. Patients with spinal cord injuries may receive heat application above the level of injury provided the sensation is normal. When there is uncertainty about the intactness of the sensation in the area to be treated with the application of heat, formal temperature testing using warm and cold objects as well as pinprick sensation should be assessed before the application of any heat process.

TABLE 2. GENERAL CONTRAINDICATIONS FOR SUPERFICIAL HEAT MODALITIES

Acute inflammation
Hemorrhage
Bleeding disorders
Insensate skin, e.g., spinal cord injury
Ischemic areas
Local areas of malignancy
Inability to communicate or respond to pain, e.g., coma, dementia

Localized areas of malignancy including metastasis are contraindicated because the heat and subsequent increase in metabolic activity may increase the growth of the tumor. Also, theoretically the increase in blood flow may increase the likelihood of metastasis.[10]

Heat therapy is contraindicated in conditions that impair a patient's ability to communicate or respond to pain, such as dementia, delirium, or other forms of cognition impairments. Again, the inability to identify correctly when the pain threshold has been exceeded and adequately convey this information to the treating provider increases the risk of burns to tissue.

THERAPEUTIC AGENTS

The response of tissue to heat is dependent on several factors: the intensity of the heat, the duration of the heat, and the area treated. The therapeutic range of temperature is typically between 40°C and 45°C. Between 45°C and 50°C, the rate at which burns occur doubles for every 1° increase.[14] The duration for superficial modalities is typically limited to 20–30 minutes. Temperatures reach a maximum after 3–5 minutes, and beyond 30 minutes, there is no significant increase in blood flow. Frequency is dependent on the condition treated and the patient response to therapy. If the patient has not had relief with a trial of 10 treatments or approximately 2–3 weeks, then a different therapeutic approach should be considered.[15] As a general precaution, repeated and prolong skin exposure to heat has been shown to result in erythema ab igne, a skin condition of brown mottled pigmentation and telangiectasia.[16]

Hot Packs

Hot packs consist of silica beads or gel encased in a canvas pack (Fig. 1). The silica can absorb several times its volume in water. Hot packs come in a variety of shapes and sizes, allowing them to be customized to fit the area to be treated, including the low back and cervical regions (Fig. 2). Because the heat source is not

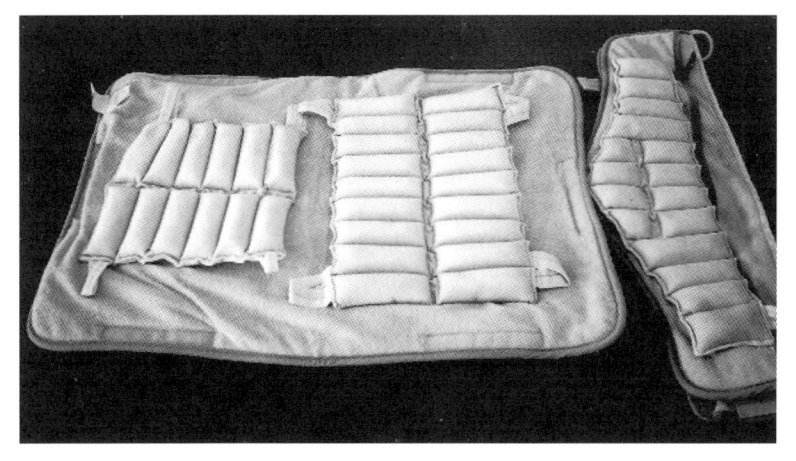

FIGURE 1. Hot packs come in a variety of shapes and sizes to accommodate various areas of the body, including the cervical and lumbar regions.

12   Superficial Heating Modalities

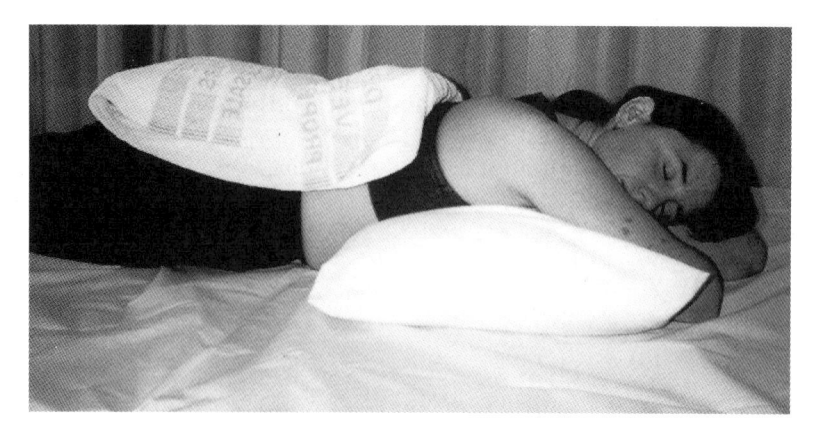

FIGURE 2. The hot pack applied over a patient.

constantly applied to the hot packs, the heat dissipates quickly as it transfers from the hot packs to the body part.

The packs are immersed in hot water tanks overnight to allow them to absorb moisture and heat. The packs are heated to a temperature of 70–80°C. The hot packs are removed from the water tanks and wrapped in six to twelve layers of towels. Some hot pack manufacturers supply terry cloth cases, providing the equivalent of three to six layers of toweling. Because of the high heat of the packs when they are removed from the water, they must be wrapped to prevent burns of the skin. The more towels applied, the greater the decrease in conduction between the hot pack and the skin and, therefore, less elevation in skin temperature. Typically, the elevation in skin temperature ranges from 37.8°C to 46.1°C.[10]

Hot packs should not be placed under the patient. This can increase the risk of burns by the increased extraction of water from the packs. Patients who cannot tolerate the weight of the hot packs can be placed on their side with the pack draped over the treatment area so the amount of direct weight on patients is minimized. Otherwise alternative heating applications should be considered.

The patient's skin should be checked at 5-minute intervals to assess for signs of excessive heat exposure such as mottling of the skin. The duration of treatment is 20–30 minutes. After treatment, the packs should be return to the tank for 30 minutes before initiating the next treatment.

An advantage of the hot pack is that it is usable where other modalities such as water immersion cannot reach, for example, the neck region. A disadvantage of the hot pack is that some people cannot tolerate the weight of the pack.

Infrared Lamps

Infrared lamps are a form of conversion heat. Radiant energy, in the form of photons, is emitted from all substances and is converted into heat. Infrared rays are located in the electromagnetic spectrum that is beyond the red portion of visible light. Infrared radiation is divided into two spectrums. **Near-infrared**, or luminous, includes some visible light and has a wavelength of 770–1500 nm; and **far-infrared** or nonluminous, has a wavelength of 1500–12,500 nm.

The depth of penetration as well as the thermal energy produced in the body surface is dependent on the wavelength.[16] As the wavelength increases, the depth of the penetration decreases. Near-infrared electromagnetic energy has a depth of penetration of 5–10 mm. Far infrared has a depth of penetration of approximately 2 mm.

The amount of energy that is absorbed and converted to heat depends on other factors as well. The angles at which the rays strike the surface influence the intensity of the thermal reaction. The amount of radiation absorbed is greatest when the rays are perpendicular to the surface. As the rays angle away from the perpendicular, the rays are refracted away from the surface and the intensity decreases in proportion to the cosine of the angle. Another factor that influences the intensity of the radiant heating is the distance of the source from the surface being treated. This is determined by the inverse square law, which states that the intensity of irradiation varies inversely with the square of the distance from the source. Therefore, as the distance is halved, the intensity increases fourfold.

The infrared generators are divided into two categories: luminous and nonluminous. Luminous rays are produced by tungsten carbon filament lamps and include portions of the visual spectrum from which visible light is located. Spiral coils of metal wire wrapped around nonconductive material produce the nonluminous rays, although some visible light is produced as indicated by the low-intensity glow. Electricity flowing over the wire meets resistance, producing rays. The luminous lamps have a deeper penetration into the subcutaneous tissue because of its smaller wavelengths.

When using infrared lamps, the patient is cleaned of all ointments, and jewelry is removed from the treating area (Fig. 3) Areas that are not treated should be covered with protective towels, especially the eyes and hair. The lamp is positioned approximately 20–45 cm from the surface to be treated. The distance is determined in part by the patient's tolerance to heat, as well as specifications of the particular piece of equipment, which is dependent on the lamp's wattage. Also, the lamp should not be adjusted while it is over the patient because of the risk of the lamp falling on the patient.[17] The skin should be checked frequently to assess for mottling and burns. Burns are more likely to occur over bony prominences or areas where the lamps are placed too close to the body. With repetitive intense treatments, skin pigmentation changes may occur.

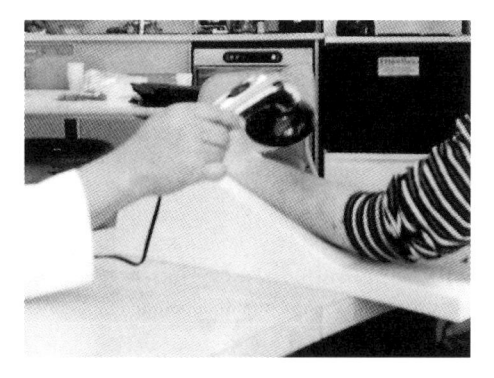

FIGURE 3. Infrared lamp used directly over.

The main advantage of infrared treatment is that it does not involve weight on the body and, therefore, is tolerated by patients who cannot tolerate direct contact or weight such as hot packs. Also, larger surfaces can be treated, particularly the thoracolumbar region. The main disadvantage of infrared treatment is the risk of burns, particularly over the bony prominences, as well as the drying effect, which may be intolerable to some patients.

Paraffin Baths

Paraffin baths are another form of conductive heat transfer. Paraffin, which typically melts at 54.5°C, stays liquid with a melting point of 47.8°C when mixed with mineral oil.[18] Mixing the wax with the mineral oil results in a substance with a lower specific heat, which allows patients to tolerate a much higher temperature than water therapy. The therapeutic temperatures of paraffin baths are typically 48–54°C.

Therapeutic effects are typically for decreasing pain or to increase soft tissue extensibility. It is used primarily for the distal extremities including the hands and feet. Although temperature penetration is limited to approximately 1 cm, in the distal extremities, this typically is sufficient.

Paraffin mixture is commercially available and is mixed in a ratio of 6:1 or 7:1 of wax to mineral oil. The mixture is heated in plastic or stainless steel tanks (Fig. 4). The units have built-in heating thermometers, which are set to a temperature of 45–57°C.[17] Before treatment the extremity must be cleaned to prevent bacterial build-up at the bottom of the paraffin bath, which may occur over time with repetitive use.

There are three principal methods of applying liquid paraffin. In the dipping technique, the body part is repetitively dipped in the paraffin bath so that layers of paraffin are applied. The first layer must completely cover the body part treated so that subsequent layers cannot get between the first layer and the skin. If this occurs, the heat will be prevented from dissipating, and a burn may occur.[19] It is also important to instruct the patient not to move the fingers or foot because the paraffin may crack and compromise the protective barrier of the first layer. The body

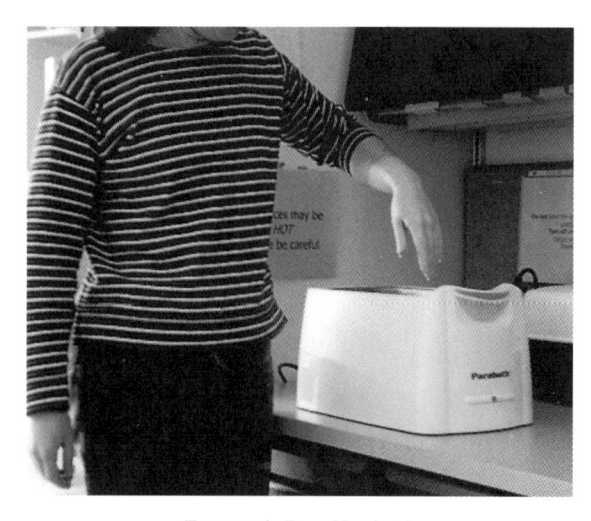

FIGURE 4. Paraffin bath.

part is then removed from the paraffin and wrapped in plastic followed by a towel. This insulates the paraffin and produces a mild to moderate amount of heat.

The second technique involves submersion of a body part, particularly the hands and feet. With this technique, the body part is initially dipped and then removed. The initial layer solidifies against the cooler skin, forming a protective barrier from higher temperatures. The body part is then reimmersed and maintained submerged in the bath for 15 minutes. This method produces a higher temperature in the skin compared with the dipping technique.[20]

The third technique involves brushing the paraffin on the desired body part with up to 10 coats. This is often done on areas of the body that are not conducive to dipping in the paraffin. This technique typically produces only slight increases in temperature. After completion of the treatment, the paraffin is then peeled off the skin.

An advantage of the paraffin bath is that it provides an even heat over irregularly shaped body areas, especially the hand, foot, and ankle region, reducing the risk of burns over the bony prominences. The disadvantage is that it is messy. Also, open wounds and infected wounds should not be immersed in a paraffin bath because heat can exacerbate the condition, and there is the risk of contamination to the tank and the wound.

Fluidotherapy

Fluidotherapy is a relatively new form of superficial heat therapy. The device has been in existence since the 1970s. Fluidotherapy is a form of dry heat, and the transfer of energy is by convection. Fine solid particles in the form of silica or cellulose such as corncob particles are heated and suspended in warm air that is forced through the particles. The properties of fluidotherapy are similar to liquid.

An evaluation of fluidotherapy compared with whirlpool and paraffin baths showed that heat absorption was greatest with fluidotherapy during a 15-minute treatment of the hand.[21] The three methods were also compared using in vivo temperature measurements of the joint capsule in the hands and feet. The temperature rises were noted to be greatest with fluidotherapy.[22]

The typical temperature range for the fluidotherapy can be varied depending on the setting of the air. Temperatures are usually between 38°C and 50.6°C, depending on the patient's tolerance.

There are variations among the fluidotherapy units, with the smaller units able to accommodate distal extremities such as the hand and foot. Larger units can accommodate proximal portions of the extremities including the thigh. The application of fluidotherapy initially involves removing all jewelry on the involved extremity. Open wounds should be protected with plastic covering to prevent particles from becoming embedded in the wound. The patient inserts the body part to be treated through a sleeve and into the unit. While the hand or foot is in the unit, exercises including stretching and ROM can be performed. The duration of the treatment is typically 15–20 minutes. On completion of the therapy, the unit is turned off and the patient removes as many particles are possible before removing the body part from the unit.

The advantage of fluidotherapy is that it is a dry heat with a lower specific heat, which allows higher temperatures to be used compared with hydrotherapy. In addition, owing to the fluid nature, irregular body surfaces such as the hands and feet can achieve uniform temperature without increased risk of burns over bony prominences. Also, the patient is able to move the limb so that exercise can be performed simultaneously, which can produce an improved stretch compared to using heat alone or stretching alone.

Heating Pads

Heating pads typically come in two forms: electric and water filled. The electric heating pad generates heat from the flow of electrical current through wires in the pad, and the temperature is regulated by the control of the current flow. The water-filled pads generate heat by circulating water through tubing in the unit. Water-filled heating pads control temperature thermostatically, allowing for safer control compared to electric heating pads.

Heating pads are pliable, which allows them to be applied or wrapped around body surfaces that are curved, such as the leg and lumbar region. Unlike the hot pack, heating pads provide a continuous supply of heat. Heating pads are used frequently in the home setting and in institutions, particularly for pain relief and muscle spasms in the back and neck region. They are readily available from a variety of manufacturers and are used in an unsupervised setting. Therefore, in addition to the general precautions and contraindications for the use of heat modalities, the patient should be instructed on the proper use of a heating pad.

Injuries do occur with improper use of electric heating pads. Annually, the Consumer Product Safety Commission receives reports of an average of eight deaths from heating pads, mostly due to fires. Fires occur when the insulation breaks or becomes worn, allowing the electrical wires in the pad to ignite the material, or when the electric cords become cracked. Burns are another concern with electric heating pads. At the low setting of an electric heating pad, the temperature can reach 51°C.[23] Also, at the lowest setting with a temperature of 42°C, second-degree burns can be produced in 12–20 hours.[23] Patients should be instructed not to use heating pads for longer than 30 minutes. The heating pad should be placed over the body part, not underneath, because this will produce increased focal heating and trapping of heat, increasing the risk of developing a burn.

Gel Packs

Gel packs are another form of superficial heat modality that is available for home use. Gel packs are filled with a gelatinous material that can be frozen or heated. They are available from a variety of manufacturers and come in various shapes and sizes. The packs are heated by placing them in water that was previously boiled for 5–10 minutes or by placing them in the microwave for 30–60 seconds. The pack is then wrapped in a towel or insulated sleeve and applied to the body part for 20–30 minutes. The gel packs are convenient and simple to use, but the heat dissipates quickly from the pack.

CONCLUSION

Superficial heating modalities, when selected appropriately and used in conjunction with other treatment options including ROM, stretching, and exercise, can be an effect treatment option for various conditions. The treating provider's understanding of the physiologic response to heat, pathophysiology of the condition to be treated, and response of the patient to the treatment are paramount to developing an appropriate treatment plan.

REFERENCES

1. Torg JS, Vegso JJ, Torg E: Modalities. In Torg TS (ed): Rehabilitation of Athletic Injuries: An Atlas of Therapeutic Exercise. Chicago, Year Book, 1987, pp 1–8.
2. Weber DC, Brown AW: Physical agent modalities. In Braddom R, (ed): Physical Medicine and Rehabilitation. Philadelphia, WB Saunders, 1996, pp. 449–463.
3. Denegar CR, Donley PB: Managing pain with therapeuticmodalities. In Prentice WE (ed): Therapeutic Modalities for Allied Health Professionals. New York, McGraw-Hill, 1998, pp 28–48.
4. On AY, Colakoglu Z, Hepguler S, Aksit R: Local heat effect on sympathetic skin responses after pain of electrical stimulus. Arch Phys Med Rehabil 78:1196–1199, 1997.
5. Lehmann JF, Brunner GD, Stow RW: Pain threshold measurements after therapeutic application of ultrasound, microwaves and infrared. Arch Phys Med Rehabil 39:560–565, 1958.
6. DonTigny R, Sheldon K: Simultaneous use of heat and cold in treatment of muscle spasms. Arch Phys Med Rehabil 43:235–237, 1962.
7. Fountain F, Gersten J, Sengir O: Decrease in muscle spasm produced by ultrasound, hot packs, and infrared radiation. Arch Phys Med Rehabil 41:293–298, 1960.
8. Abramson DI, Chu LSW, Tuck S: Effect of tissue temperatures and blood flow on motor nerve conduction velocity. JAMA 198:1082–1088, 1966.
9. Warren C, Lehmann J, Koblanski J: Heat and stretch procedures: An evaluation using rat tail tendon. Arch Phys Med Rehabil 57:122–126, 1976.
10. Lehmann JF, Warren CG, Scham SM: Therapeutic heat and cold. Clin Orthop Rel Res 99:207–245, 1974.
11. Wright V, Johns RJ: Quantitative and qualitative analysis of joint stiffness in normal subjects and in patients with connected tissue diseases. Ann Rheum Dis 20:36–45, 1961.
12. Lehman JF, Masock AJ, Warren CG: Effects of therapeutic temperatures on tendon extensibility. Arch Phys Med Rehabil 51:481–487, 1970.
13. Weisberg J: Pain. In Hecox B, Mehreteab TA, Weisberg J (eds): Physical Agents. East Norwalk, CT, Appleton & Lange, 1994, pp 37–48.
14. Moritz A: Studies of thermal injury. Part 2: The relative importance of time and surface temperature in the causation of cutaneous burns. Am J Path 23:695–720, 1947.
15. Weber DC, Stillwell GK: Therapeutic Heat and Cold. In Sinaki M (ed): Basic Clinical Rehabilitation Medicine. St. Louis, Mosby-Year Book, 1993, pp 435–440.
16. Dover JS, Phillips TJ, Arndt KA: Cutaneous effects and therapeutic uses of heat with emphasis on infrared radiation. J Am Acad Dermatol 20:278–286, 1989.
17. Fond D, Hecox B: Superficial heat modalities. In Hecox B, Mehreteab TA, Weisberg J (eds): Physical Agents, East Norwalk, CT, Appleton & Lange, 1994, pp 125–142.
18. Michlovitz SL: Biophysical principles of heating and superficial heating agents. In Michlovitz (ed): Thermal Agents in Rehabilitation, 3rd ed. Philadelphia, FA Davis, 1996, pp 88–107.
19. Bell GW, Prentice WE: Infrared modalities. In Prentice WE (ed): Therapeutic Modalities for Allied Health Professionals. New York, McGraw-Hill, 1998, pp 201–262.
20. Abramson DL, Tuck S, Chu LSW, Agustin C: Effects of paraffin baths and hot formentations on local tissue temperature. Arch Phys Med Rehabil 45:87–94, 1964.
21. Borrell RM, Henley EJ, Ho P, Hubbell MK: Fluidotherapy: Evaluation of a new heat modality. Arch Phys Med Rehabil 58:69–71, 1977.
22. Borrell RM, Parker R, Henley EJ, et al: Comparison of in vivo temperatures produced by hydrotherapy, paraffin wax treatment, and fluidotherapy. Phys Ther 60:1273–1276, 1980.
23. Diller KR: Analysis of burns caused by long-term exposure to a heating pad. J Burn Care Rehabil 12:214–217, 1991.

Chapter 3
Deep-Heating Modalities

Kevin Ochs, MPT, STS, Upinder Pal Singh, MD, and Kamala Shankar, MD

The goal of early investigators in the field of deep heating modalities was to identify methods of heating that would penetrate the skin and subcutaneous tissues (muscles, tendons, ligaments) to produce therapeutic temperatures of 40–45°C. In this pursuit, three identifiable deep-heating modalities were discovered: short-wave diathermy (SWD), microwave diathermy (MWD), and ultrasound. The use of microwave heating for therapeutic applications was popular in the United States in the late 1940s. In 1955, the Council of Physical Medicine and Rehabilitation of the American Medical Association recommended the use of ultrasound for the treatment of pain, and soft tissue and joint dysfunction.

All three deep-heating modalities work on the principle of conversion techniques. SWD and MWD are commonly used to heat large areas by using nonionizing electromagnetic waves that produce heat, and ultrasound uses acoustic energy to heat relatively small areas. Unlike superficial heating agents, such as moist hot packs, which produce temperature elevation in the skin and subcutaneous tissue at a depth no greater than 1 cm, ultrasound is able to produce temperature elevations in deep subcutaneous tissue and superficial muscle that lie at a depth of 3 cm or more. Ultrasound has gained popularity for both its thermal and non-thermal effects and is by far the most commonly used deep-heating modality.

This chapter focuses primarily on a review of the physics, biophysical effects, uses and controversies of ultrasound treatment. An additional section is devoted to SWD and MWD.

THERAPEUTIC ULTRASOUND

Physical Properties of Ultrasound

Ultrasound is mechanical radiant energy derived from the application of an electric current on a crystal, which results in a vibratory motion. This motion is then applied to particles of the medium, through which it travels in the frequency range beyond the upper limits of sound perception. See Table 1 for the various applications of ultrasound energy.

TABLE 1. Various Applications of Ultrasound Energy

Application	Frequency	Intensity
Internal structure imaging	0.1 W/cm2	
Echocardiography		5 MHz
Doppler blood flow		8.2 MHz
Fetal scanning		2.25 MHz
Surgical tissue destruction	10 W/cm2	
Tumor irradiation due to thermal effects		> 5 MHz
Therapeutic effects	0.25–2.0 W/cm2	
Thermal and nonthermal		850 kHz–3 MHz

The human ear is capable of perceiving sound frequencies between 16 Hz and 20,000 Hz. Sound with a frequency greater than 20,000 Hz is called *ultrasound*. As the frequency increases from a given sound source, the sound beam diverges less. Audible sounds tend to spread in all directions, whereas ultrasound beams with their higher frequency are well collimated, similar to the light beam emerging from a flashlight. As a result, ultrasound beams at typical treatment frequencies are sufficiently collimated to selectively sonicate a limited target area for a physical therapy treatment.

As the ultrasound beam travels through the treated tissue, its energy decreases secondary to absorption and scattering, which is collectively referred to as *attenuation*. *Scattering* refers to the deflection of sound out of the beam that occurs when the sound contacts a reflecting medium, whereas *absorption* refers to the conversion of the mechanical energy of an ultrasonic wave into heat. Tissues with high collagen and protein content will absorb large amounts of the ultrasound energy and thus are more reactive to ultrasound energy. For instance, bone and cartilage, which have a high collagen content, absorb most of the ultrasound energy, whereas skin and fat will absorb minimal ultrasound energy owing to their low collagen content.

Absorption occurs partly because of the internal friction in tissue that needs to be overcome in the passage of sound. The higher the frequency, the more rapidly the molecules are forced to move against this friction. Attenuation, or weakening, of the sound beam occurs as the energy is absorbed, resulting in less available energy to propagate further to the deeper tissue. At frequencies greater than 20 MHz, superficial absorption predominates because less than 1% of the energy passes through the first centimeter. A frequency of 1.0 MHz is commonly used for physical therapy treatments because it offers an adequate compromise between depth of penetration of the ultrasound energy and heating of tissue. Many ultrasound units are also equipped to provide sonication at frequencies of 3 MHz for treatment of superficial tissues.

Continuous Versus Pulsed Waves

Sound waves that are produced by ultrasound units are either continuous or pulsed. A *continuous wave* is one in which the sound wave intensity remains the unchanged, whereas a *pulsed wave* is intermittently interrupted. Pulsed waves are further classified by specifying the fraction of time the sound is present over one pulse period. This fraction is called the *duty cycle* and is calculated by using the following equation:

Duty cycle = duration of pulse (on time)/pulse period (total cycle time)

Most ultrasound units have the capability to adjust their duty cycle, ranging from 0.05 (5%) to 0.5 (50%), with the most common duty cycle being 20%.

Intensity and Effective Radiating Area

Another factor that effects ultrasound conduction is intensity. *Intensity* refers to the strength of the ultrasound beam or, in other terms, the rate at which the ultrasound energy is delivered per unit area. Intensity is typically expressed in terms of watts per centimeter squared (W/cm^2). If all other variables are left constant, increases in intensity will result in increases in tissue temperature.

The measurement of intensity is made by dividing the total power output (in watts) of the ultrasound applicator by the area (in square centimeters) of the ultrasound head or applicator, also known as the effective radiating area (ERA). The ERA is determined by using an underwater microphone (acoustic hydrophone) that scans the transducer at a distance of 5 mm from the radiating surface and records all the areas in excess of 5% of the maximum power output found at any location on the surface of the transducer. The ERA is always smaller than the transducer surface. Common ERA measurements found on ultrasound heads are 0.5 and 5 cm^2 (Fig. 1). However, it should be noted that the ultrasound beam is not truly homogeneous under the ERA, which creates relative hot spots. Therefore, the intensity measurement is typically an average intensity and is also referred to as the *spatial average intensity*. The relative hot spots where the greatest intensity can be found are referred to as the *spatial peak intensity* and should be known by the therapist.

To ensure that these relative hot spots do not cause tissue damage to the sonicated area by exposing any one area to high intensity ultrasound energy, the therapist must use a moving applicator technique. The term *beam nonuniformity ratio* (BNR) is used to describe the homogeneity of the ultrasound beam and is measured as the ratio of peak intensity to average intensity. The greater the ratio difference of the BNR, the less homogeneous the ultrasound beam, resulting in the above-mentioned hot spots. For example, if an ultrasound beam has a 7:1 BNR with a desired intensity of 1.0 W/cm^2, the true intensity could be as high as 7 W/cm^2. A desirable BNR should be as low as possible, between 2 and 6 W/cm^2. In the United States, ultrasound units made after 1979 are required by the Food and Drug Administration to have labels indicating the BNR.

One must consider other variables of intensity when using pulsed or interrupted ultrasound. When the pulse is off, the intensity will be zero, and when it is on, the intensity will be at its peak. This maximum intensity is referred to as the *temporal peak intensity*, or the pulse average intensity. The temporal average intensity meas-

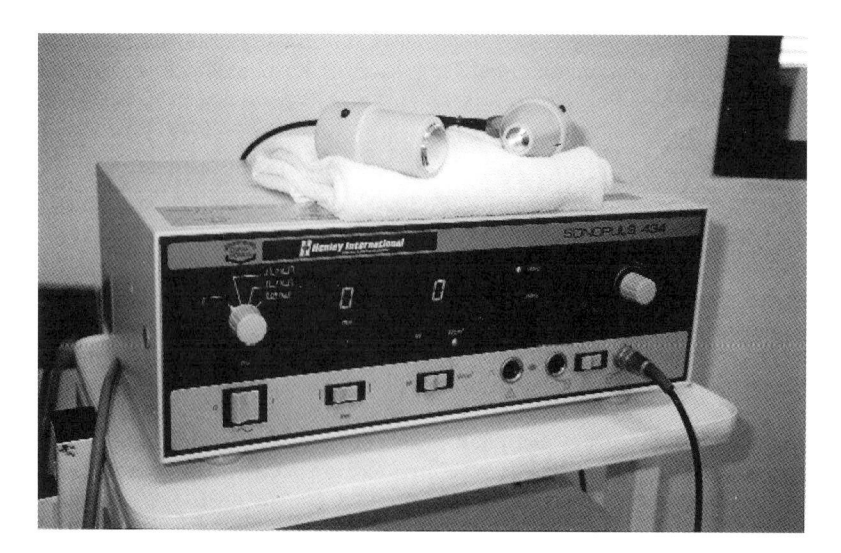

FIGURE 1. An ultrasound unit with 0.5- and 5-cm^2 ultrasound heads.

ures the average intensity over the entire pulse period, including both the on and off times. For example, a pulsed beam of 1.5 W/cm^2 with a duty cycle of 50% would have a temporal average intensity of 0.75 W/cm^2 (1.5 W/cm^2 × 0.5 = 0.75 W/cm^2). By manipulating the duty cycle, the amount of energy delivered to the treatment area can be controlled, even though the temporal peak intensity is held constant. This method can be used to ensure less heating of the tissues when a nonthermal effect of ultrasound is desired.

When documenting an ultrasound treatment, the therapist must clearly specify the ultrasound variables used, including frequency, intensity, duty cycle, total duration of treatment, and location of treatment with anatomic landmarks. For example, 1 MHz / 1.0 W/cm^2 / pulsed 20% / 7 minutes / to the R subacromial space. When using continuous ultrasound, one must include the frequency, the spatial average intensity, the continuous wave, the duration, and treatment area, for example, 1 MHz / 2.0 W/cm^2 / cont / 5 min to the lumbar spine, left of L5.

Spatial average intensities used for therapeutic purposes range from 0.25 to 2.0 W/cm^2. The World Health Organization limits the spatial average intensity to 3.0 W/cm^2.

Generation of Ultrasound through the Piezoelectric Effect

As mentioned, ultrasound is derived from an oscillating electrical current applied to a crystal, typically synthetic crystals such as barium titanate or lead zirconate titanate (PZT), causing the crystal to expand or contract. These crystals are said to possess the property of piezoelectricity. There are two types of the piezoelectric effect: direct and reverse (indirect). The **direct piezoelectric effect** is the generation of an electric voltage across a crystal when the crystal is compressed. If the crystal is expanded, a voltage of opposite polarity is induced. A sound wave that contacts the crystal will cause the crystal to expand and contract at the same frequency of the sound wave and, in turn, will induce an oscillating voltage across the crystal surface. This direct piezoelectric effect is used for converting ultrasound into an electric signal that replicates the sound pattern, which can then be processed and analyzed.

The **reverse piezoelectric effect** is the contraction and expansion of the crystal in response to an electrical current applied to the crystal surface. An alternating current causes the crystal to vibrate at the frequency of the electrical oscillation. In this manner, ultrasound can be generated at any desired frequency. The ultrasound crystal is consequently referred to as a *transducer*, because it converts electrical energy into sound energy. The crystals are sliced into thin, fragile wafers, approximately 2–3 mm thick, and then placed in an applicator to protect them. The entire applicator is commonly referred to as the transducer or the ultrasound head. A coaxial cable connects the ultrasound head to the console, where the various ultrasound parameters can be adjusted to the desired settings.

Biophysical Effects

The biophysical effects produced by ultrasound can be grouped into two categories:
1. Thermal—effects produced by ultrasound elevating tissue temperature
2. Nonthermal—effects believed to be caused by mechanisms other than tissue temperature elevation

The mechanism of some of the biophysical changes that are produced by ultrasound may be thermal, nonthermal, or a combination of both. Many responses to ultrasound, such as pain reduction, are poorly understood and their mechanisms are purely speculative.

Thermal Effects

Therapeutic ultrasound has been used extensively for its thermal effects to elevate tissue temperatures approximately 5 cm or more.[1-3] Typically, the thermal effects are used for the treatment of subacute or chronic inflammation, muscle spasm, pain, and stretching of collagenous tissue contracture. The physiologic responses attributed to a thermal mechanism include increase in collagen tissue extensibility, alterations in blood flow, changes in nerve conduction velocity[4,5] producing a decreased sensitivity of the neural elements, increase in pain threshold, increased enzymatic activity, and changes in the contractile activity of skeletal muscle.[6]

In order to achieve ultrasound's thermal benefits, specific tissue temperatures must be reached. Based on studies by Lehman[7] and Lehman et al.[8,9] an increase of 1°C (mild heating) accelerated metabolic rate in healing tissue. An increase of 2–3°C (moderate heating) reduces muscle spasm, pain, and chronic inflammation, and increases blood flow. More vigorous heating (≥ 4°C) decreases viscoelastic properties and inhibits sympathetic activity.

As discussed, ultrasound attenuation or absorption and the consequent tissue temperature elevation are frequency dependent. At 3.0 MHz, the majority of the ultrasound energy is absorbed at depths less than 2.5 cm, whereas at 1.0 MHz, tissue temperature elevation can be measured up to 5 cm.[10] Therefore, when treating relatively superficial injuries such as tennis elbow or ankle sprains, a 3-MHz setting is preferred. Another consideration when using different frequencies is the rate at which the tissue temperature is elevated. Draper and colleagues found that, at 3 MHz, the heating rate is three times faster than at 1 MHz, which may support the use of shorter duration of treatment times when using 3 MHz.[11]

Ultrasound can be used to selectively heat periarticular structures[12] and the muscle at the muscle bone interface.[8,9] Intensities of 1.0–2.0 W/cm^3 with treatment times of 5–10 minutes were required to elevate the tissue temperature higher than 4°C to allow significant stretching of tendons when a stretch was applied while the tendon was at an elevated temperature.

When attempting to increase the tissue temperature, one must also consider the possibility of blood flow-induced cooling and tissue thermal conduction that may reduce thermal efficiency.[13] A baseline threshold ultrasound intensity and duration is required to overcome this cool down, which may be significantly different than the standard treatment time of 5 minutes at 1.5 W/cm^2.[11]

When the primary goal of a treatment is to increase the blood flow, ultrasound is thought to create a mild inflammatory response. However, the research is mixed. It does appear that treatment times and intensities that produce the desired result of increased blood flow are far larger than what is clinically performed. Treatment times of 10–20 minutes at intensities greater than 2 W/cm^2, continuous wave, 1 MHz showed increases in blood flow and skeletal muscle temperature.[14,15] Without these duration and intensity levels, the blood flow increases were inconsistent or nonexistent.

The pain threshold has also been shown to be increased by elevating tissue temperature from ultrasound at 0.8 MHz, continuous wave, at 1.5 W/cm².[16] This is what is commonly expected when using thermal agents for tissue temperature elevation and may also help reduce muscle spasm.

Nonthermal Effects

When ultrasound is used with a pulsed duty cycle, the thermal effects are minimized. Pulsed ultrasound at 20% is commonly used to achieve nonthermal effects or "healing" effects, effects that cannot be explained by a thermal mechanism. Note that if one were to use 20% pulsed ultrasound and increase the duration fivefold, one may achieve thermal heating, as if continuous ultrasound were used. These nonthermal effects include cavitation, acoustic streaming, microstreaming, and chemical reactions. The effects of nonthermal ultrasound are numerous, including increases in cell membrane permeability and diffusion; increases in intracellular Ca^{2+}; mast cell degranulation; histamine and chemotactic factor release; increases in rate of protein synthesis and fibroblast stimulation leading to increased collagen synthesis and strength; changes electrical activity in nervous tissue; increases in enzymatic activity; and increases in angiogenesis.[4,6,17–20]

Cavitation refers to various kinds of sonically generated activity of gas or vapor-filled bubbles. The vibrational effect of ultrasound can cause expansion or contraction of gas bubbles that may be found in tissue fluid or blood. This cavitation may be stable or transient, having the potential to cause tissue damage. If the bubbles are in the field pulse, with a limited change in overall amplitude, stable cavitation is thought to occur, which is thought to result in diffusional changes along the cell membrane, consequently altering cell function.[4] Transient or unstable cavitation refers to the violent collapse of bubbles within the tissue fluid or blood, resulting in tissue destruction and possibly blood vessel damage, with the safe range for peak intensity to prevent unstable cavitation being < 8 W/cm².[21]

Acoustic streaming is thought to be another mechanism that causes nonthermal effects of ultrasound. *Acoustic streaming* refers to the steady flow of cellular fluids along the cell membrane induced by ultrasonic pulses or waves. Consequent changes in ion fluxes across the cell membrane and resultant changes in cellular activity are thought to occur. Noted increases in cell membrane and vascular permeability have been found within normal treatment intensities with ultrasound.[17–19]

Similar to acoustic steaming, *microstreaming* refers to microscale eddying that takes place near any small vibrating objects, such as gas bubbles, that have been set into oscillation by a sound field, but appear to have a more adverse effect. This process affects cells more directly, causing cell lysis, alteration of cellular function, degradation of DNA, and inactivation of certain enzymes.

Indications and Contraindications

Ultrasound is commonly used in rehabilitation for a variety of musculoskeletal dysfunctions including muscle spasms and pain, joint contractures, bursitis and tendinitis, neurofibromas, and pain following sprains and strains (Table 2). There has been increased popularity of the use of ultrasound for wounds, both open and closed, and bone healing. Other uses of ultrasound include treatment of plantar

24 Deep-Heating Modalities

TABLE 2. INDICATIONS AND CONTRAINDICATIONS OF ULTRASOUND

Indications of Ultrasound
Muscle spasm
Pain from immobilization, rheumatic processes, degenerative joint disease, trauma
Joint contracture
Bursitis
Tendinitis
Neurofibromas
Plantar warts
Scar tissue remodeling
Wound healing
Tendon healing
Bone healing
Transdermal drug delivery

Contraindications of Ultrasound
Over the eye
Over open spinal cord (e.g., s/p laminectomy)
Over the heart, over pacemakers
Areas of malignancies or suspected malignancies
Thrombophlebitis
Over pregnant uterus

Ultrasound Applications Warranting Special Caution
Over areas of epiphysis of growing bone in children
Areas of vascular insufficiency
Areas of dysthesia, hypothesia
Areas with pins (surgically implanted)
Areas with glue and artificial joints

---

warts, remodeling of scar tissue, and noninvasive techniques to allow transdermal drug delivery (phonophoresis; see Chapter 4). Copious amounts of research are reported on the clinical applications for ultrasound; however, much of the results present contradictory conclusions.[22]

Although there is contradictory information regarding the efficacy of ultrasound, the contraindications of ultrasound are less ambiguous. Ultrasound should not be used over the eye because temperature elevations at the poorly vascularized lens can lead to cataract production.[23] Sonication over the spinal column was once contraindicated, but researchers now know that the bones surrounding the spinal cord prevent the ultrasound beam from reaching the neural tissue. However, irradiation over an open spinal cord (e.g., pt. s/p laminectomy) is contraindicated because the spinal cord is not protected.

Ultrasound performed over the heart should also be avoided, because there is evidence of electrocardiographic (ECG) changes, namely ST-segment elevation, following application of ultrasound. Furthermore, as with electrical modalities, care must be taken to avoid ultrasound exposure to the heart of persons with cardiac pacemakers because the ultrasound beam may interfere with the electrical circuitry of the pacemaker.

It is commonly known that ultrasound should not be used on malignant tissue or in areas where malignancies may be located. It has been suggested that ultrasound has the potential of increasing cellular detachment, resulting in the possibility of metastasis.[24,25] If there is any uncertainty about whether an area has some malignant tissue based on the patient's past medical history and clinical signs, it is best to avoid ultrasound. This same principle applies to areas of thrombophlebitis, in which a thrombus could be released.

Under no circumstances should ultrasound be used over the pregnant uterus. Temperature elevation in fetuses has been shown to result in low birth weight, brain size reduction, and orthopedic deformities in guinea pigs.[26] It is probably best to avoid ultrasound over the low back and abdominal region of women during their reproductive years, unless reassured by the patient that there is no chance of her being pregnant. In men, ultrasound should be avoided over the testes because it may produce temporary sterility.

Ultrasound over areas of epiphysis of growing bone in children should be used with caution, although it is believed that therapeutic levels of ultrasound are safe.[27] However, there is evidence of retardation of bone growth at intensities greater than 3.0 W/cm^2 and using a stationary transducer.

Similar to heating pads and cold packs, caution must be taken when using ultrasound on poorly vascularized areas or areas of impaired temperature or pain sensation. Poor vascularization, as in patients Reynard's syndrome, may result in overheating of the tissue because of inadequate heat dissipation. Patients with reduced sensation may be unable to detect pain or changes in temperature, increasing their risk of injury from ultrasound.

When treating patients with metal implants or pins, ultrasound can be safely incorporated into the treatment if the moving transducer technique is used.[28,29] However, most of the materials used for joint replacements have high-density polyethylene components and use methyl methacrylate cement, which have not been thoroughly tested for safety or integrity in response to ultrasound sonication.

Tissue Healing

Ultrasound has been proposed as a treatment to facilitate the healing of tissues. It is used in the treatment of many types of tissue injuries ranging from tendon injuries to open wounds. Numerous articles have been written on ultrasound's effect on tissue healing; however, the ultrasound parameters vary considerably among the studies. Furthermore, it is difficult to study tissue healing because of the complexity of the healing process and because there are many steps in the healing process for which the regulatory mechanisms are still undefined.

Since the late 1960s, Dyson and associates at Guy's Hospital in London have conducted numerous studies on pulsed, low-intensity ultrasound at 3 MHz on the healing of skin lesions. In 1968, Dyson noted accelerated healing of lesions in the ears of rabbits with TIW treatments.[19] In 1978, chronic varicose ulcers were treated with TIW ultrasound for a month. Those treated with ultrasound had a significant reduction in ulcer size (66% of the original size) compared with the control group that received mock ultrasound (92% of original size).[30] A later study demonstrated increased protein synthesis of fibroblasts in vitro and in vivo.[31]

Fyfe et al. studied the vascular permeability and release of histamine in rats following one treatment of ultrasound at the ankle.[32] Histologic sections showed increased degranulation of mast cells. Also, evaluation of the leakage of a dye from the blood indicated that ultrasound induced an increase in vascular permeability.

In 1988, Dyson continued her work with another study using low-intensity, pulsed ultrasound showing increased calcium transport in fibroblast cell membranes in culture.[33] Later in 1990, ultrasound was used to treat skin lesions in rats, with daily ultrasound treatments for 5 days. Results showed increased blood vessels per area of granulation tissue, increased granulation tissue, fewer polymorphonuclear (PMN) leukocytes and macrophages, and more fibroblasts.[34,35]

The study of ultrasound's effect on tendon and ligament has evolved from the work of Dyson et al. In most of these studies, ultrasound intensities are higher (1.5 W/cm^2), frequencies are 1.0 MHz, and duty cycle is either pulsed or continuous. Roberts et al. showed potential harmful effects of ultrasound after treating induced lesions of forepaw flexor profundus tendons in rabbits.[36] Ultrasound was used 5 days/week through a window in the splint that was used to protect the lesion. Treatment interfered with healing, demonstrated by the fact that the breaking strength of all ultrasound treated tendons was 0 newtons (N), whereas the nontreated tendon strength was 1 N. Later, Stevenson and colleagues studied the effect of ultrasound (3 MHz, 0.75 W/cm^2 × 20 days starting 4 weeks after surgery) on surgically repaired profundus tendons in chickens.[37] After 6 weeks of treatment, there was no difference in the tensile strength of the tendons between the treated and control groups; however, it was reported that the treated chickens were able to flex their toes better than the control group. Enwemeka treated surgical repairs of rabbit Achilles tendons with daily ultrasound for 9 days beginning the day after surgery.[38] Exposure to ultrasound induced significant increases in the tensile strength and energy absorption capacity of the tendons. Furthermore, Jackson et al. administered ultrasound to the Achilles tendon lesions in rats daily for 8 days, then four times a day until sacrifice at 15 or 21 days.[39] Collagen synthesis and tendon breaking strength were both increased in the sonicated group.

The healing of muscle and nerve injury has also been studied. In 1989, Gillett et al reported that continuous ultrasound at 1.5 W/cm^2 every 12 hours following injection of lidocaine into the anterior tibialis resulted in an accelerated rise in the activity of the muscle enzyme ornithine decarboxylase (ODC) and a subsequent decrease in the activity by 48 hours after injury (ODC activity is an index of cell proliferation and differentiation).[40] This study supports the theory that ultrasound accelerates early inflammation and repair. Hong et al. studied the effects of ultrasound on crushed tibial nerves in rats.[41] They used continuous ultrasound at 0.5 or 1.0 W/cm^2 TIW for 35 days beginning 5 days after injury. The recovery rates of motor nerve conduction velocities and the amplitude of the evoked compound muscle action potentials (measured by electromyography [EMG]) were faster when ultrasound was used at 0.5 W/cm^2, but the recovery rate was slower with the group treated at 1.5 W/cm^2.

Recent interest has developed in the potential role of ultrasound to facilitate healing in fractures. However, in the past, ultrasound was thought to interfere with the healing process of fractures or the break up of calcified tissue. Early studies by Dyson indicated that pulsed ultrasound at 0.5 W/cm^2 performed four times per week would accelerate the repair process during the inflammatory and early proliferative phases of repair.[42] More recent studies by Heckman and Kristiansen reported acceleration of tibial and Colles' fractures in humans.[43] Treatments were begun within 7 days of fracture and given through windows in the cast. Frequencies around 1.5 W/cm^2, intensities of 30 mW/cm^2, and durations of 20 minutes were used.

In summary, ultrasound can facilitate healing in several ways. Probably the most important effect of ultrasound is its ability to increase oxygen delivery to the wound. In addition, it is thought that ultrasound can increase collagen deposition and protein synthesis, which is enabled by the piezoelectric effect. Other factors include increased mast cell degranulation (initiating vasodilation), increased blood flow to the wound, and the possibility of decreased infection, which may be related to increasing oxygen.

Other Commonly Treated Conditions

Joint contractures due to trauma, immobilization, surgery, or even insidious onset, as is frequently found in cases of adhesive capsulitis of the shoulder (frozen shoulder), are commonly treated in physical therapy. The restricted joint motion can be the result of degenerative arthritis, muscle tone, or cartilage dysfunction. If motion is restricted by periarticular connective tissue changes, ultrasound may be of benefit. As described in the section on thermal effects of ultrasound, ultrasound can be used to heat these collagen tissues to allow increased extensibility of tissues. It is important to note that ultrasound alone will not cause increased range of motion (ROM); stretching during or after the application of ultrasound is required. One component of joint contractures may be scar tissue, which can also be heated and stretched because of the high collagen content of scars. To achieve the necessary temperature increases in the selected tissue, the intensities must be of sufficient energy (> 1.0 W/cm^2), the time of treatment sufficient (typically > 7 minutes), and the treatment area small enough to allow selective sonication.

Research on the effect of ultrasound on bursitis and tendinitis is mixed, with some studies showing enhanced recovery with ultrasound.[44,45] However, most studies tend to show little *statistically significant* benefit of ultrasound, although ultrasound is commonly used to treat these conditions.[46,47]

Treatment Considerations

Although some conditions (e.g., plantar warts) were treated in the past with a stationary ultrasound applicator, the consensus today calls for the moving applicator technique. The stationary technique has been noted to cause hot spots that can be responsible for stasis of blood flow, venular endothelial damage, and platelet aggregation, in addition potential tissue damage.[6] By moving the applicator at the recommended speed of approximately 4 cm/second, the ultrasound energy is distributed evenly throughout the sonicated tissue.[2]

To ensure that the ultrasound energy is transmitted from the applicator to the treated tissue, a coupling agent must be used. This approach ensures that the ultrasound energy is not totally reflected at the air–tissue interface before it even reaches the tissue and will eliminate "overheating" of the ultrasound crystal owing to the fact that ultrasound waves are unable to travel through air. The objective of the coupling agent is to eliminate as much air as possible between the applicator and tissue to ensure maximal energy entering the selected tissue. Most commercially available ultrasound gels are adequate. For patient comfort, it is best to preheat the gel slightly.

When sonicating irregular, bony surfaces, several options exist to ensure proper coupling. Some ultrasound units have the capability to switch sound heads, which

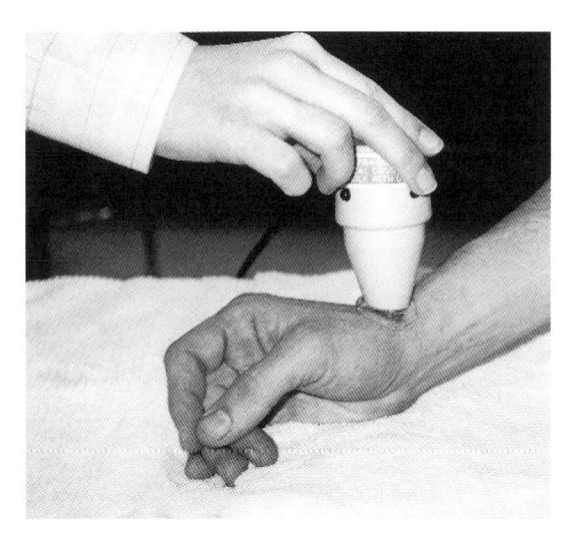

FIGURE 2. Application of ultrasound to a bony, irregular surface with a small 0.5-cm^2 ultrasound head surface.

allows the therapist to use a smaller sound head (Fig. 2). This method can ensure more direct contact with the tissue being treated. Another option, which can work well with open wounds to minimize trauma from contact with the applicator, is the use of a closed rubber balloon filled with water (Fig. 3).[48] The balloon is placed between the applicator and the tissue being treated with ultrasound gel at the skin–balloon and balloon–applicator interfaces. Another option when treating a distal extremity is to immerse the extremity to be treated in a basin filled with water

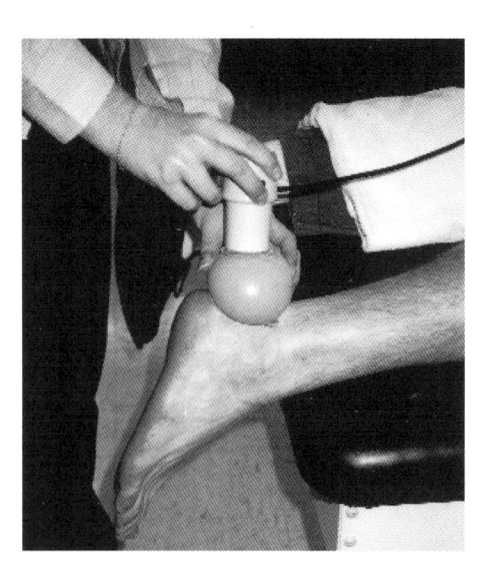

FIGURE 3. Using a water-filled balloon to treat an open wound that would otherwise be harmed by moving the ultrasound head directly on the wound. Note the ultrasound gel at the balloon–skin and balloon–ultrasound head interfaces.

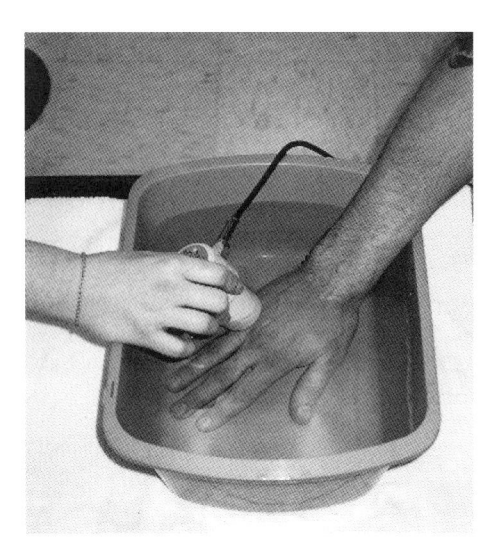

FIGURE 4. A water-filled, plastic wash basin is used to treat a distal extremity. The distal tip of the ultrasound head must be submerged under water to ensure the crystal is not damaged.

(Fig. 4). The ultrasound head should be held 0.5–3.0 cm from the skin, using the moving ultrasound technique. To ensure proper coupling, accumulated air bubbles on the patient's skin and applicator head should be wiped off. If it is available, a plastic or rubber basin should be used instead of a metal basin because some of the ultrasound energy will be reflected off the metal, potentially increasing the intensity in treated areas near the metal.

When determining the intensity for an ultrasound treatment, consideration must be made to the desired effect of ultrasound and the tissue or condition being treated (Table 3). For treatment of chronic disorders, vigorous heating may be desired. To ensure maximal heating, Lehman recommended turning the intensity up until the patient senses a dull ache, and then decreasing the intensity slightly below pain threshold. In areas of deep soft tissue, such as in the hip and back, intensities greater than 1.5 W/cm^2 may be required. In areas of thin, soft tissue with bony prominences, it may be prudent to reduce the intensity to 0.5–1.0 W/cm^2 and use a 3-MHz frequency.

As noted, a smaller sized applicator may be desired; however, special considerations need to be made. Because of the size of the sound head (ERA), there is a reduced amount of ultrasonic energy emitted from the applicator head. For instance, if the size

TABLE 3. GENERALIZED ULTRASOUND PARAMETERS IN COMMONLY TREATED CONDITIONS

CONDITION	INTENSITY	PULSED (20%)/ CONTINUOUS
Acute injury	0.25–0.5 W/cm^2	Pulsed
Scar tissue remodeling	1.0–1.5 W/cm^2	Continuous
Increased blood flow	1.5–2.0 W/cm^2	Continuous
Increased oxygen	0.5–2.0 W/cm^2	Continuous or pulsed
Wound healing	0.5 W/cm^2	Pulsed

of the applicator head is 5 cm^2, it will emit half the amount of energy as a 10 cm^2 head at the same intensity. Therefore, to ensure an adequate dose with the smaller sound head, the therapist may be required to double the treatment time.

Another consideration when using ultrasound is to ensure proper maintenance of the ultrasound unit. Units should be checked annually for homogeneity of the beam shape (measured by the BNR) to reduce the risk of hot spots, intensity, and power. The transducer assembly should also be checked periodically for water tightness because this part is prone to deterioration. All electrical components should also be checked periodically, including the cable assembly. These tests are typically performed in a biomedical instrumentation department.

Controversies Concerning Ultrasound

Although the effects and mechanisms of ultrasound are not clearly understood, ultrasound is a widely used modality in rehabilitation. The use of ultrasound tends to be based on empirical experience, although the research on ultrasound provides contradictory information. Recent work by Gam and van der Windt involved extensive reviews of the research on ultrasound in the treatment of musculoskeletal disorders. Much of the research was found to be lacking information regarding the description of drop-outs, randomization methods, ultrasound apparatus, sham-ultrasound apparatus, control of apparatus, mode of delivery, size of sound head, treated area, and treatment time. In research studies that could be statistically analyzed, there was little evidence to support the use of ultrasound in the treatment of musculoskeletal disorders. It is clear that further well-designed research studies need to be conducted to clearly justify the use of ultrasound and to determine the appropriate parameters that should be used for common dysfunctions.

Summary

Therapeutic ultrasound is one of the most common modalities used in rehabilitation today. Ultrasound can generate acoustic energy capable of affecting tissues to depths of 5 cm, either through its thermal or nonthermal effects. Ultrasound can be used to treat a variety of musculoskeletal disorders by elevating the pain threshold, increasing collagen extensibility, increasing oxygenation and blood flow to tissues, increasing cell membrane permeability, enhancing transdermal drug delivery, and facilitating tissue healing.

Although numerous studies have been performed on ultrasound, the benefits of ultrasound are not clearly justified secondary to contradictory research. Aggressive research with properly designed studies needs to be performed to improve our ability to offer effective treatment. Ultimately, these research studies not only will empower therapists to more carefully match treatment variables with specific musculoskeletal disorders but also should encourage therapists to stop using treatment procedures that are not effective.

DIATHERMY

Over the years, much experimentation and research have been conducted on electromagnetic radiation. It was only as a result of much, initially crude and later scientific, experimentation that it was found how diathermies actually work. Through conversion of electrostatic or electromagnetic wave energy, heat energy is produced. With this capability, deep tissues inside the body can be warmed for therapeutic purposes. The word *diathermy* is from the Greek, meaning "through heat." Although the therapeutic modality of diathermy became popular in the 1940s, not much work has been done after the initial enthusiasm in the medical world. Its indications, procedures, and types of machines have not changed very much from the time of it inception.

In many countries, long before SWD and MWD were used by physiatrists, doctors used them as one of the modalities of radiation therapy. The indications for the radiation therapy were not always clear; however, it is believed that the primary use was for treatment of malignancies, using the principles of hyperthermia. It was a popular modality in management of aches and pains in 1930s and 1940s. Since 1950, diathermy has lost popularity and declined in usage, because of the large bulky equipment, high cost, and difficulty with shielding and eliminating electromagnetic interference with other electronic equipment. These authors do not often use this modality, and most of the information presented here has been obtained from other publications. Potential health hazards from stray electromagnetic radiation for both the user and the applicator have always been a concern. There are, however, advantages of SWD and MWD. One being that little time is required for set up. Additionally, the treatment can be administered without the therapist being in direct contact for the entire treatment session.

The electromagnetic waves with wavelengths that can penetrate the body are short-waves and microwaves. The SWD and pulsed magnetic field frequencies (pulsed short-wave diathermy [PSWD]) approved by the Federal Communications Commission (FCC) are 13.56 MHz (22 m wavelength), 27.12 MHz (11 m), and 40.68 MHz (7.5 m). The 27.12 MHz band is the most commonly used because it is relatively easy to generate. The FCC has approved MWD of following frequencies for therapeutic use: 915.00 MHz (33 cm wavelength), and 2450.00 MHz (12 cm). Both SWD and MWD create increased tissue temperatures in deeper tissues, significantly in muscle tissues. PSWD can be used when nonthermal effects are desired. Several articles have noted that the nonthermal therapeutic effects are achieved by increasing microvascular tissue perfusion or by mechanisms of alternations at the cellular level. Some of the beneficial effects of diathermy include increase in blood flow due to vasodilation, improvement in tissue oxygenation, increased capillary pressure and cell membrane permeability, and increased concentration of white blood cells and antibodies. Other benefits include relaxation of muscles, relief of muscle spasms, decreased tension of the collagenous tissue, and increased ROM of collagenous tissues such as found in tendons and joint capsules.

Both SWD and MWD are nonionizing, so there is no danger of mutation. SWD and MWD are therapeutically capable of depolarizing motor nerves and eliciting a contractile response from innervated or denervated skeletal muscle. With SWD and MWD, electrical shock is not a concern, except when a person has a direct contact with the metallic portion of the machine. Dosimetry is subjective, and the patient's feeling of warmth helps guide the dosage.

Physical Principle and Methods of Application

SWD units can be capacitive or inductive. For capacitive applicators, the patient may be placed between two metal condenser plates (Fig. 5). The plates and the patient's intervening tissue act as a capacitor, and heat is generated by rapid oscillations in the electric field from one plate to the other and a strong electrostatic field (with weak electromagnetic field) is produced. The predominate electrostatic energy tends to conjugate in the skin and fat, which provides the greatest resistance; thus, the maximum heating occurs in the skin and fat, with little occurring in the muscle. Depending on the part to be heated (e.g., condenser plate or pancake coils for shoulder, space plates for hands, internal metal electrodes for pelvic organs), various types of electrodes could be used.

Inductive applicators use induction coils that apply a magnetic field to induce circular electrical field in the tissue (e.g., wraparound coils used for knee, elbow, or ankles). These applicators may have a cable or drum conjugation. An induction coil electrode may produce the most even heating of tissues that possess greater conductivity, such as muscles. In inductive application, more electromagnetic energy output electrostatic shielding is used. Pulsed electromagnetic frequencies (PMF), or PSWD, for the treatment of diseases were developed in the 1960s. They have an average power of 40 W. All PSWD devices use an inductive coil applicator in a drum form. It is important to note that inductive applicators produce more heat in deeper tissues compared with capacitive plates because the magnetic fields can achieve greater penetration to induce an electrical field.

SWD units take many forms, but they all have three basic components: the power supply, the oscillating circuit, and the patient circuit. The machine is

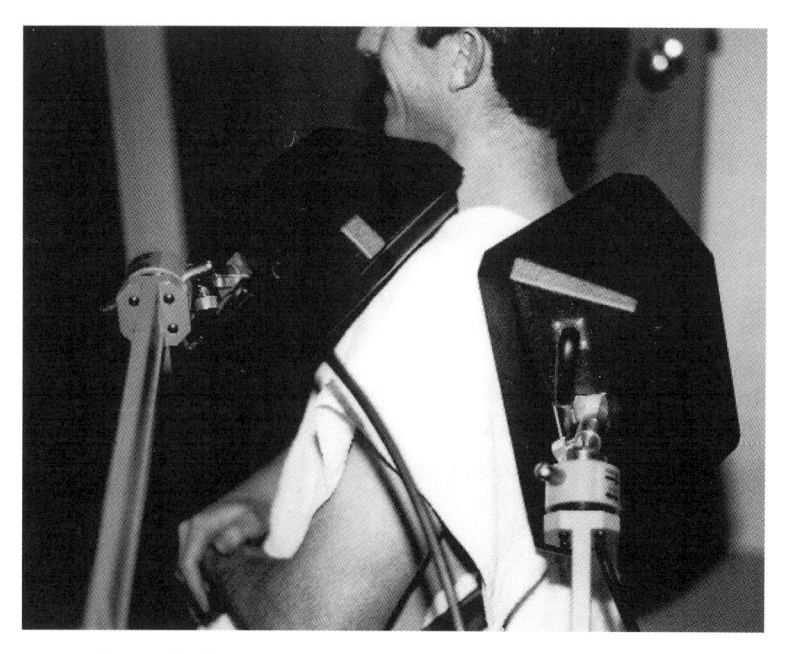

FIGURE 5. Shortwave diathermy treatment to the shoulder.

retuned after each patient is inserted into the circuit so that the frequency of patient circuit is made equal to the frequency of oscillatory circuit of the machine. Latest models have two independent drum applications, designed to treat one area from two directions or treat two separate areas at the same time. Portable and mobile units are becoming available.

Microwave Diathermy

MWD units have the basic components of power supply and magnetism tube (which is the specialized amplifying component). With MWD applications, the electrical fields predominate with only a minor amount of magnetic field being generated or transmitted. MWD also uses conversion as its primary form of heat production. The temperature distribution in a particular tissue is largely affected by its water content.

The higher frequency, shorter wavelength transmissions are focused and beamed into the tissues from varying distances through specifically designed treatment heads. With this capability, specific areas can be localized, including small joints of the hand for the treatment of rheumatoid arthritis. Another example is a focal treatment for malignant tumors by hyperthermia.

Indications

Both SWD and MWD are used to produce heat in tissues deeper than superficial layers. They are most commonly used for heating joints, muscles, pelvic regions, the thoracic cavity, and ear conditions. Recently, microwave technology has been used by urologists at Duke University for shrinking benign prostate hypertrophy. Also, diathermies are being used to treat dysmenorrhea. Diathermies not only help with relieving pain but also can help decrease inflammation and edema. Di Massa et al. conclusively found that patients with postherpetic pain and patients simultaneously suffering from neck and lower back pain improved with treatment of pulsed electromagnetic fields.[53]

Some of the common indications for diathermy include:

> Joint contractures
> Muscle contracture
> Degenerative joint diseases
> Ankylosing spondylitis
> Rheumatoid arthritis
> Bursitis, tendinitis
> Nonspecific pelvic inflammatory diseases
> Prostatitis, sinusitis, otitis media

Contraindications

Both MWD and SWD are contraindicated in the presence of acute inflammations, hemorrhage, and tumors. High-frequency heat treatments should be avoided in the presence of a pacemaker. Although the metal itself will not become hot enough to produce damage, heat trapped in tissue–metal interfaces can cause deep-seated burns. MWD is not recommended around the eyes or testicles because of the hypersensitivity of these structures. Common contraindications and special precautions include:

>Acute inflammation, hemorrhage
>Metal objects
>Presence of surgical implants
>Intrauterine contraceptive device (IUD)
>Contact lenses
>Pregnant women
>Inadequate vascular supply
>Anesthetized or insensate areas
>Malignancy
>Bleeding tendency, hemorrhage

Summary

Diathermy was once a popular physical agent that has been used not only for musculoskeletal inflammatory conditions but also for various infectious illness. However, in the recent days, SWD is making a comeback in the field of sports medicine.

REFERENCES

1. Byl NN, McKenzie A, Wong T, West J, Hunt TK: Incisional wound healing: A controlled study of low and high dose ultrasound. J Orthop Sports Phys Ther 18:619–628, 1993.
2. Kramer JF: Ultrasound: Evaluation of its mechanical and thermal effects. Arch Phys Med Rehabil 65:223, 1984.
3. Oakley EM: Application of continuous beam ultrasound at therapeutic levels. Physiotherapy 64(6):169–172, 1978.
3a. Paul ED, et al: Temperature and blood flow studies after ultrasonic irradiation. Am J Phys Med 34:370, 1955.
4. Currier DP: Sensory nerve conduction: Effect of ultrasound. Arch Phys Med Rehabil 59:181, 1978.
5. Halle JS, et al: Ultrasound's effect on the conduction latency of superficial radial nerve in man. Phys Ther 61:345, 1981.
6. Michlocitz S: Thermal agents in rehabilitation. In Contemporary Perspectives in Rehabilitation, 2nd ed. Philadelphia, FA Davis, 1990, pp 134–169.
7. Lehman JF: Therapeutic Heat and Cold, 4th ed. Baltimore, Williams & Wilkins, 1990, pp 437–442
8. Lehman JF, et al: Therapeutic temperature distribution produced by ultrasound as modified by dosage and volume of tissue exposed. Arch Phys Med Rehabil 48:662–666, 1967
9. Lehman JF, et al: Bone and soft tissue heating produced by ultrasound. Arch Phys Med Rehabil 48:397–401, 1967.
10. Gann N: Ultrasound: Current concepts. Clin Manag 11:64–69, 1991.
11. Draper DO, et al: Rate of temperature increase in human muscle during 1 MHz and 3 MHz continuous ultrasound. J Orthop Sports Phys Ther 22:142–150, 1995.
12. Lehman JF, et al: Heating of joint structures by ultrasound. Arch Phys Med Rehabil 49:28, 1968.
13. Baker RJ, et al: The effect of therapeutic modalities on blood flow in the human calf. J Orthop Sports Phys Ther 13:23–27, 1991.
14. Paul ED, Imig CJ: Temperature and blood flow studies after ultrasonic irridation. Am J Phys Med 34:370, 1955.
15. Abramson DI, et al: Changes in blood flow, oxygen uptake and tissue temperatures produced by therapeutic agents. I. Effect of Ultrasound. Am J Phys Med 39:51, 1960.
16. Lehman JF, et al: Pain threshold measurements after therapeutic application of ultrasound, microwave and infared. Arch Phys Med Rehabil 39:560, 1958.
17. Dyson M, et al: The response of smooth muscle to ultrasound [abstract]. In Proceedings from an International Symposium on Therapeutic Ultrasound. Winnipeg, Manitoba, September 10, 1981.

18. Harvey W, et al: The stimulation of protein synthesis in human fibroblasts by therapeutic ultrasound. Rheumatol Rehabil 14:237, 1975.
19. Dyson M, Pond JB, Joseph J, Warwick R: The stimulation of tissue regeneration by means of ultrasound. Clin Sci 35:273–285, 1968.
20. Lehmann JF, Bieglar R: Changes in potentials and temperature gradients in membranes caused by ultrasound. Arch Phys Med Rehabil 35:287, 1954.
21. Lehman JF, et al: Biologic reaction to cavitation: A consideration for ultrasonic therapy. Arch Phys Med Rehabil 34:86, 1953.
22. McDiarmid T, et al: Clinical applications of therapeutic ultrasound. Physiotherapy 73:155, 1987.
23. Sokoliu A: Destructive effect of ultrasound on ocular tissues. In Reid JM, Sikov MR (eds): Interaction of Ultrasound and Biological Tissues. Washington, DC, DHEW, 1972, publication 73-8008.
24. Conger AD, et al: Ultrasonic effects on mammalian multicellular tumor spheroids. J Clin Ultrasound 9:167, 1981.
25. Siegal E, et al: Cellular attachment as a sensitive indicator of the effects of diagnostic ultrasound exposure on cultured human cells. Radiology 133:175, 1979.
26. Edwards MJ: Congenital defects in guinea pigs: Prenatal retardation of brain growth of guinea pigs following hyperthermia during gestation. Teratology 2:329, 1969.
27. Vaughen JL, et al: Effects of ultrasound on growing bone. Arch Phys Med Rehabil 40:158, 1959.
28. Gerston JW: Effects of metallic objects on temperature rises produced in tissues by ultrasound. Am J Phys Med 37:75, 1958.
29. Lehman JF: Ultrasonic effects as demonstrated in live pigs with surgical metallic implants. Arch Phys Med Rehabil 40:483, 1959.
30. Dyson M, Suckling J: Stimulation of tissue repair by ultrasound: A survey of the mechanisms involved. Physiotherapy 64:105–108, 1978.
31. Webster DF, Harvey W, Dyson M, Pond JB: The in vitro stimulation of collagen synthesis in human fibroblasts by ultrasound induced cavitation. Ultrasonics 16:33, 1980.
32. Fyfe MC, Chahl LA: Mast cell degranulation and increased permeability induced by 'therapeutic' ultrasound in the rat ankle joint. Br J Exp Pathol 65:671–676, 1984.
33. Mortimer AJ, Dyson M: The effect of therapeutic ultrasound on calcium uptake in fibroblasts. Ultrasound Med Biol 14:499–506, 1988.
34. Young SR, Dyson M: Effect of therapeutic ultrasound on angiogenesis. Ultrasound Med Biol 16:261–269, 1990
35. Young SR, Dyson M: Effect of therapeutic ultrasound on the healing of full-thickness excised skin lesions. Ultrasonics 28:175–180, 1990.
36. Roberts M, Rutherford JH, Harris D: The effect of ultrasound on flexor tendon repairs in the rabbit. Hand 14:17–20, 1982.
37. Stevenson JH, Pang CY, Lindsay WK, Zuker RM: Functional, mechanical and biochemical assessments of ultrasound therapy on tendon healing in the chicken toe. Plast Reconst Surg 77:965–72, 1986.
38. Enwemeka CS: The effects of therapeutic ultrasound on tendon healing: A biomechanical study. Am J Phys Med Rehabil 68:283–287, 1989.
39. Jackson BA, Schwane JA, Starcher BC: Effect of ultrasound therapy on the repair of Achilles tendon injuries in rats. Med Sci Sports Exerc 23:171–176, 1991.
40. Gillett JH, Mitchell JLA: Acceleration of repair of damaged skeletal muscle using ultrasound [abstract]. Presented at the 1990 APTA Annual Conference, Aneheim, CA.
41. Hong CZ, Lie HH, Yu J: Ultrasound thermotherapy effect on the recovery of nerve conduction in experimental compression neuropathy. Arch Phys Med Rehabil 69:410–414, 1988.
42. Dyson M: Therapeutic applications of ultrasound. In Nyborg WL, Ziskin MC (eds): Biological Effects of Ultrasound. New York, Churchill-Livingstone, 1985, p 129.
43. Kahn J: Electrotherapy, ultrasound enjoy publicity in healing of fractures. P.T. Bulletin 37:4, 1991. Cited studies by Heckman JD, Creighton MG: Acceleration of tibial fractures by noninvasive low intensity pulsed ultrasound, and Kristiansen T: Acceleratory effect of ultrasound on the healing time of Colles' fractures.
44. Bundt FB: Ultrasonic therapy in supraspinatus bursitis. Phys Ther Rev 38:826, 1958.
45. Echternach JL: Ultrasound: An adjunct treatment for shoulder disability. Phys Ther 45:865, 1965.
46. Downing DS, Weinstein A: Ultrasound therapy of subacromial bursitis [abstract]. Phys Ther 66:194, 1986.

47. Lundberg T, Abrahamsson P, Haker E: A comparative study of continous ultrasound, placebo ultrasound and rest in epicondylagia. Scand J Rehab Med 20:99, 1988.
48. Summer W, Patrick MK: Ultrasonic Therapy. New York, Elsevier, 1964.
49. Lehmann JF, deLateur BJ: Diathermy and superficial heat and cold. In Kottke FJ, Stillwell GK, Lehmann JF (eds): Krusen's Handbook of Physical Medicine and Rehabilitation, 3rd ed. Philadephia, W.B. Saunders, 1982, pp 275–304.
50. Klotis LC, Ziskir MC: Diathermy and pulsed electromagnetic fields. In Micholovitz SL (ed): Thermal Agents in Rehabilitation, 2nd ed. Philadelphia, F.A Davis, 1986, pp 170–197.
51. Weber DC, Brown AW: Physical agents and modalities. In Braddom RL (ed): Physical Medicine and Rehabilitation. Philadelphia, W.B. Saunders, 1996, pp 449–463.
52. Cameron MH, Perez D, Otano-Lata S: Electromagnetic radiation. In Physical Agents in Rehabilitation: From Research to Practice. Philadelphia, W.B. Saunders, 1999, pp 321–338.
53. Di Massa A, Misuriello I, Olivieri MC, Rigato M: Pulsed magnetic fields. Observations in 353 patients suffering from chronic pain. Minerva Anestesiol 55(7–8):295–299, 1989.
54. Draper DO, Knight K, Fujiwara T, Castel JC: Temperature change in human muscle during and after pulsed short-wave diathermy. J Orthop Sports Phys Ther 29:13–18; discussion 19–22, 1999.
55. Gray RJ, Quayle AA, Hall CA, Schofield MA: Physiotherapy in the treatment of temporomandibular joint disorders: A comparative study of four treatment methods. Br Dent J 176:257–261, 1994.
56. Vanharanta H: Effects of short-wave diathermy on mobility and radiological stage of the knee in the development of experimental osteoarthritis. Am J Phys Med 61:59–65, 1982.
57. Stuchly MA, Repacholi MH, Lecuyer DW, Mann RD: Exposure to the operator and patient during short wave diathermy treatments. Health Phys 42:341–366, 1982.
58. Goats GC: Microwave diathermy. Physiotherapy treatment modalities. Br J Sports Med 24:212–218, 1990.

Chapter 4

Iontophoresis and Phonophoresis

Nirmala Nayak, MD, and Kenneth D. Randall, MPT, GCS, ATC

IONTOPHORESIS

Iontophoresis has been described as a method of facilitating the transfer of ions by means of an electrical potential into soft or hard tissues of the body for therapeutic purposes.[1,2] It is a noninvasive procedure whereby free ions are applied topically into the skin using direct current. Iontophoresis is based on Faraday's law of electrolysis: $M = nIT/ZF$, where M is the number of moles of a given ion that will be released by the passage of I amperes of charge of the same polarity as the drug molecule during each second of the ejection time (T). The number of ions delivered depends on the valence of the charged ion (Z) and the Faraday constant (F). The relationship between the passage of charge and the passage of charged ions depends on the complex factor *n*, known as the transport number, which varies for individual compounds as an expression of their solubility, polarity, and type of media into which the molecules are ejected. Simply put, the basis of iontophoresis is that an electrically charged electrode will repel a similarly charged ion.

Historical Background

The uses of iontophoresis have been studied by professionals from different backgrounds—physicians, dentists, pharmaceutical scientists, chemical engineers, biologists, and physical therapists. It was found to be useful not only for local conditions but also for systemic delivery of drugs, in particular proteins and peptide drugs.[3]

In 1747, Veratti described the application of electric current to increase penetration of drugs into surface tissues.[4] The first controlled study was done in 1900 by LeDuc using strychnine and cyanide ions in rabbits.[5] One of the well-known applications of iontophoresis is for treatment of hyperhidrosis based on studies done by Ichihashi in 1936.[6] The sweat test used to diagnose cystic fibrosis, first used by Gibson and Cooke, is performed using iontophoresis with topically applied pilocarpine to induce sweating.[7]

Mechanism of Action

Acids, bases, salts, and alkaloids are ionizable substances that dissociate into their component charged ions when dissolved in water. The resulting solution with electrolytes is capable of conducting electric current by virtue of migration of the dissociated ions. When a continuous direct galvanic current (DC) is passed between two electrodes in an electrolyte solution, the cathode (negative pole) will attract positive ions, and the anode (positive pole) will attract negative ions. Iontophoresis is the transfer of ions into the body by this method for therapeutic purposes. Membrane barriers made up of lipids and proteins are present in the skin and other surface tissues; thus, ionized compounds are less easily absorbed than nonionized compounds. The rate of membrane penetration of ionized drugs may be increased by means of an electrical source. The process of iontophoresis provides this electrical energy source for passage across the membrane. The skin has an isoelectric point of around 3–4. When in contact with solutions with a pH of less than 3, it carries a net positive charge. When in contact with solutions with a pH of greater than 4, it carries a net negative charge.[8] A negative charge on the skin during iontophoresis causes electro-osmotic movement of water from within the body toward the outer surface of the skin, anode to cathode. This water movement may result in pore shrinkage at the anode and pore swelling at the cathode.[9] Thus cation transfer may occur during anodal iontophoresis in the same direction as the water flow.

Factors Affecting Iontophoretic Transport

Ionic Strength

The ionic strength of a solution is related to the concentration of the various ions in the solution. Migration of a particular ion requires that an ion of the opposite charge should also be present in close proximity. The pH of the delivery medication is often controlled by the addition of buffering agents, in which the ions are usually more mobile than the ions meant for iontophoretic delivery. This has a retarding effect on the protein of the ion, which should be delivered iontophoretically into a tissue. Ideally, the use of a buffer system should be avoided in iontophoresis, but if that is not possible, buffers containing ions with low mobility or conductivity are preferred. The drug transport in skin always is less than unity owing to the pressure of endogenous ions, such as bicarbonate, potassium, chloride, which carry a sizable fraction of ionic current.

Vehicle pH

Vehicle pH is important for drugs whose degree of ionization is pH dependent. The optimum pH for iontophoretic delivery is where the compound exists in an ionized form. Siddiqui and colleagues studied the effect of pH on the rate and extent of lidocaine iontophoresis through the skin.[10] The rate of penetration was highest at the pH where lidocaine existed in the ionized form. The pH changes become significant for protein and other drugs because the pH of the solution changes the charge on these molecules. For example, greater skin permeability has been shown at a pH below its isoelectric pH for drugs such as insulin.[11]

Current Strength

A linear relationship between the applied current and the movement of the compound has been observed. However, the maximum strength that can be used is limited by consideration for patient safety. The maximum tolerable current increases with the electrode area. The upper limit of current strength for clinical use has been suggested to be 0.5 mA/cm^2.[12]

Concentration

The effect of the solute concentration may be determined by the Nerst-Planck equation. However, it is possible that at higher concentrations, the transport may become independent of concentrate owing to the saturation of the boundary layer relative to the saturation of the donor solution.[13]

Electro-osmotic Transport

An electrically driven flow of ions across a membrane with a net charge can produce a flow of solvent called electro-osmosis. Delivery of compounds through the anode has been observed to be higher than those delivered through the cathode.[14]

Continuous versus Pulsed Current

Use of continuous direct current may result in skin polarization, which can reduce the efficiency of the iontophoretic delivery system. A pulsed direct current delivered periodically can overcome this problem.[15]

Physiologic Factors

Limited studies have suggested that iontophoretic delivery may be independent of the type of skin studied. Iontophoresis using lithium and pyridostigmine through human, pig, and rabbit skin have been found to be comparable. Insulin delivery through hairless rat skin was comparable to fuzzy rat skin.[16] Factors such as age, race, skin thickness, degree of hydration, and normal versus diseased skin have yet to be studied. The effect of dermal blood flow on iontophoresis has been shown in pigs using lidocaine delivery in the presence of vasoactive chemicals (epinephrine). There was a decrease in lidocaine flux because of lidocaine's vasoconstrictor effect compared with use of tolazoline, which increased the iontophoretic lidocaine flux caused by its vasodilator effect.[17,18]

Therapeutic Applications of Iontophoresis

Iontophoresis has many advantages that render it a desirable modality for drug delivery. Some of the advantages are similar to those of phonophoresis, including the noninvasive nature of the procedure, low risk of infection, systemic absorption, and enhanced drug penetration. Additionally, the iontophoresis unit is available for home use and provides a simplified therapeutic regimen, which helps with compliance. Disadvantages of the procedure are that it can be time consuming, and minor skin irritation and burning can occur with treatment.

Inflammatory conditions such as bursitis, tendinitis, strains, and sprains have been successfully treated using dexamethasone sodium phosphate combined with lidocaine (Xylocaine) iontophoresis.[19,20] Glass and associates demonstrated effectiveness of iontophoresis in a series of animal studies with rhesus monkeys by introducing radio-labeled dexamethasone sodium phosphate into tissues surrounding major joints including tendons and cartilage.[21] Iontophoresis using acetic acid has been reported to treat successfully calcifying tendinitis of the shoulder in humans and traumatic myositis ossificans in the quadriceps femoris muscle.[22,23] Banta found outstanding results with his patients with carpal tunnel syndrome using dexamethasone. In this study, more than 58% of the subjects had a positive response to iontophoresis, and he suggested that this is an excellent alternative to steroid injections.[24]

Other conditions found useful for treatment are skin conditions such as hyperhidrosis,[25,26] small open ulcers,[27,28] and fungal infections.[29] Iontophoresis has also been used to administer local anesthetics for dental, ear, nose, throat, and eye procedures.[30–32] Edema reduction using hyaluronidase, which appears to increase absorption of fluid from skin and subcutaneous tissue, has been attempted, but as

TABLE 1. COMMONLY USED IONS WITH IONTOPHORESIS

Ion	Polarity	Indication
Dexamthasone	−	Musculoskeletal inflammatory conditions
Acetate	−	Calcium deposits
Lidocaine	+	Analgesic agent
Hyaluronidase	+	Edema reduction
Zinc	+	Ischemic ulcers
Copper	+	Fungal infections of feet

with other edema-reduction techniques, the effect is short-lived.[33,34] Table 1 contains a list of the most commonly used ions and their respective polarity.[35]

General Principles of Application

Identification of the appropriate ion and its polarity for treating the presenting pathology is paramount for successful treatment. Some ions, such as those in iron, silver, copper, and zinc, form insoluble precipitates as they pass into the tissues and should be avoided. Other important factors that influence outcome are the (1) depth of penetration, (2) number of ions transferred, and (3) whether vascular transportation of the ions carry away from the application site. The number of ions transferred into the body is dependent on three factors: the current density, duration of the current flow, and the concentration of ions in the solution. The current density is determined by the size of the electrode used—the smaller the electrodes, the higher the density. To decrease the caustic alkaline reaction in the body tissue that occurs under the cathode, the surface area of the cathode is always at least twice that of the anode. Normal intact skin is intolerant of current densities greater that 1 mA/cm^2. This impedance is further lowered in abraded or lacerated skin, fair skin, and scarred skin. The anesthetic effect produced under the electrodes poses a high risk for electrical burns. Therefore, close monitoring and caution is advised during treatment. Research on the penetration and distribution of ions with iontophoresis has demonstrated effectiveness. Several studies have indicated that ions penetrate and have therapeutic effects on deep structures.[36,37] More recently, Costello found penetration of at least 1 cm into the gluteal muscles of rabbits when using lidocaine with iontophoresis. His ideal parameters for ion penetration were current of 4 mA for 10 minutes, with a 4% lidocaine solution.[38]

Equipment

Three types of equipment are available for iontophoresis: line-operated units, simple battery-operated units, and rechargeable power units. Line-operated units are used mostly for the pilocarpine iontophoresis sweat test in cystic fibrosis.[39] Because of the potential for electric shock from the wall outlets, battery-operated units were developed.

Battery-operated units are available for commercial and home use. A more sophisticated multipurpose unit, called the Phoresor, is popular in dentistry and physical therapy. The Phoresor runs on a 9-volt battery with a 45-volt DC transformer. It delivers a constant current and adjusts to change in resistance in the external circuit during the procedure. It is equipped with safety features including a limited maximal rate of current of 2 mA/sec to prevent shock. The actual procedure entails massaging the chosen drug solution or cream into the bare skin over the area to be treated or placing a towel soaked with the drug solution on the skin to be treated. The active pad electrode made of tin, aluminum foil, or commercial metal electrode that has the same polarity as the ions is placed over the towel. Avoiding direct contact between the pad and skin is essential to prevent chemical burns. On the other hand, good contact between the electrode and towel and between the towel and skin is needed to avoid "hot spots" from increased current density. A second electrode pad, moistened with tap water or saline solution, is placed at a distance on the same side as the active electrode. The lead wires from the pads are connected to the appropriate generator terminals. The amplitude of the current is set to achieve current density between 0.1 and 0.5 mA/cm^2. The duration of treatment can be up to 15 minutes, depending on the patient's comfort.

Today, several brands of electrodes are available that allow for simple drug delivery. With these modern electrode systems, the ion solution is simply injected onto the drug delivery electrode, saturating it. The pads come in various sizes, each with their respective drug fill volume. This pad is placed over the treatment area, and a separate dispersive pad is placed over a muscle group at least 6 inches away. The lead clips are attached to the appropriate electrodes, and the unit is turned on. For inflammatory musculoskeletal conditions, these authors typically use dexamethasone with the following settings:

Dose: 40 mA-min
Current: 2 mA
Treatment time: 20 minutes

The newer Phoresor units automatically calculate the treatment time once the dose and current variables have been selected. These units sound an audible alarm and shut down once the treatment time is complete. Figure 1 shows a Phoresor in use with electrode placement for treatment of lateral epicondylitis.

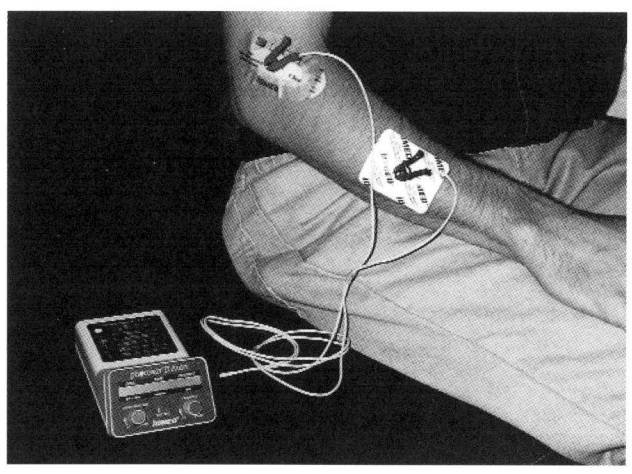

FIGURE 1. A typical electrode placement for treatment of lateral epicondylitis using the Iomed Phoresor II.

Summary

Iontophoresis has enjoyed considerable success in the treatment of musculoskeletal and dermatologic conditions. With use of appropriate parameters, it has proven to be a safe and effective modality. As knowledge of the mechanism and physiology of the iontophoretic process increases, the potential for its use for drug delivery in the treatment of musculoskeletal conditions expands.

PHONOPHORESIS

Phonophoresis may be defined as ultrasonic energy used to enhance skin permeability, allowing uncharged or charged molecules of drugs into dermal tissues. Ultrasound refers to sound waves with frequencies beyond the human audible range of 20 kHz. High-frequency waves in the 800–1000-kHz range are generated by applying alternating current to a crystal, usually quartz or silicone dioxide. Through a phenomenon known as the **piezoelectric effect**, the electric current causes the crystal to undergo rhythmic deformation producing ultrasonic vibrations. The vibrations are then transferred through a coupling medium to tissue surface.[40,41] In phonophoresis, the coupling agent (water or gel) is replaced with the drug to be delivered. Phonophoresis can thus be used as a transdermal drug delivery system.

Historical Background

In 1954, Fellinger and Schmid first reported use of phonophoresis to enhance drug delivery in treatment of arthritis using hydrocortisone ointment.[42] In 1963, Griffin and Touchstone used cortisol to demonstrate percutaneous penetration into paravertebral nerve and skeletal muscle.[43,44] Hydrocortisone has been used successfully for treatment of sprains, strains, tendinitis, bursitis, and epicondylitis.[45]

Mechanism of Action

Phonophoresis is different from simple ultrasound therapy in that the drug is delivered to deep tissue by ultrasound energy and the clinical effect is associated with the pharmacologic effect of the drug. The exact mechanism of action of phonophoresis is still unknown, but several theories hold that ultrasound may cause intracellular diffusion from high-speed vibration of drug molecules along with vibration of the cell membrane and its components.[46] Other theories involve the cavitation effect of ultrasound. Cavitation may cause mechanical stress. Temperature elevation or enhanced chemical reactivity causes drug transport.[47,48] Brown suggested that ultrasound increased cell permeability and drug absorption by raising skin temperature.[49] Increased tissue permeability has been attributed to mechanical "stirring" and increased pore size.[50] Other studies suggest that changes in stratum corneum lipid structure enhance percutaneous absorption.[51]

Applications of Phonophoresis

Transcutaneous drug delivery through use of topically applied agents is a well-known treatment for conditions such as angina, hypertension, motion sickness, and local musculoskeletal injuries. Anti-inflammatory agents and local anesthetics have been used to treat pain and inflammation. Steroid phonophoresis generally has been used in conditions for which steroid injection is considered.

Advantages of using phonophoresis over injections include:

1. The method of delivery is noninvasive.
2. There is little or no systemic absorption, minimizing the risk of hepatic and renal injury from drug elimination. Studies that substantiate this finding document absence of dexamethasone, hydrocortisone, and salicylates after phonophoresis in humans.[52-54]
3. Patient comfort is increased.
4. Drug delivery can be terminated rapidly through termination of ultrasound.
5. There is a low risk of infection when used on intact skin.
6. Delivery of selected drugs is enhanced.

Phonophoresis should be limited or is contraindicated in the following conditions:

1. Broken skin surface and skin infections
2. Allergy to the drug used for phonophoresis
3. Conditions with reduced temperature and light touch sensation
4. Peripheral vascular diseases
5. Malignancies
6. Pregnancy
7. Presence of cemented prosthesis
8. Weak and unstable joints
9. Presence of keloid or exuberant scar formation

Equipment

Performance of phonophoresis requires an ultrasound machine that is AC powered, has two or more frequencies of operation, and has outputs that are easily adjusted. The treatment head is sized to treat irregular body surfaces and has a transducer that senses poor coupling. There is total contact between the gel and transducer that is constantly moved at a rate of 1 inch per second. The pulsed mode of ultrasound is preferred to minimize thermal injury. The usual treatment dose is 1.0–1.5 watts/cm^2 for 5 minutes.

Review of Drugs Used for Treatment of Musculoskeletal Conditions

The most frequently used and most studied drug for phonophoresis in musculoskeletal conditions is hydrocortisone. Ten percent hydrocortisone has been shown to be more effective than 1% hydrocortisone in the treatment of humeral epicondylitis, subdeltoid bursitis, and bicipital tendinitis.[55] Byl and associates studied the effects of phonophoresis with corticosteroids on collagen deposition in pigs under controlled conditions.[56] Collagen activity, as measured by level of hydroxyproline, showed decreased levels in the subcutaneous tissues but not in the submuscular or tendinous tissue. This highlights the limitations of phonophoresis for conditions deeper than subcutaneous tissue. This observation was substantiated by Muir and colleagues, who studied phonophoresis of hydrocortisone in canine knees.[57] Compared with intra-articular steroid injection, phonophoresis was shown to be ineffective in delivering the hydrocortisone into the knees. However, phonophoresis has been shown to be superior to ultrasound alone using 10% cortisol solution in the hind leg joints of dogs.[58] Because of the potential for adverse effects, systemic effects of hydrocortisone phonophoresis have been studied. Ten percent hydrocortisone did not appear to suppress adrenal function in patients who received phonophoresis with dexamethasone every other day for 2 weeks over the shoulder area.[59] Similarly, no increase in blood levels of cortisol was found in a blinded study of healthy human volunteers who received 1.0 watts/cm^2 ultrasound treatment using either 10% hydrocortisone gel or Aquasonic gel for a total of two treatments, 1 week apart.[60] Many PT clinics use dexamethasone in Aquasonic $1/_3$% gel. There are many anecdotal reports of benefits in using this for treating lateral epicondylitis. To date, there is no clear scientific data available to verify which medication or dose of medication works best and how much of the active ingredient is actually absorbed. Oziomek and associates, who studied effects of phonophoresis on serum salicylate level, suggest that phonophoresis is substrate specific. Topical application of salicylates with and without use of ultrasound resulted in no increase in serum salicylate level. Thus, they concluded that perhaps no appreciable absorption of salicylates occurred in subdermal tissues.[54] A double-blind study by Benson et al. using benzydamine, a nonsteroidal anti-inflammatory drug for phonophoresis, also found no percutaneous absorption.[61]

Summary

Phonophoresis as a modality for transdermal drug delivery in the treatment of selected musculoskeletal disorders appears to be useful. Inflammatory conditions such as tendinitis bursitis and epicondylitis are some of the conditions that have been successfully treated, and phonophoresis could be considered a viable modality before the use of invasive procedures such as surgery or injections.

REFERENCES

1. Walton RE, Leonard LA, Sharawy M, Gangarosa LP: Effects on pulp and dentin of iontophoresis of sodium fluoride on exposed roots in dogs. Oral Surg 48:545–547, 1979.
2. Pashley DH: Strategies for clinical evaluation of drugs and for devices for the alleviation of hypersensitive dentin. In Rowe NH (ed): Proceedings of Symposium on Hypersensitive Dentin: Origin and Management. Ann Arbor, MI, University of Michigan, 1985.
3. Lee VHL: Peptides and protein drug delivery: Opportunities and challenges. Pharm Int 7:208–212, 1986.
4. Turnell WJ: Therapeutic action of constant current. Proc Royal Soc Med 14:41–52, 1921.
5. LeDuc S: Electric Ions and Their Use in Medicine. Liverpool, Rebman, 1903.
6. Ichihashi T: Effect of drugs on the sweat glands by cataphoresis and an effective method for suppression of local sweating. J Orient Med 25:101, 1936.
7. Gibson LE, Cooke RE: A test for concentration of electrolytes in sweat in cystic fibrosis of the pancreas utilizing pilocarpine by iontophoresis. Pediatrics 23:545–549, 1959.
8. Rosendal T: Studies on the conducting properties of the human skin to direct current. Acta Physiol Scand 5:130, 1942–43.
9. Harris R: Iontophoresis in therapeutic electricity and ultraviolet radiation. In Stillwell GK (ed). Baltimore, Williams & Wilkins, 1967, p 156.
10. Siddiqui O, Roberts MS, Polack AE: The effect of iontophoresis and vehicle pH on the in vitro penetration of lignocaine through stratum corneum. J Pharm Pharmacol 37:732–735, 1985.
11. Siddiqui O, Sun Y, Liu JC, Chen YW: Facilitated transport of insulin. J Pharm Sci 76:341–345, 1987.
12. Abramson HA, Gorin MH: Skin reactions. X. Preseasonal treatment of hay fever by electrophoresis of ragweed pollen extracts into the skin: Preliminary report. J Allergy 12:169, 1941.

13. Phipps JB, Padmanabhan RV, Lattin GA: Iontophoretic delivery of model inorganic and drug ions. J Pharm Sci 78:365, 1989.
14. Green PG, Hinz RS, Cullander C, et al: Iontophoretic delivery of amino acids and derivatives across the skin in vitro. Pharm Res 8:1113–1120, 1991.
15. Banga A, Chien YW: Iontophoretic delivery of drugs: Fundamentals, developments, and biomedical applications. J Cont Rel 7:1, 1988.
16. Siddiqui O, Chien YW: Nonparenteral administration of peptide and protein drugs. Crit Rev Ther Drug Carrier Syst 3:195–208, 1987.
17. Riviere JE, Sage B, Williams PL: Effects of vasoactive drugs on transdermal lidocaine iontophoresis. J Pharm Sci 80:615, 1991.
18. Riviere JE, Riviere NA, Inman AO: Determination of lidocaine concentration in skin after transdermal iontophoresis: Effects of vasoactive drugs. Pharm Res 9:211, 1992.
19. Harris PR: Iontophoresis: Clinical research in musculoskeletal inflammatory conditions. J Orthop Sports Ther 4:109, 1982.
20. Bertolucci LE: Introduction of anti-inflammatory drugs by iontophoresis: Double-blind study. J Orthop Sports Ther 4:103, 1982.
21. Glass JM, Stephen RL, Jacobsen SC: The quantity and distribution of radiolabeled dexamethasone delivered to tissues by iontophoresis. Int J Dermatol 19:519, 1980.
22. Perron M, Malouin F: Acetic acid iontophoresis and ultrasound for the treatment of calcifying tendinitis of the shoulder: A randomized, control trial. Arch Phys Med Rehabil 78:379–384, 1997.
23. Weider DL: Treatment of Traumatic Myositis Ossificans with Acetic Acid Iontophoresis. Physical Therapy 72(2):133–137, 1992.
24. Banta CA: A prospective, nonrandomized study of iontophoresis, wrist splinting, and anti-inflammatory medication in the treatment of early-mid carpal tunnel syndrome. J Occup Med 36: 166–168, 1994.
25. Kahn J: Clinical Electrotherapy. Syosset, NY, Joseph Kahn, 1973.
26. Levit F: Simple device for treatment of hyperhidrosis by iontophoresis. Arch Dermatol 98:505, 1968.
27. Cornwall MW: Zinc iontophoresis to treat ischemic ulcers. Phys Ther 61:359, 1981.
28. Falcone AE, Spadaro JA: Inhibitory effects of electrically activated silver material on cutaneous wound bacteria. Plast Reconstr Surg 77:455, 1986.
29. Haggard HW, Strauss MJ, Greenberg LA: Fungus infectious of hand and feet treated by copper iontophoresis. JAMA 112:1229, 1939.
30. Gangarosa LP: Iontophoresis for surface local anesthesia. J Am Dent Assoc 88:125, 1974.
31. Sisper HA: Iontophoresis local anesthesia for conjunctional surgery. Ann Ophthalmol 10:597 1978.
32. Comean M, Brummet R, Vernon SJ: Local anesthesia of the ear by iontophoresis. Arch Otolaryngol 98:114, 1973.
33. Magistro CM: Hyaluronidase by iontophoresis. Phys Ther 44:169, 1964.
34. Schwartz MS: The use of hyaluronidase by iontophoresis in the treatment of lymphedema. Arch Intern Med 95:662, 1955.
35. Costello CT, Jeske AH: Iontophoresis: Application in transdermal medication delivery. Phys Ther 75:559, 1995.
36. Harris PR: Iontophoresis: Clinical research in musculoskeletal inflammatory conditions. J Orthop Sports Phys Ther 4:109–112, 1982.
37. Kahn J: Acetic acid iontophoresis for calcium deposits. Phys Ther 57:658–660, 1977.
38. Costello CT: Optimization of Drug Delivery with Iontophoresis [dissertation]. Houston, TX, Texas Women's University, 1993.
39. Denning CR, Huang NN, Cuasay LR et al: Cooperative study: Comparing three methods of performing sweat test to diagnose cystic fibrosis. Pediatrics 66:757, 1980.
40. Wells PN: Biomedical Ultrasonics. New York, Academic Press, 1977, pp 421–430.
41. Newman JT, Nellermoe MD, Carnett JL: Hydrocortisone phonophoresis. A literature review. J Am Pediatr Med Assoc 82(8):432–435, 1992.
42. Fellinger K, Schmid J: Klinik and therapic des Chronischen Gelenkhuematismus. Vienna, Mandrich, 1954, pp 549–551.
43. Griffin JE, Touchstone JC: Ultrasonic movement of cortisol into pig tissue I. Movement into skeletal muscle. Am J Phys Med 42:777–785, 1963.
44. Griffin JE, Touchstone JC: Ultrasonic movement of cortisol into pig tissue II. Movement into paravertebral nerve. Am J Phys Med 44:20–25, 1965.

45. Griffin JE, Eternach JL, Price RE: Patients treated with ultrasound driven hydrocortisone and with ultrasound alone. Phys Ther 47:594–601, 1967.
46. Byl NN: The use of ultrasound as an enhanced for transcutaneous drug delivery: Phonophoresis. Phys Ther 75:6539–6553, 1995.
47. Baldes EJ, Herrick JF, Strobel CF: Biologic effect of ultrasound. Am J Phys Med 37:111–121, 1958.
48. Griffin JE: Physiologic effects of ultrasonic energy as it is used clinically. J Am Phys Ther Assoc 46:18–26, 1966.
49. Brown SA: Transdermal delivery of drugs I: Relationship of drug agents and carriers in skin penetration. Dermatol Rep 6:1, 2, 8, 1987.
50. Saxena J, Sharma N, Makoid MC: Ultrasonically mediated drug delivery. J Biomat Appl 7:277–96, 1993.
51. Tyle P, Agrawala P: Drug delivery by phonophoresis. Pharm Res 6:355–361, 1989.
52. Franklin ME, Smith ST, Chenier TC, Franklin RC: Effect of phonophoresis with dexamethasone on adrenal function. J Orthop Sports Phys Med 22:103–107, 1995.
53. Bare AC, Caristie DS, McAnaw MB, et al: Phonophoretic delivery of 10% hydrocortisone through the epidermis of humans as determined by serum cortisol concentrations. Phys Ther 76:738–749, 1996.
54. Oziomek RS, Perrin DH, Herhold DA, Denger CR: Effect of phonophoresis on serum salicylate levels. Med Sci Sports Exerc 23:397–401, 1991.
55. Kleinkort JA, Wood F: Phonophoresis with 1% versus 10% hydrocortisone. Phys Ther 55:1320–1324, 1975.
56. Byl NN, McKenzie A, Halliday B: The effects of phonophoresis with corticosteroids: A controlled pilot study. J Sports Phys Ther 18:590–600, 1993.
57. Muir MS, Magee FP, Longo JA: Comparison of ultrasonically applied vs. intraarticular injected hydrocortisone levels in canine knees. Orthop Rev 19:351–356, 1990.
58. Davick JP, Martin RK, Albright JP: Distribution and deposition of tritiated cortisol using phonophoresis. Phys Ther 68:1672–1675, 1988.
59. Franklin ME, Smith ST, Chenier TC, Franklin RC: Effect of phonophoresis with dexamethasone on adrenal function. J Orthop Sports Phys Ther 22:103–107, 1995.
60. Bare AC, McAnaw MB, Pritchard AE, et al: Phonophoretic delivery of 10% hydrocortisone through the epidermis of humans as determined by serum cortisol concentrations. Phys Ther 76:738–745, 1996.
61. Benson HAE, McElnay JC, Harland R: Use of ultrasound to enhance percutaneous absorption of benzydamine. Phys Ther 69:113–118, 1989.

# Chapter 5
Cryotherapy

Kirstin Young, MD, MPH, and Eugenie Atherton, MSPT

Cryotherapy, or cold therapy, has been used for centuries to treat many ailments. Superficial cooling is a basic tool for all rehabilitation practitioners owing to its simplicity, low cost, safety, and effectiveness. Most forms of cryotherapy are based on superficial cooling agents, with energy transfer occurring through conduction. Conduction involves the transfer of energy through direct contact. The cold surface (usually ice or other cold modality) extracts energy or heat from the warmer surface (usually skin). The larger the temperature difference between the two surfaces, the larger the drop in tissue temperature.[1,4]

Although conduction is the primary mechanism of energy transfer in most cryotherapy techniques, exceptions to this rule exist. Vapocoolant spray extracts energy or heat through evaporation. As the liquid spray is emitted and comes in contact with the skin, it vaporizes, which requires heat or energy. The skin temperature drops as the spray is applied due to energy loss in the evaporative process.

Hydrotherapy is another exception to the conduction rule. The transfer of energy or heat through convection occurs during hydrotherapy. The temperature of the skin and underlying tissue drops as the cool water current passes by the warm skin extracting heat in an attempt to equalize the two temperatures.

MECHANISMS OF ACTION

Cold acts through several mechanisms to produce the desired therapeutic effects. First, cold results in immediate arteriole vasoconstriction, which decreases the delivery of blood to the cooled area. This occurs through sympathetic fibers and by a direct effect on the blood vessels.[18,31] In addition, the use of cold can decrease the delivery of substances carried in the blood. Some of these agents may be undesirable vasoactive agents such as histamine. Without the delivery of large amounts of histamine, inflammation and fluid filtration are kept to a minimum.[27]

Another substance that is retarded by cooling is cytochrome oxidase. This can cause mitochondrial damage; therefore, its decrease as a result of cooling can be beneficial in retarding secondary injury.[25] The **hunting response** has been described as a delayed vasodilation of arterioles after cooling. This protects the peripheral tissues from cold induced damage.[19]

Neuromuscular effects of cooling are well documented. The cooler the muscle, the slower the rate of firing. The site of the thermal effect is the sensory terminal itself.[10] With cooling, the tendon jerk is diminished. This is due to the decreased tone of the muscle at the spindle level.[14,17,26] The motor nerve fibers display prolonged twitch in both contraction and relaxation. The nerves demonstrate conduction slowing with cooling and effectively become blocked at the neuromuscular junction. As temperature decreases, the amplitude and duration of the motor unit end plate potentials increase, and the frequency of their firing decreases.[20]

The peripheral nerves are affected by cryotherapy as well. The duration of action potential recovery is increased after cooling,[7] and the action potential duration itself increases inversely as the temperature decreases.[20] The rate of stimulation required to obtain fusion of the twitches to complete tetanus drops as the temperature decreases.[33] The cooling effect on spasticity lasts long after application of ice (up to at least 30 minutes).[32]

The threshold at which patients experience pain has been found to be decreased with the use of cryotherapy. This is thought to be due to a direct effect of temperature reduction on nerve fibers and receptors.[18] The diminished sensitivity of the muscle-spindle afferent fibers to discharge may contribute to this decrease in pain and also to muscle spasms.

However, cryotherapy also causes some effects that may be less desirable, such as increased tissue and blood viscosity, which can result in decreased elasticity of the tissue and increased resistance to motion. This could hamper therapeutic efforts,[27] because it becomes progressively more difficult to perform skilled motor tasks as cooling takes effect.[11,12]

As cold compresses are applied, skin temperature drops first, then the subcutaneous adipose tissue temperature slowly decreases, the intra-articular region (synovium) is cooled, and finally the rectal (core) temperature drops. As little as 5 minutes of cooling can produce a decrease in intra-articular temperature, and the decrease is linear until 30 minutes. Rewarming takes longer than 1 hour, perhaps because of vasoconstriction.[2,34] Compared with compresses, ice baths cool superficial tissues faster and have a more dramatic cooling effect, but they exert a lesser effect in the deep tissues.[35]

INDICATIONS

The most common indications for cryotherapy are:

- To decrease muscle tone
- To decrease spasticity in upper motor neuron lesions
- To facilitate muscle contraction and muscle reeducation
- To decrease bleeding
- To decrease edema
- To alleviate thermal burns
- To increase pain threshold
- To decrease inflammation
- To decrease joint pain and edema
- To decrease collagenolysis
- To decrease synovial inflammation

In patients with increased muscle tone, application of cryotherapeutic agents have been shown to decrease tone and spasticity through reflex decreases in motor neuron activity and muscle spindle discharge.[14,28] Not only does abnormal muscle tone diminish through the application of cryotherapy, but muscle strength and endurance increase, facilitating muscle re-education and contraction.[18]

In an acute musculoskeletal injury, cold has been found to decrease bleeding, edema, and delivery of inflammatory cells.[15,18,24,27,31] In addition, cryotherapy is believed to increase the pain threshold in both chronic and acute conditions through direct and indirect mechanisms.[6,18,24] The pain receptors are impaired by cold directly, and the reduction of spasticity, edema, and inflammation contribute to the relief of pain.

The use of cold has been shown to inhibit the development of burns, shorten healing time, and decrease severity of the burn. The more quickly the cold is applied after the initial burn, the better the therapeutic effects.[8,36]

Cryotherapy may also decrease collagenolysis and synovial inflammation and, therefore, slow joint destruction in patients with rheumatoid arthritis.[13,30]

PRECAUTIONS

Cryotherapy is contraindicated:

- In areas with absence of sensation
- In patients with cold hypersensitivity
- In patients with arterial insufficiency
- In patients with cryopathies, such cryoglobulinemia, paroxysmal cold hemoglobinuria, and Raynaud's phenomenon

Prolonged joint cooling with topical ice can lead to nerve palsy and extensive axonotmesis. Ulnar and peroneal nerve damage have been reported in the literature.[5,9,29] To prevent these complications, avoid compression of nerves that lie relatively superficially, avoid the use of gel packs, which produce temperatures below freezing, and do not ice areas where patients may be insensate and unable to feel a cold "burn."

The nerve injury thought to be caused by cold is likely a result of direct injury to the nerve membrane as well as secondary injury due to neural ischemia, edema, and suspension of axoplasmic transport.[5] Some patients have been reported to have "hypersensitivity" to cold. The release of histamine or histamine-like substances causes cold urticaria. Symptoms include erythema, itching, and sweating. These cases are rare but do constitute a contraindication to cold therapy.[16]

Additionally, patients with arterial insufficiency should not receive prolonged cold therapy because of the already compromised delivery of blood.

Additional precautions for the use of cold include cryopathies such as cryoglobulinemia, paroxysmal cold hemoglobinuria, and Raynaud's phenomenon.

SPECIAL CONSIDERATIONS

The major component of vapocoolant spray, fluoromethane, is made of dichlorodifluoromethane and trichlorofluoromethane, both of which harm the environment by destroying ozone in the upper atmosphere. This product is still used in some locations and is still sold in the United States. However, it does require a medical prescription by a physician for use.

The amount of subcutaneous adipose tissue directly relates to the rate of temperature decrease when ice is applied and rewarming when ice is removed due to the depth of the tissue, poor conductivity, and insulatory characteristic. In practice, a client who has little adipose tissue will benefit from a 10-minute ice pack application, whereas a client with a greater adipose layer may require as much as a 30-minute cold pack application to receive benefit.[18,21]

Cryotherapy can alter a client's true range of motion (ROM) and strength. This can result in a skewed evaluation or re-evaluation. Ice increases the viscosity and decreases the elasticity of muscle and, therefore, can decrease the potential ROM for a given muscle.[27] Clinically, measurements taken after cryotherapy is applied can appear more restricted than their actual values. Therefore, measurements should always be made before the application of cryotherapy. Performance can be diminished as well, and fine motor skills or activity involving full ROM may be impaired by the application of cryotherapy techniques.

Additional confounding occurs with strength measurements. Strength of a given muscle group appears to increase temporarily after cryotherapy.[23] Thus, true strength measurements should be taken before cryotherapy. In addition, greater work can be accomplished after cryotherapy because the client may be able to perform therapeutic exercise with greater weight than without cryotherapy. This factor needs to be taken into consideration when prescribing or directing therapeutic exercises.

Ice is used to prevent inflammation in the first 24–48 hours after an acute injury. After that time, if swelling has been prevented, ice is to be discontinued because it can delay the healing process.[18,22]

Ice immersion, chipped ice in a bag, ice massage, and applying frozen vegetables to the involved site are inexpensive and easy for the client to perform as part of his or her home exercise program.

CHOOSING A TYPE OF CRYOTHERAPY

The size and type of the area to be treated and time constraints are factors to consider when selecting a cryotherapeutic agent. A large treatment site requires a larger agent; therefore, a large commercial ice pack, chipped ice, or iced towel would be appropriate. Ice massage is used if a small region, such as a small muscle, tendon, or joint, is involved. If a distal extremity is involved, ice immersion is the treatment of choice. If time is limited and a muscle region is small, ice massage provides quicker results for cooling than an ice bag.[35]

METHOD OF ADMINISTRATION

Commercial Gel Ice Packs. Commercial gel ice packs are applied to the entire region with a layer of towels placed between the client's skin and the pack (Fig. 1).

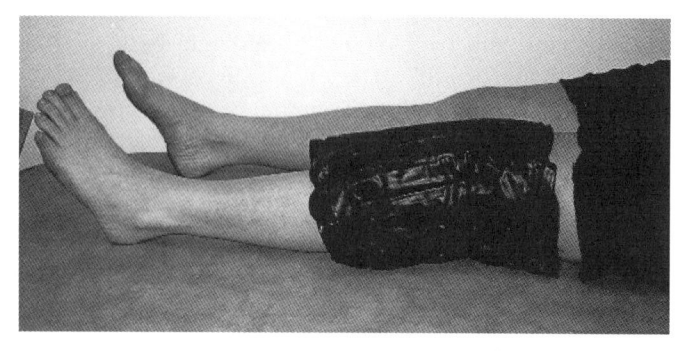

FIGURE 1. Commercial gel ice pack applied to the knee.

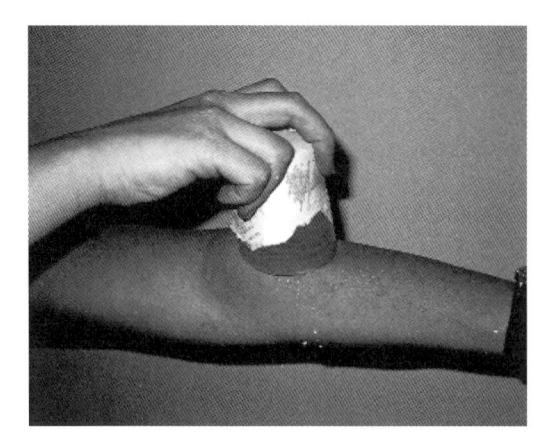

FIGURE 2. Ice massage applied to wrist extensors.

For increased cooling effect, the towel is moistened with water and then placed on the treatment area and secured with a strap. The treatment time is 10–15 minutes, depending on the amount of adipose tissue.

Chipped Ice Bag. Scoop chipped ice into a plastic bag. To decrease the temperature more significantly, add one part water to three parts ice. Secure opening, and place on treatment site for 10–15 minutes.

Ice Massage. Water is frozen in paper cups, and the paper is partially peeled back to expose the ice. The therapist grasps the cup and rubs the ice in quick sweeping circular movements over the target area for 5–10 minutes (Fig. 2).[3,34] The patient should report analgesia of the region after the session.

Iced Towels. A towel that has been submerged in ice water or chipped ice is placed over the joint or muscle and secured with a strap (Fig. 3). This is beneficial when performing the contract/relax method during therapeutic exercise. The

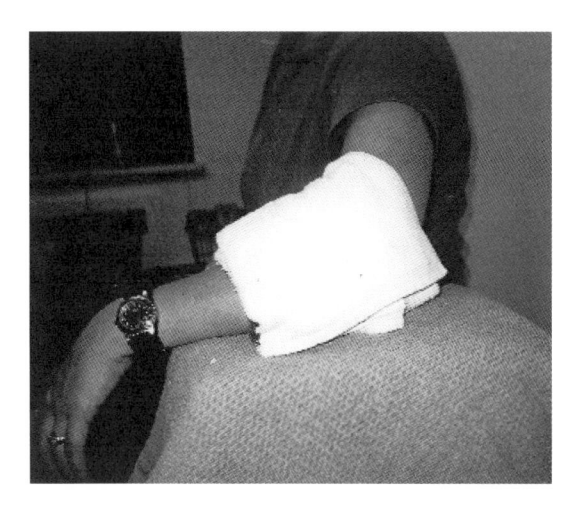

FIGURE 3. Iced towel applied to the elbow.

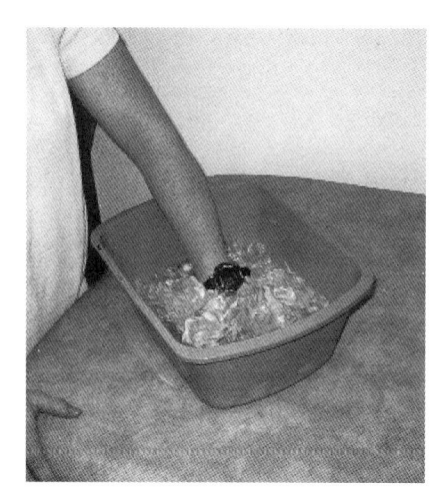

FIGURE 4. Iced bath immersion of the left hand.

towels will need to be reapplied throughout the session because the iced towels warm quickly. The duration of application is the duration of the exercise session.

Iced Bath Immersion. The muscle or joint to be treated is placed in a basin or a whirlpool filled with crushed ice and water at a temperature around 13(C–27°C for 10–20 minutes (Fig. 4). The duration is dependent on the temperature: the lower the temperature, the shorter the duration of treatment. Immersion is beneficial when treating an extremity and circumferential cooling is needed.

Vapocoolant Spray (Fluoromethane). The glass bottle of vapocoolant spray is held with the nozzle down approximately 12–18 inches above the treatment site, so that the stream will directly contact the skin (Fig. 5). Spray the site at a rate of 4 inches/second in one direction. Perform PROM while spraying and have the client

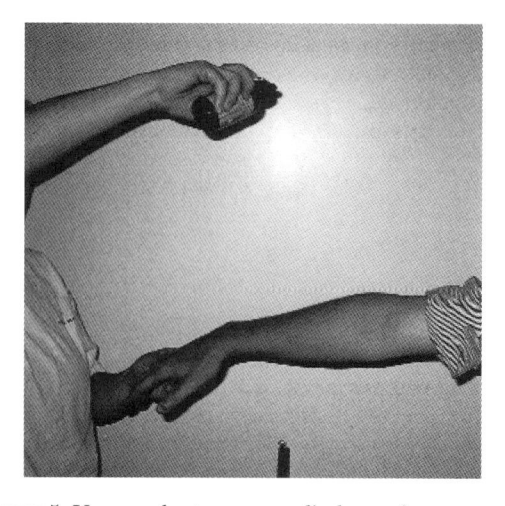

FIGURE 5. Vapocoolant spray applied to wrist extensors.

perform active ROM immediately afterwards. The entire process can be repeated three to four times. Rewarm the skin manually or with a hot pack, if necessary.

REIMBURSEMENT

At the time of this writing, Medicare, Medicaid, and most large insurance companies are not reimbursing providers for cryotherapy treatment. Many hospitals and clinics continue to provide this service to the client pro bono. Some clinicians may instruct clients to perform the ice treatment at home after their session is complete, because many types of cryotherapy are easy to perform independently and are inexpensive.

REFERENCES

1. Abramson DI: Physiologic basis for the use of physical agents in peripheral vascular disorders. Arch Phys Med Rehabil 46:216, 1965.
2. Bocobo C, Fast A, Kingery W, Kaplan M: The effect of ice on intra-articular temperature in the knee of the dog. Am J Phys Med 70:181–185, 1991.
3. Bugaj R: The cooling, analgesic, and rewarming effects of ice massage on localized skin. Phys Ther 55:11–19, 1975.
4. Clarke RJ, Hellon RF, Lind AR: Vascular reactions of the human forearm to cold. Clin Sci 17:165, 1958.
5. Collins K, Storey M, Peterson K: Peroneal nerve palsy after cryotherapy. Phys Sportsmed 14:105–108, 1986.
6. Curkovic B, Vitulic V, Babic-Naglic D, Durrigl T: The influence of heat and cold on the pain threshold in rheumatoid arthritis. Z Rheumatol 52:289–291, 1993.
7. Douglas WW, Malcolm JL: The effect of localized cooling on conduction in cat nerves. J Physiol 130:53–71, 1955.
8. Demling RH, Mazess RB, Wolberg W: The effect of immediate and delayed cold immersion on burn edema formation and resorption. J Trauma 17:56–60, 1979.
9. Drez D, Faust DC, Evans JP: Cryotherapy and nerve palsy. Am J Sports Med 9:256–257, 1981.
10. Eldred E, Lindsley DF, Buchwald JS: The effect of cooling on mammalian muscle spindles. Exp Neurol 2:144–157, 1960.
11. Fox RH: Local cooling in man. Br Med Bull 17:14–18, 1961.
12. Gaydos HF, Dusek ER: Effects of localized hand cooling versus total body cooling on manual performance. J Appl Physiol 12:377–380, 1958.
13. Harris ED, McCroskery PA: The influence of temperature and fibril stability on degradation of cartilage collagen by rheumatoid synovial collagenase. N Engl J Med 2:154–158, 1974.
14. Hartviksen K: Ice therapy in spasticity. Acta Neurol Scand 38:79–84, 1962.
15. Ho SSW, Illgen RL, Meyer RW, et al: Comparison of various icing times in decreasing bone metabolism and blood flow in the knee. Am J Sports Med 23:74–76, 1995.
16. Juhlin L, Shelley WB: Role of mast cell and basophil in cold urticaria with associated systemic reactions. JAMA 117:371–377, 1961.
17. Knutsson E, Mattsson E: Effects of local cooling on monosynaptic reflexes in man. Scand J Rehabil Med 1:126–132, 1969.
18. Lehmann JF: Heat and Cold, 4th ed. Baltimore, Williams & Wilkins, 1990.
19. Lewis T: Observations upon the reactions of the vessels of the human skin to cold. Heart 15:177, 1930.
20. Li C-L: Effect of cooling on neuromuscular transmission in the rat. Am J Physiol 194:200–206, 1958.
21. Lowdon BJ, Moore RJ: Determinants and nature of intramuscular temperature changes during cold therapy. Am J Phys Med 54:223, 1975.
22. Lundgren C, Mureen A, Zederfeldt B: The effect of cold-vasoconstriction on wound healing in the rabbit. Acta Chir Scand 118:1–4, 1959.
23. McGown HL: Effects of cold application on maximal isometric contraction. Phys Ther 47:185, 1967.

24. Mennell JM: The therapeutic use of cold. JAMA 74:1146–1157, 1975.
25. Merrick MA, Rankin JM, Andres FA, Channing LH: A preliminary examination of cryotherapy and secondary injury in skeletal muscle. Med Sci Sports Exerc 31:1515–1521, 1999.
26. Michalski WJ, Seguin JJ: The effects of muscle cooling and stretch on muscle spindle secondary endings in the cat. J Physiol 253:341–356, 1975.
27. Michlovitz SL: Thermal Agents in Rehabilitation. Philadelphia, F.A. Davis, 1990.
28. Miglietta O: Action of cold on spasticity. Am J Phys Med 52:198–205, 1973.
29. Nukada H, Pollack M, Allpress S: Experimental cold injury to peripheral nerve. Brain 104:779–811, 1981.
30. Pegg SMG, Littler TR, Littler EN: A trial of ice therapy and exercise in chronic arthritis. Physiotherapy 55:51–56, 1969.
31. Perkins JF Jr, Li M-C, Hoffman F, Hoffman E: Sudden vasoconstriction in denervated or sympathectomized paws exposed to cold. Am J Physiol 155:165–178, 1948.
32. Petajan JH, Watts N: Effects of cooling on the triceps surae reflex. Am J Phys Med 41:240–251, 1962.
33. Walker SM: Potentiation of twitch tension and prolongation of action potential induced by reduction of temperature in rat and frog muscle. Am J Physiol 157:429–435, 1949.
34. Waylonis GW: The physiologic effects of ice massage. Arch Phys Med Rehabil 48:37–42, 1967.
35. Zemke JE, Anderson JC, Guion WK, et al: Intramuscular temperature responses in the human leg to two forms of cryotherapy: Ice massage and ice bag. JOSPT 27:301–307, 1998.
36. Zitowitz L, Hardy JD: Influence of cold exposure on thermal burns in the rat. J Appl Physiol 12:147–154, 1958.

Chapter 6
Aquatic and Hydrotherapy in Rehabilitation

Sandra L. Symons, PTA, and Maynard M. Tabachnick, MSPT

HISTORY OF AQUATIC AND HYDROTHERAPY

Humans have used water for healing and spiritual rituals since ancient times. One of the earliest known instances were the hygeinic installations found in proto-Indian culture around 2400 B.C.[15,40] There has also been mention of the use of the therapeutic properties of water in ancient Mesopotamia, Egypt, India, China, Rome, and Greece. Many religions including Judaism, Christianity, Hinduism, and Islam hold ceremonies involving water.

Medieval Europeans built religious structures around thermal springs such as the Benedictine Abbey at Pfaefers, Switzerland, erected around A.D. 740. Using thermal springs as their source, healing pools were built in Aachen and Baden-Baden, Germany; Bath, England; and Spa, Belgium. Some of these baths have evolved into the well-known European health resort spas of today.

Native Americans have long used hot air sweat lodges, followed by a cold plunge, for medical and spiritual purposes. English, Dutch, and French settlers built their settlements near some of these springs in the 1600s placing wooden tubs next to their stone huts for bathing. In the 1700s, John de Normandie and Benjamin Rush sought out colonial mineral springs to analyze their chemical and medicinal value. Thomas Jefferson built the Sweet Springs spa in West Virginia based on diagrams of ancient Roman baths.

The use of water's therapeutic and healing properties gained popularity among the Western medical community in the 1800s. The American Medical Association (AMA) Committee on Sanitaria and Springs published their first report in 1880, classifying the nation's 646 known springs and mineral water pools. Not long after this, Albert Charles Peale classified 2822 active therapeutic springs. One of the better-known larger thermal pools was constructed in Hot Springs, Arkansas, and at its peak in 1896, 19 spa doctors were working there. Together they collaborated to publish medical theories and cases in the *Hot Springs Medical Journal.*[22]

Until the beginning of the 20th century, spas and their pools had not often been used for therapeutic exercise. Charles LeRoy Lowman, who founded the Orthopedic Hospital for Children (now Rancho Los Amigos) in 1913, observed paralyzed patients exercising in a wooden tank at the Spaulding Hospital for Crippled Children in Chicago. Afterward, he returned to California and converted the hospital's lily pond into two therapeutic pools. One was a fresh water pool used for therapy with patients who had been paralyzed or had poliomyelitis; the other pool contained saline water and was used to treat patients with infectious diseases.[41]

PHYSICAL PROPERTIES OF WATER

Aquatic and hydrotherapy have evolved considerably in this century, taking advantage of increased knowledge of the physical properties of water and the physiologic responses of the human body to immersion. Much of this research came from the push to send man into space because water's buoyancy made it the most convenient environment on earth in which to mimic the weightlessness found outside our atmosphere.[6] Knowledge of the physical properties of water and the physiologic responses of patients when submerged is vital to the proper and safe treatment of patients in aquatic therapy.

Density, Specific Gravity, and Buoyancy

Density (represented by the Greek letter ρ is the ratio of a substance's mass (m) to its volume (v) as stated in the formula: Density (ρ) = m/v.

As substances can exist in a solid, gaseous, or liquid state, density is temperature dependent.

The **specific gravity** of a substance is the ratio of the density of a substance to the density of water. Water's specific gravity is defined as 1.00 at 4°C. The average human has a specific gravity of 0.974. Bone, muscles, connective tissue, and organs, which are considered lean body mass, have a specific gravity close to 1.10. Fat mass, which is essential body fat combined with fat in excess of essential needs, has a density of approximately 0.90.[8]

Any object with a specific gravity less than 1.00 floats in water. This is explained by Archimedes' Principle, which states that there is an upward force on any body, that is submersed that is equal to the volume of water it has displaced. Thus, the average human will be at floating equilibrium when 97.4% of his or her body's volume has been submerged.

Buoyancy is the upward force generated by a liquid that enables submerged objects to have decreased apparent weight compared with their weight on land. Buoyancy acts opposite the force of gravity resulting in the off-loading benefit that the aquatic therapeutic environment offers. This decreased weight bearing can be measured in humans in relation to the level their body has been submersed (Fig. 1).[6,37]

It is important to consider the center of gravity (COG) in relation to the center of buoyancy (COB) when working with patients in the water. The point where all force moments are in equilibrium is the COG. Similarly, the COB is defined as the center of all buoyancy force moments summating each body segment.[6] Because the lower limbs of humans are denser than the chest, which contains the air-filled lungs, the COG and the COB are at different locations in the body. The COG is found slightly posterior to the midsagittal plane of the second sacral vertebra, and the COB is located in the midchest. Because the force of buoyancy opposes the force of gravity if these two centers are not maintained in alignment, a torque or rotational force can result, causing instability and the possibility of a weak dependent patient or a patient with paralysis being forced into a face down-position (Fig. 2).[6]

Hydrostatic Pressure

Measured at a specific point, fluids exert an equal pressure in all directions. Water pressure or hydrostatic pressure (P) is measured in force (F) per unit area (A): P = F/A.

The pressure exerted by a fluid is proportional to the density of the fluid and its depth. The earth's atmosphere also exerts pressure on water's surface, adding to the force of hydrostatic pressure. Every foot depth of water exerts a pressure of 22.4

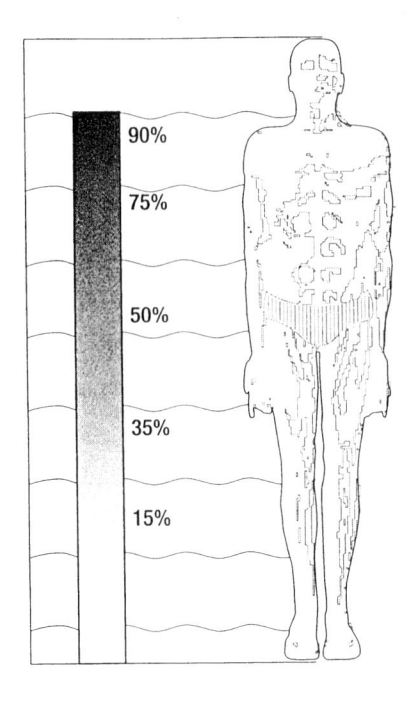

FIGURE 1. Percentage of body weight off-loaded with increasing immersion depth. (From Becker BE: Biophysiologic aspects of hydrotherapy. In: Comprehensive Aquatic Therapy. Woburn, MA, Butterworth–Heinemann, 1997, with permission.)

mmHg, so that at a depth of 4 feet, a pressure of 89.6 mmHg is experienced. This is much greater than the average venous or lymphatic pressure, and is slightly greater than the average diastolic pressure on land, allowing hydrostatic pressure to promote edema resolution.

Water Flow

The flow of water can be either laminar or streamline, resulting in a smooth flow with all layers at equal speed. As the speed of water flow increases, minor oscillations develop, creating uneven flow that disturbs the parallel alignment of the path of water and results in turbulence.

The molecular attraction of a fluid also contributes to resistance to movement through viscosity. This occurs through the internal friction of the fluid, resulting in a disruption or decrease in flow. Thus, the major factors in water motion are viscosity, turbulence, speed, fluid density, and if enclosed, the radius of the enclosure.

Drag

Objects moving in a fluid or water environment are subject to the force created by the turbulence that develops behind the moving object and is known as drag. Drag develops in two ways:
1. Form drag, which provides an additional resistance to movement through the water or fluid's direction opposite that of the moving object
2. Surface drag, which develops through friction between the boundary layer of water or fluid and the moving object

The force of drag is dependent on the frontal area of the submersed object, its size, shape, velocity, and the coefficient of drag.

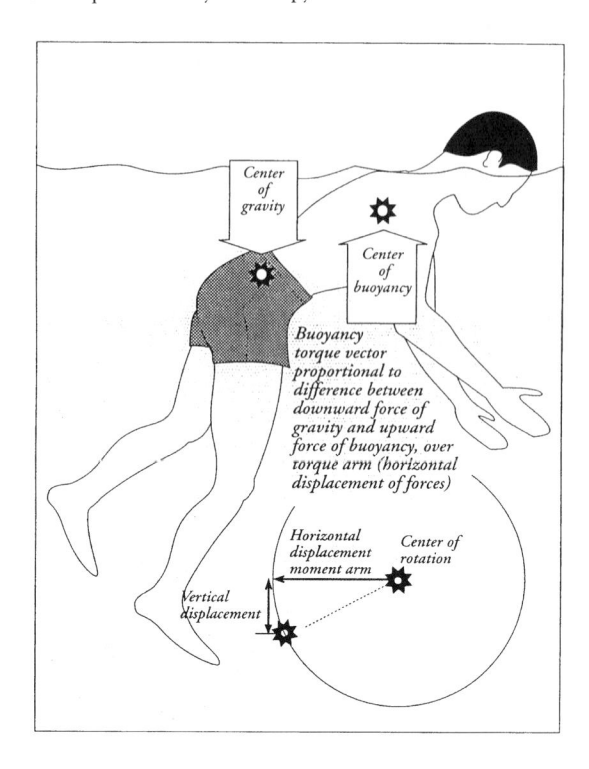

FIGURE 2. Buoyancy torque. (From Becker BE: Biophysiologic aspects of hydrotherapy. In: Comprehensive Aquatic Therapy. Woburn, MA, Butterworth–Heinemann, 1997, with permission.)

Specific Heat Capacity

Water is used as a therapeutic modality in all its forms: water, ice, and steam. The specific heat capacity of a substance is a measure of the energy that it has stored as heat. Water has a specific heat capacity of 1.00, which is much greater compared with that of air, which is 0.001. This allows water to store heat 1000 times more easily than an equal volume of air.

Water also is a superior conveyor of heat compared with air. Thermal energy transfer from heat occurs in three ways:
1. Through conduction, which is a result of molecular collisions over a small distance
2. Through convection, which is the result of the mass movement of large numbers of molecules over great distance
3. Through radiation, which is the heat transfer resulting from electromagnetic wave transfer

Water conducts heat well, transferring heat 25 times faster than air. Water's thermal conductivity and high specific heat allow it to retain and transfer heat to an immersed body part for therapeutic treatment.

THE PHYSIOLOGY OF IMMERSION

Circulatory System Effects

Venous and lymphatic pressure develop as a result of a vertical system of columns with valves to prevent backflow. Pressure within these systems varies depending on location, with the greatest pressures being found peripherally (~ 30 mmHg) and the lowest at the right atrium (~ –2 to –4 mmHg). These one way valves divide the columns into many shorter ones of decreased height in order to convey blood or lymph using lower pressure gradients.

When a human subject is immersed to the neck, the surrounding pressure of water causes an increase in venous pressure of ~ 14–18 mmHg, resulting in a pressure of ~ 14–17 mmHg at the right atrium. This increased venous pressure results in displacement of a large quantity of blood upward through the thighs, abdominal cavity vessels, great vessels of the chest, and finally into the heart. Overall. a 60% increase in central blood volume is appreciated.[1]

Cardiac volume increases by ~ 30%, producing greater stretch of the myocardium.[49] Increased stretch is a healthy response to increased blood filling and results in a greater force of contraction owing to the improved actin myosin filament relationship in the myocardium.[28] This improved myocardial efficiency from greater cardiac filling consequently increases stroke volume and is known as Starling's law. The average increase in stroke volume is ~ 35%, which is close to the exercise maximum for sedentary, deconditioned individuals on land and equivalent to ~ 71–100 ml/beat.[1,23] Increased stroke volume (SV) (Fig. 3) is a factor in increased cardiac output (CO), as seen in their relationship represented by the equation: CO = SV × HR (heart rate).

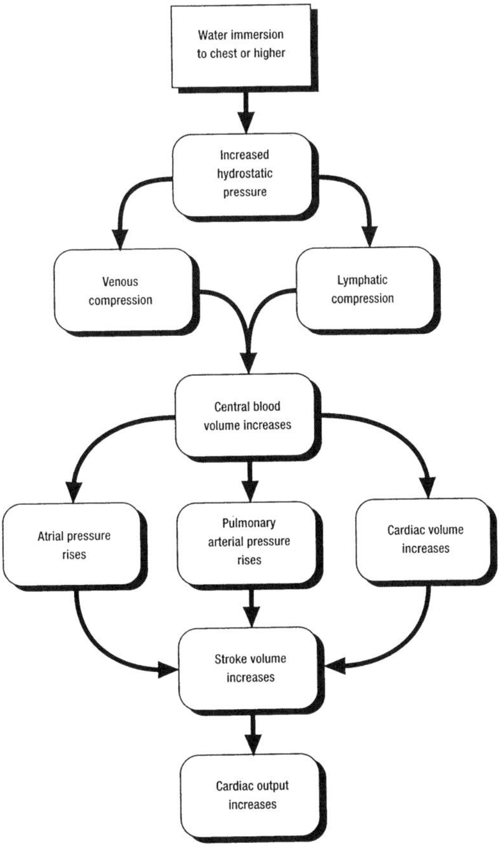

FIGURE 3. Schematic of cardiovascular changes following immersion. (From Becker BE: Biophysiologic aspects of hydrotherapy. In: Comprehensive Aquatic Therapy. Woburn, MA, Butterworth–Heinemann, 1997, with permission.)

Changes in CO and heart rate are temperature dependent, with a 30% increase in CO seen at 30°C and 121% at 39°C. HR decreases 12–15 bpm at 25°C, and a 15% decrease is seen at thermoneutral temperatures. HR increases are experienced in warmer water, possibly due to decreased peripheral resistance at increased temperatures and increased vagal effects.[23,59]

Pulmonary System Effects

Compression of the chest wall by water pressure results in altered respiratory function and an increase in the work of breathing after immersion.[9] The rib cage shrinks approximately 10% when submersed, resulting in decreased lung volumes and expiratory flow rates and an increase in the time it takes to move air.[33] Chest wall compliance is also reduced by water pressure resulting in an increase in pleural pressure from −1 to +1 mmHg.[1] Overall, the water pressure on the chest is responsible for 25% of the greater work of breathing required after submersion to the neck.

The larger factor that accounts for the remaining 75% of the increased work of respiration after immersion results from the shift of blood to the thorax, which allows for less lung volume to be filled by air.[9] Diffusion capacity, or the ability of the alveolar membrane to exchange gases, is also decreased slightly after to-the-neck immersion reducing blood oxygen concentration. This occurs because the lung beds are overly distended with blood displaced from the abdomen and extremities. The overall result is a 60% increase in the work of breathing when immersed to the neck (Fig. 4). The result is that water presents an outstanding workload challenge to the respiratory system beyond that found on land and is an excellent medium in which to train and increase the efficiency of breathing. However, consequently, caution must be used with respiratory compromised patients and it is not recommended to allow a patient with a vital capacity of less than 1.0–1.5 L to participate in aquatic therapy.

Musculoskeletal System Effects

The compressive effects of water pressure and reflex regulation of blood vessel tone combine to increase blood flow after immersion. Research shows that most of the increased cardiac output is directed to skin and muscle.[27] Resting baseline muscle blood flow on land has been measured at 1.8 ml/min/100 gm tissue compared with 4.1 ml/min/100 gm tissue after submersion up to the neck. The same research found tissue perfusion to increase 30% with submersion to heart level, an equivalent amount as cardiac output increase during immersion.[4] In summary, increases in blood flow seen with immersion translate into increased metabolic waste removal, edema reduction, and increased oxygen delivery to muscle tissue.

Conditioning Effects

Cardiorespiratory conditioning can be accomplished in water with highly fit athletes and deconditioned patients. Deep water running with a buoyant vest and no ground contact has been found to be equal to running on land in highly fit subjects when training intensity and frequency are equal, allowing athletes to maintain their VO_2max in an unweighted environment after injury.[31] This is also found with deconditioned subjects and can be accompanied by a decreased heart rate when the exercise is performed at lower temperatures.[3] For deconditioned or geriatric patients, water's supportive quality can also help to improve postural capabilities and bal-

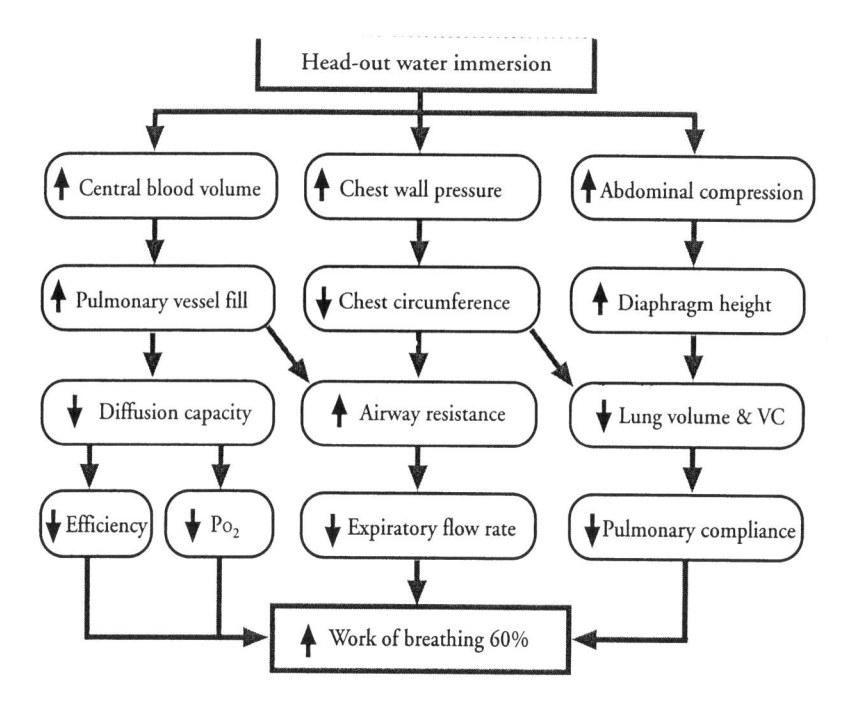

FIGURE 4. Schematic of immersion effects on respiration. (VC = vital capacity; Po_2 = partial pressure of oxygen.) (From Becker BE: Biophysiologic aspects of hydrotherapy. In: Comprehensive Aquatic Therapy. Woburn, MA, Butterworth–Heinemann, 1997, with permission.)

ance, decreasing the risk of falls.[52] Other studies also confirm the benefits of water exercise training in maintaining and improving cardiorespiratory performance in comparison to land.[35,55] Thus, water provides an excellent and often superior alternative to training on land when decreased weight bearing on injured limbs or the ability to produce movement errors without suffering a fall are desired.

AQUATIC THERAPEUTIC EXERCISE

Indications

Throughout the history of hydrotherapy, forms of treatment consisted of more passive techniques, such as soaking in mineral springs. More recently, research has proven exercise to be an important component of a healthy lifestyle, and as a result, more active forms of aquatic therapy have developed.

Aquatic therapeutic exercise can prove beneficial in improving flexibility, range of motion (ROM), strength, balance, coordination and proprioception for patients with a variety of diagnoses.[35,52,56] These diagnoses include, but are not limited to, rheumatic diseases, chronic pain, neurologic conditions, stable cardiorespiratory pathology, and injuries that necessitate decreased weight bearing such as sprains and fractures or after orthopedic surgeries (Table 1).

As with conventional land-based physical therapy, the ultimate goal is to discharge the patient with an independently performed exercise program in order to maintain strength, conditioning, and functional gains. In the case of aquatic exer-

TABLE 1. GOALS OF AQUATIC THERAPEUTIC EXERCISE PERFORMANCE

Decrease:	Increase:
Pain	ROM and flexibility
Edema	Strength and endurance
	Proprioception and balance
	Cardiorespiratory capacity

Ultimate goal—improve function as a consequence of gains experienced in one or more of the above.

cise, the patient typically must locate a community swimming pool where he or she may continue the exercise program independently or join one of the many aquatic exercise classes sponsored by local gyms, YMCAs, and community pools. For many geriatric patients and patients suffering from rheumatic diseases, the Arthritis Foundation offers an excellent standardized aquatic exercise program with instructors who must be certified by the Arthritis Foundation and follow their protocol.[2] It may be helpful for health-care practitioners to compile a list of community pools or programs in the patient's area to provide him or her with a smoother transition to a pool in the community after discharge.

All aquatic therapy exercise programs must be initiated only after a complete evaluation of the patient by a licensed therapist. The patient's program should include an on-land component, except in some cases in which reports of pain have made it impossible for the patient to perform any exercise outside of the pool. In those cases, the goal will still be to progress exercise eventually to land-based forms.

Aquatic Therapeutic Exercise Progression

Cole et al. identified three scenarios for aquatic therapeutic exercise progression[17,18]:

1. **Wet to dry transition**. This begins with aquatic therapy and then transitions to a land-based exercise program. It is recommended when musculature chosen for strengthening and the associated joint(s) are affected by axial and compression forces. An example would be after orthopedic surgeries, when weight bearing is decreased. Water-based exercise allows a more gradual return to full weight bearing with progression to land-based activities as permitted by the referring physician's protocol and as tolerated by the patient.

2. **Dry to wet transition**. Therapy begins with a land-based program but results in aggravation of the patient's condition. After the exacerbation has resolved and the patient demonstrates sufficient strength and functional gains, the patient may return to performance of a land-based exercise program.

3. **Wet only**. Exclusive performance of aquatic therapeutic exercise is recommended only for those patients who cannot tolerate any form of land-based exercise or prefer to perform aquatic exercise only. These patients still should be reassessed periodically in the physical therapy clinic for functional gains resulting from their aquatic exercise program and the possibility of eventually tolerating some form of out-of-pool exercise.

It is extremely important to consider that, because most patients will tolerate a greater amount of exercise earlier in water than on land, the patient risks overexertion and irritation of the injured body part during their first few sessions. Therefore, the therapist must monitor the new aquatic therapy patient closely, encouraging him or her to begin slowly and allow a comfortable level of exercise to develop initially. This is best accomplished through emphasizing gait and gentle ROM during the first few sessions, with a gradual progression to more strenuous aquatic exercise. The therapist must diligently record the types of exercise, duration or quantity of repetitions, and the intensity level (if equipment is used to increase resistance). This will assist the therapist and the patient through a smoother increase in intensity of the aquatic exercise program.[47]

Aquatic Therapeutic Exercises

Six types of therapeutic aquatic exercise were identified by Genuario et al to create a well rounded program with the possibility for progression in difficulty.[32]
1. Water walking or slow jogging at varying depths, emphasizing normal gait
2. Slow, gentle, rhythmic ROM and stretching to emphasize flexibility
3. Vigorous movement with increased speed to increase strength and endurance
4. Dynamic rhythmic movement or altering gait patterns to increase proprioception and improve balance and neuromuscular coordination
5. Walking or running at increased speed at various depths to improve cardiorespiratory fitness and conditioning
6. Swimming

The major determinants of resistance when exercising in the water are buoyancy, speed of movement, the resistance afforded by the water's viscosity, and the surface area of the body parts, moving through the water. During aquatic exercise, buoyancy can assist, support, or resist movement, depending on the positioning of the patient and the limb(s) he or she is/are moving. If the extremity is moving toward the surface, as with shoulder abduction, the movement will be buoyancy assisted. When an extremity moves across the surface, as during horizontal shoulder abduction or adduction, the movement will be buoyancy supported. Resistance afforded by buoyancy can be encountered with movement away from the water's surface as with shoulder extension, which begins with the arm resting on the surface of the water.

Because buoyancy acts in the direction opposite gravity, movement in buoyancy-resisted planes offers an interesting advantage over exercise performed outside the water. Conventional land-based strengthening ROM exercises are normally in planes against gravity, thus strengthening the antigravity musculature. However, water-based exercise can be used to strengthen gravity-assisted musculature while standing upright and without the use of pulleys or other exercise equipment. Through the use of buoyant equipment, such as foam hand buoys the force of buoyancy and the work of the musculature that is normally assisted by gravity is increased.

Stretching can be aided by buoyancy. Many patients find it more comfortable and effective to stretch soft tissue in a gravity free environment, allowing them to improve their kinesthetic sense and awareness of an injured body part.[36] Stretching should be performed after an initial warm-up session of walking for the safest, most comfortable, and effective results.

Aquatic Exercise Equipment

Exercise equipment may be used in the water to increase the resistance against movement by using objects that enlarge the surface area of the limb being moved or by using buoyant objects to work in buoyancy-assisted, supported, or resisted planes. There are many types of aquatic exercise equipment available. Examples

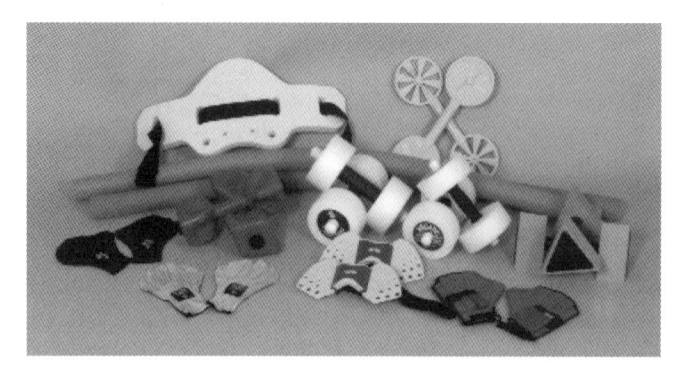

FIGURE 5. Equipment for aquatic exercise.

include webbed gloves with or without weights, hand paddles with blades that may be adjusted in graded amounts to increase surface area. Foam dumbbells (hand buoys) or foot cuffs of varying sizes may be used to alter buoyancy (Fig. 5).

Equipment can also be used to increase the buoyancy of the patient, such as flotation vest, long foam tubes ("noodles") or belts similar to those worn on boats or for water-skiing. One device that may be used to assist with deep water exercise is the Aquajogger™. Buoyant equipment can prove helpful for patients who cannot tolerate full weight bearing. In addition to buoyant waist belts during deep water exercise the patient may also use buoyant hand buoys or foot cuffs until he or she can progress to a level at which less assistance is required to keep the head above water.

Masks and snorkels may be beneficial for performing a variety of swimming and exercise techniques in the prone position. Patients requiring cervical spine stabilization exercises may perform them using a mask and snorkel together with the assistance afforded by the buoyancy of the water.

Aquatic Therapy Contraindications and Precautions

Each facility needs to establish procedures regarding contraindications and precautions to ensure the safety of patients and staff. The aquatic environment is unique and requires specific procedures to be implemented. These procedures vary depending on the comfort and skill level of the health-care professional. Education of referring practitioners is extremely important to ensure that appropriate patients are referred who can safely participate in aquatic therapy (Table 2).

Precautions

The aquatic environment is one with its own specific set of precautions and considerations. Following are areas to exercise caution and special handling at times. Patients with the following medical conditions or related care need not be excluded from aquatic therapy.

Urinary. Treatment of urinary problems includes the use of indwelling, external, or suprapubic catheters. Leg bags, sport bags, or bed bags may be worn in the water. Empty the collection bag before participation to avoid spills. Sports bags are smaller and more discreet, and can increase a patient's comfort level but need to be emptied more frequently.

TABLE 2. CONTRAINDICATIONS TO AQUATIC THERAPY

1. Bowel or bladder incontinence
2. Open wounds, including IV sites
3. Uncontrolled seizures
4. Uncontrolled autonomic dysreflexia or blood pressure
5. Fever > 100°F within 24 hours
6. Tracheostomy
7. Infectious diseases. (HIV and hepatitis are *not* contraindicated. Observe universal precautions during aquatic activity)
8. Vital capacity of less than 1–1.5 L
9. Unstable angina or atrial fibrillation

Bowel. Continence is important for sanitation and patient comfort. Colostomies may be worn in the water if they are secured properly and emptied before participation. A shirt or one-piece bathing suit may be worn to increase patient comfort. Consistent bowel programs for patients with spinal cord injuries is a necessity. There can be no episodes of incontinence between each scheduled program. Once a program results in incontinence, it may require a week to be re-established, during which time a patient will not be allowed to use the pool.

Menstruation. An internal collection device is required.

Open wounds. Superficial wounds must be covered with a waterproof dressing. Patients with open areas created by intravenous (IVs) or subclavian lines may participate as long as these are located on areas of the body that can be easily kept out of the water, such as the upper arm or neck. Some facilities permit patients with halo cervical stabilization devices to participate in aquatic therapy if the pin sites remain dry. Sheepskin liners on some vests can be changed after the session.

Orthotic Stabilization Devices. It is important to allow patients the freedom to participate in aquatic therapy without splints or braces. This may be the only environment where they can move freely without these devices. Orthotic stabilization devices that must be worn by patients and are permitted in the pool include soft collars, Philadelphia collars, Somi braces, Minerva braces, Aspen collars and thoracic lumbar sacral orthoses (TLSOs). After the aquatic session, these orthotics can be dried or patients can have an extra set of pads to replace wet ones after the session.

Autonomic Dysreflexia. Autonomic dysreflexia is a specific life-threatening medical condition that affects spinal cord–injured patients with lesions at T6 or above. Symptoms may include severe pounding headache, sweating, nausea, and blurred or spotted vision. Immediately loosen any restrictive clothing, check catheter tubing for obstruction, empty urine bags, and elevate the patient's head. If symptoms persist, remove the patient from the pool and keep the head elevated. Seek medical assistance immediately if a cause is not identified. Facility policies must be established for treatment should this occur during an aquatic therapy session.

Respiratory Problems. Patients with respiratory compromise must have a minimum vital capacity of 1.0–1.5 L. These patients may experience shortness of breath in chest-deep water secondary to the effects of hydrostatic pressure. Patients requiring oxygen may participate in aquatic therapy using extension tubing with an oxygen cannister on deck. Patients with asthma who experience sudden changes in temperature in the aquatic environment may experience an asthma attack. Gradually introduce these patients into the water and be careful when exiting the pool that they do not become overly chilled. Refer to the previous section on hydrostatic pressure and pulmonary system effects for more information.

Thermoregulation. Many patients' thermoregulatory systems are affected after injury or illness. Water and air temperatures need to be considered depending on the condition being treated. In therapeutic pools, with water temperature at 88°F or above, patients need to be monitored for overheating and dehydration. Drinking water must be available. Other patients may be susceptible to excessive chilling and need to be monitored for hypothermia during and after the aquatic session.

Circulatory. Immersion of patients in water above thermoneutral temperatures (98°F [36.5°C]) has been shown to accelerate heart rate and increase blood pressure.[59] Patients with cardiac conditions must be approved by their physician before treatment.

Medical Conditions Exacerbated by Fatigue/Heat. Therapeutic water temperatures can cause fatigue in patients who are deconditioned or have a medical condition such as multiple sclerosis or Guillain-Barré syndrome. It is imperative that individuals with multiple sclerosis and Guillain-Barré syndrome be monitored closely during aquatic therapy. The patient's energy level should be monitored before, during and after sessions. Begin therapeutic pool treatments with lower intensity workouts of shorter duration (~ 15 minutes initially). Increase the level of intensity and treatment length gradually. Many individuals with multiple sclerosis and Guillain-Barré syndrome can successfully participate and maximize the benefits of therapeutic aquatics if temperatures are monitored closely. If significant fatigue lasting more than 2 hours after the session is experienced, then aquatic therapy is not an appropriate modality for these individuals and should be discontinued.

Therapeutic Pool Selection and Maintenance

Ideally the therapeutic pool should allow a variety of depths so that buoyancy maybe varied depending on the patients' needs. Water temperatures vary from 82–98°F, depending on the patient population served. Athletes and fit individuals who tolerate a higher intensity workout will require a lower water temperature because heart rate is directly influenced by water temperature (Table 3).[23,49,59]

Patients who are deconditioned, are neurologically impaired, have spinal cord injuries above the sixth thoracic vertebrae level, or are diagnosed with rheumatic disease require warmer temperatures. This may be due to thermoregulatory system impairment or their tendency to have a lower exercise output. Thus, they will not usually increase their heart rates through exercise at the same rate as the more fit or athletic patients.

The environment surrounding the therapeutic pool requires consideration as well. Air temperatures should not be more than 10°F below water temperature. Pool decks, entries and exits, and bathroom facilities are mandated by the Americans with Disabilities Act to provide the public with accessible accommodations for all individuals.

TABLE 3. POOL WATER TEMPERATURE RANGES

Pool Type	Temperature Range
Lap swimming (most community pools)	78–84°F
Therapeutic pools (e.g., Arthritis Foundation aquatic exercise classes, water shiatsu (watsu))	88–96°F
Hot tubs, Jacuzzis, spas, whirlpools	98–104°F

Pool sanitation is extremely important because infection or skin irritation can occur depending on the type and quantity of chemicals used. Respiratory, gastrointestinal, urinary tract, and, rarely, central nervous system infections have been associated with pools. However, in almost all cases, the pool used was found to be contaminated as a result of poor or no disinfection.[20] To ensure that a safe and sanitary environment exists for aquatic therapy, chemical levels must be monitored daily. A staff member must be knowledgeable in the appropriate and safe chemical levels for sanitation. Certification of an employee as a pool operator (CPO) or a contract with a pool maintenance company to assist with monitoring the pool sanitation is recommended.[39] Policies must be established for incidents involving pool contamination, such as blood, feces, and vomitus. It is advisable for the pool facility manager to be in contact with the state's agency of public recreation or health department to determine requirements that exist in his or her jurisdiction.

AQUATIC THERAPY TREATMENT TECHNIQUES

Water Shiatsu (Watsu)

Watsu was developed by Harold Dull in 1980 at Harbin Hot Springs, California, and is based on his studies in Japan of zen shiatsu which is practiced on land. Watsu is a combination of shiatsu and warm water therapy originally created to attain wellness in all individuals. Eastern philosophy embraces a mind–body relationship that is not always accepted in traditional aquatic rehabilitation. Zen shiatsu and Watsu incorporate passive stretches, joint mobilization, and acupoints to balance the flow of energy through the meridians (pathways of energy) as the therapist cradles the patient. Centering and connecting with the breath are essential components of Watsu.[25] Therapists learn to adapt Watsu movements to physical restrictions or limitations and outline a program designed on individual goals. Patients are passive participants as the therapist gently floats, rocks, and swirls them through warm water. Patients experience a profound relaxation from the water's support and the continual rhythmic movement, working through a specifically designed transition and sequence of movements that are learned and applied in treatments. Therapists stabilize or move individual body segments through the water, resulting in a passive stretch to another segment as a result of the drag forces encountered by the water. The treatment usually lasts for 1 hour, but can be adjusted depending on individual tolerance. Warm water is essential for the patient to achieve a state of relaxation. Water temperatures should never exceed 98°F (37°C).

Watsu precautions include all aquatic therapy precautions that were previously stated in this chapter. There are some specific precautions related to Watsu treatments: Watsu is a physically close, intimate, non-sexual technique, and it is important to know your comfort level in performing these techniques and to be aware and respect your patient's feelings. The close physical contact necessary to perform Watsu can release deep emotions in patients. Hypersensitivity to vestibular stimulation may cause symptoms of motion sickness. Use movements that are slow and smooth, and that involve less turning and rotation of the head.

Initial sessions can begin at 5 minutes and gradually increase to 60 minutes in length.

Limiting factors of Watsu are that it is a close patient-to-therapist technique and a warm water environment is essential.

Watsu is practiced worldwide. Harold Dull has established the not-for-profit Worldwide Aquatic Bodywork Association to explore the benefits of giving and receiving aquatic bodywork, and to make it available to everyone.[26]

Bad Ragaz Ring Method

The Bad Ragaz ring method was developed in Bad Ragaz, Switzerland, in the 1960s. Current techniques have been significantly influenced by proprioceptive neuromuscular facilitation (PNF). These diagonal ROM exercises have been used to simulate normal functional movement patterns. The patterns used have been adapted to be performed in a horizontal position in the water. The method is used for muscle re-education, strengthening, spinal rotation and elongation, relaxation, and tone inhibition in the water. The patient is floated at the surface of the water using flotation devices to support the neck, trunk, and extremities. Resistance is provided by negative pressure produced behind the patient as he or she is dragged through the water. There are three ways in which the therapist acts in relation to the patient:

1. Isokinetically. The therapist provides fixation while the patient moves through the water either toward, away from or around the therapist. The resistance is determined by the speed of movement by the patient.
2. Isotonically. The therapist acts as a movable fixed point. Patients can be pushed or swung in the opposite direction of their movement, increasing the resistance encountered. Conversely, a therapist moving the patient in the opposite direction of the intended movement can assist movements.
3. Isometrically. The patient holds a fixed position while being pushed through the water by the therapist, promoting muscle stabilization.[30]

Patients can also be moved passively through the water to promote relaxation and tone inhibition through trunk rotation and elongation techniques.

Sessions can begin at 5 minutes, increasing to 45 minutes with breaks incorporated. Passive relaxation techniques may be used to increase relaxation and decrease hypertonicity in the neurologically involved patient at the beginning or end of a session. Techniques that increase spasticity should be avoided. Resistance can be increased as the patient becomes stronger by:

- Adding flotation devices to the trunk or extremities
- Changing the direction of movement
- Incorporating quick reversals
- Providing more distal than proximal handholds causing the patient to control more body segments
- Increasing the level of difficulty or speed at which movements are performed

Some specific precautions related to the Bad Ragaz ring method include all aquatic therapy precautions mentioned previously and hypersensitivity to vestibular stimulation, and care must be taken not to overstretch weak joints, causing further damage.

A limiting factor of the Bad Ragaz method is that it requires 1:1 therapist-to-patient interaction to be performed (Fig. 6).

Halliwick Method

The Halliwick method was developed by James McMillan in the 1950s at the Halliwick School for Crippled Girls in England. Although McMillan had no medical

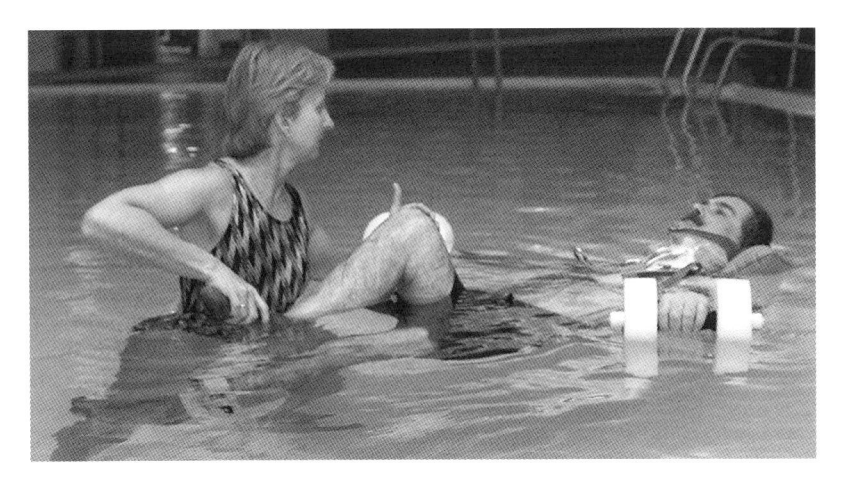

FIGURE 6. Bad Ragaz ring method (American style).

training, his background was in engineering, including the field of fluid mechanics, and his method is based on the principles of hydromechanics and human development that are used in swimming and therapy.

Four principles of instruction were established:

1. **Mental adaptation** is the recognition of two forces acting on the body in water: gravity and up-thrust. In combination, these result in rotational movement.

2. **Balance restoration** emphasizes the use of large patterns of movement, particularly with the arms, to restore or maintain balance. Instruction involves the use of wide-ranging body movements to move the body into different postures while maintaining balance control. The most important of these postures is the immediate response around midline.

3. **Inhibition** is the ability to create and hold a desired position or posture and the ability to contain all unwanted movement.

4. **Facilitation** is the ability to create a mentally desired and physically controlled movement (e.g., swimming) by any means without flotation aids. These phases of learning are in an order by which the cerebral cortex learns all physical movement. Known as the developmental sequence, these phases are set out in a structure know as the Ten Point Program:

1. Mental adjustment and disengagement
2. Sagittal rotation (control)
3. Simple progression
4. Basic swimming movement
5. Vertical rotation (control)
6. Lateral rotation (control)
7. Combined rotation
8. Mental inversion/up-thrust
9. Turbulent gliding
10. Balance in stillness

Instruction takes place in groups of no more than seven swimmers, each with his or her own assistant who guides them through series of games and water activities that are lead by an experienced Halliwick instructor. The Halliwick method is learned in an atmosphere where fun and games are encouraged. There are two main purposes to this method: (1) to teach swimmers about themselves and their balance control in water and (2) to teach swimming.[19] A limitation to the Halliwick approach is that it requires close therapist-to-patient interaction to be performed.

Ai Chi (Aquatic Tai Chi)

Developed by Jun Konno from Tokyo, Japan, ai chi, or aquatic tai chi, uses tai chi techniques. The benefits include increased flexibility and ROM, improved circulation of energy along important acupoint meridians, decreased stress, increased mental alertness, improved kinesthetic awareness, and enhanced breathing through learned yogic breathing techniques. Diagnoses treated with ai chi include orthopaedic injuries, neurologic diseases, anxiety or depressive disorders, rheumatic diseases, fibromyalgia, cardiac conditions, respiratory diseases, and prenatal and chronic pain.[38]

A benefit to ai chi is that it can be performed independently once the patient has learned a safe program that is appropriate for his or her needs.

Burdenko Method

The Burdenko method, developed by Igor Burdenko, is a combination of water and sports therapy. The methods are an application of water and land based exercises to maintain health and quality of life and to enhance physical performance. His method combines the advantages of both water and land, using both shallow and deep-water activities. The Burdenko method is based on six qualities: balance, coordination, flexibility, endurance, strength, and speed.

This method challenges the COG on land and COB in water. Water characteristics include working in a vertical position in deep water, exercising in multiple directions, exercising at different speeds, and beginning in deep water and progressing to shallow water. This interaction between the two environments is believed to be the key to faster, safer, and more efficient body function. The Burdenko method works on the body as a whole, not just the injured part. The goal is to establish harmony of function in the body using a holistic approach. The water and land programs each consist of three stages: (1) warmup (walking, stretching, running), (2) working out sports qualities (coordination, balance, flexibility, endurance, strength, and speed), and (3) cool-down (e.g., stretching, breathing and shaking).[13]

HYDROTHERAPY: METHODS OF APPLICATION

Wound Healing and Hydrotherapy

There continues to be much controversy and research regarding the effectiveness of whirlpool and Hubbard tank therapy in the management of wound healing. The Agency for Health Care Policy and Research (AHCPR) Clinical Practice Guidelines for the Treatment of Pressure Ulcers consider the use of whirlpool and Hubbard tank treatments for the cleansing of pressure ulcers that contain thick exudate, slough, or necrotic tissue. Whirlpool or Hubbard tank treatment should be discontinued when the ulcer is determined to be clean.[7] Caution must be taken so that wound trauma does not occur from the high pressure water jets in the whirlpool. The water turbulence can damage granulation tissue and migrating epidermal cells. As a result, the water jets should not be positioned close to the wound. Treatment assessment is essential, and whirlpool use should be discontinued once exudate, slough, and necrotic tissue are cleared to prevent further damage.

Whirlpool Baths

There are basically two types of whirlpool tanks: fixed and portable tanks. "Lowboy" and "highboy" tanks are for extremity or trunk immersion. This treatment provides heat, gentle massage, debridement, and relief of joint pain and stiffness and promotes relaxation of muscles. The immersed body parts can perform active, active-assistive, or passive ROM exercises while the body parts are submerged.

Hubbard Tanks

Full-body immersion whirlpools are known as Hubbard tanks. An overhead lift with a stretcher is usually used to get the patient into the water. Water temperature should not exceed 1° above normal body temperature. Patients with burns requiring debridement of necrotic tissue, slough, or thick exudate may benefit from full-body immersion treatments. Burn patients may also benefit from dressing removal in water and from active exercise assisted by the water.

Certain patients with open wounds may also be suitable candidates for Hubbard tank therapy. A study of postabdominal surgical patients found a decreased gas build-up after surgery in the intestines, facilitated wound healing, and decreased anxiety with tank therapy.[44]

The advantages of the Hubbard tank are its ability to obtain full-body immersion, achieve wound debridement, facilitate active exercise, and decrease pain and anxiety in patients who have contraindications to participating in the therapeutic pool (Table 4).

Duration

Physiologic effects are generally achieved in 20 minutes when used as a heating modality. Borrell and colleagues demonstrated that 20 minutes was long enough to increase skin, muscle, and joint capsule temperature in the hand and foot.[10]

Entries

For whirlpools, a standard whirlpool chair that sits outside of the tub to allow lower extremities to be immersed or a whirlpool bench that sits inside a tank to fully immerse the lower half of the body is available.

For Hubbard tanks, stretchers with mechanical lifts are available.

TABLE 4. WATER TEMPERATURE RANGE FOR WHIRLPOOLS AND HUBBARD TANKS

Whirlpools	Temperature
Lower extremity	100–102°F (38–39°C)
Upper extremity	< 105°F (40°C)
Hubbard tank	92–98°F (33.5–36.5°C)

*Hubbard tanks must be no greater than 1° above normal body temperature.

Precautions

Tables 5 and 6 list contraindications and precautions of whirlpool and Hubbard tank use.

Disinfection of Hydrotherapy Tanks

Currently, there are no universal standards for cleaning and disinfecting hydrotherapy tanks. The Centers for Disease Control and Prevention recommend that sodium hypochlorite 70% per 100 gallons of water be added to the tank before the patient enters to produce free chlorine residual of about 15 mg/L.[16] These concentrations have been found to reduce the microbial contamination in water from 104 to less than 10 colony-forming units per milliliter in a controlled study with patients with burns.[45]

Pulsed Lavage

Pulsed lavage offers an alternative or adjunct to hydrotherapy for wound healing. Pulsed lavage is described as a system delivering an irrigation solution under pressure by an electrically powered device. This pressure cleanses the wound of debris, increases tissue perfusion, and enhances a clean wound bed for granulation to occur. Pulsed lavage delivers a pulsating stream of fluid that loosens necrotic tissue from the wound and may concurrently be used with suction to remove debris and irrigating solutions. The AHCPR guideline suggest that irrigation pressures less than 4 psi may be inefficient to remove surface pathogens and debris, and that irrigation pressures greater than 15 psi may cause wound trauma and drive bacteria into wounds. These pressure range recommendations were derived from studies conducted by Brown et al., Rodeheaver et al., Wheeler et al., and Stewart et al. and a series of studies performed at Walter Reed Army Hospital. Normal saline is the preferred cleansing agent because it is physiologic, will not harm tissue, and adequately cleanses most wounds.[42]

Advantages

Pulsed lavage can be used for treatment of patients who need to remain in their room secondary to isolation or medical compromise. Patients with tracheostomies

TABLE 5. WHIRLPOOL AND HUBBARD TANK CONTRAINDICATIONS

Incontinence of bowel or bladder
Unstable blood pressure
Uncontrolled seizure disorders
Acute febrile illness
Infectious disease

TABLE 6. WHIRLPOOL AND HUBBARD TANK PRECAUTIONS

Increased edema in extremities
Cardiac disease
Peripheral vascular disease
Decreased cognitive status
Decreased vital capacity (<1.0–1.5 L)
Controlled seizure disorders

Patients should never be left unattended during a whirlpool or Hubbard tank treatment.

or ventilators may receive pulsed lavage treatments for wound care with significantly decreased risk of water aspiration and increased safety regarding electrical equipment during treatment with water. Pulsed lavage treatments can continue after discharge in the home and may promote shorter hospital stays.

Contraindications and Precautions

Pulsed lavage is contraindicated near exposed blood vessels, eyes, or dura. The skill of the professional or caregiver performing the treatment is important to prevent spray from contaminating the surrounding treatment area, the patient, or the person administering the treatment. The irrigation fluid should be suctioned as fast as it is sprayed to decrease the risk of contamination. Two people may perform the technique, with one administering the fluid stream and the other suctioning the debris and remaining fluid. Caution must be taken when using pulsed lavage near exposed muscle.

Research comparing the effectiveness of pulsed lavage and whirlpool on wound cleansing is scant. Additional clinical studies comparing the effects of the two on wound cleansing and healing are needed. Recognizing the progressive financial restrictions facing the clinician, future comparisons should also include cost analyses of the two methods. Total cost per incident, number of treatments required to achieve wound closure, and per-treatment costs should be included in future research.[42]

Contrast Baths

Contrast baths are an alternating application of hot and cold generally applied to distal extremities, using a 3:1 ratio of hot to cold, applied with compresses or immersion. Contrast baths are used primarily for increasing blood flow through an area. Contrast baths promote a type of vascular exercise causing alternate constriction and dilation of the local blood vessels, which stimulates increased peripheral circulation. This process aids in removing wastes that accumulate in areas of inflammation and assists in bringing nutrients and oxygen to the area.

Indications

Contrast hydrotherapy is an effective treatment for subacute, postacute, and chronic cases of tendinitis, bursitis, and arthritis. It is also effective for desensitization of neuropathic or sympathetic pain syndromes, such as reflex sympathetic dystrophy (RSD). Contrast baths can assist in the treatment of RSD by reducing edema and normalizing sympathetic neuroregulation of blood vessels.

Contraindications and Precautions for Contrast Baths

Advanced atherosclerosis and advanced peripheral vascular disease should be treated with extreme caution to avoid the exacerbation of ischemia. In the presence of open wounds, the containers should be sterilized before and after use. Pad the edges of containers to avoid constriction of the circulatory or lymphatic system. Watch skin coloration and monitor patient's pulse. Adhere to those precautions and contraindications relating to other applications of heat and cold.

Contrast Bath Procedures

Begin with hot water immersion (Table 7) for 10 minutes then begin alternating with:

TABLE 7. TEMPERATURES FOR CONTRAST BATHS

Bath	Temperature
Hot bath	100–110°F (38–43°C)
Cold bath	50–61°F (10–16°C)

- Cold water immersion for 1 minute
- Hot water immersion for 4 minutes
- Cold water immersion for 1 minute
- Hot immersion water for 4 min

Repeat the procedure for 3–5 repetitions per treatment session.

For edema reduction, begin with cold water immersion for 1 minute, followed by hot water immersion for 4 minutes, continuing for 3–5 repetitions, ending with cold water immersion.

Sitz Baths

A sitz bath is a bath in which the pelvis is immersed in hot aor cold water. Traditionally, hot sitz baths have been used for relief of postpartum perineal pain, and one of the most routine orders for postpartum patients is the warm sitz bath. Studies have investigated the effectiveness of hot versus cold sitz baths, intermittently, to relieve postpartum perineal pain. Scientific observation would suggest a change to ice therapy to decrease edema and hemorrhage, thus decreasing the length and severity of postpartum pain.[24] Alternative medicine treatments include hot, cold, and contrasting (hot/cold) sitz baths to decrease pelvic discomfort. Further research appears warranted in this area. Warm sitz baths are effective in treating hemorrhoids and anorectal pain.[12] Naturopathic hydrotherapy uses sitz baths for pelvic disorders, as well as indications for treating sciatica, insomnia, headache, congestion, constipation, and incontinence.[11]

SUMMARY

Humans have used hydrotherapy for healing and spiritual rituals for centuries. The use of water's therapeutic properties gained popularity in the medical community in the 1800s, but its frequency of use by the medical establishment has varied since then. The field of aquatic therapy has grown tremendously in the late 20th century, serving as an adjunct to land-based therapies. Water's physical properties, including buoyancy and increased resistance to movement compared to air, provide advantages that cannot be found in land-based programs.

Aquatic therapy techniques need continued development as health-care professionals acquire skill and comfort in performing them and continue to note the important role the therapeutic use of water can have in a patient's rehabilitation. Research on pulsed lavage techniques and hydrotherapy immersion in the treatment of wound care remains scant. Further research is needed to support the effectiveness of aquatic and hydrotherapy procedures and to promote evidence-based health-care practice within the financial constraints now faced in the 21st century.

REFERENCES

1. Arborelius M, Balldin UI, Lilja B, Lundgren CE: Hemodynamic changes in man during immersion with the head above water. Aerospace Med 43:593, 1972.
2. Arthritis Foundation YMCA Aquatic Program: Guidelines and procedures manual. Atlanta, Arthritis Foundation, 1996.
3. Avellini BA, Shapiro Y, Pandloff KB: Cardiorespiratory physical training in water and on land. Euro J Appl Physiol 50:255, 1983.
4. Balldin UI, Lundgren CEG, Lundvall J, Mellander S: Changes in the elimination of ^{133}xenon from the anterior tibial muscle in man induced by immersion in water and shifts in body position. Aerospace Medicine 42:489, 1971.
5. Basford J: The physical agents. In O'Young B, Young MA, Stiens SA (eds): PM&R Secrets. Philadelphia, Hanley & Belfus, 1997, pp 525–526.
6. Becker B, Cole A: Aquatic rehabilitation. In DeLisa JA, Gans BM (eds): Textbook of Rehabilitation Medicine. Philadelphia, Lippincott-Raven, 1998, pp 887–901.
7. Alvarez O, Bennett M, Bergstrom N, Allman R, et al: Clinical Guidelines Treatment of Pressure Ulcers. Rockville, MD, AHCPR, 1994, pp 51–53.
8. Bloomfield J, Fricker P, Fitch K: Textbook of Science and Medicine in Sport. Champaign, IL, Human Kinetics Books, 1992, p 5.
9. Borg GAV: Psychophysical bases of perceived exertion. Med Sci Sports Exerc 14:377, 1992.
10. Borrell R, et. al: Comparison of in vivo temperatures produced by hydrotherapy, paraffin wax treatment and fluidotherapy. Phys Ther 60:1273, 1980.
11. Boyle W, Saine A: Sitz bath, alternate baths. Naturopathic Hydrotherapy 16:87–90, 1988.
12. Braddon R: Hydrotherapy. Physl Med Rehabil 22:459-460, 1966.
13. Burdenko I: The Burdenko Method-Water and Land Program. From Burdenko I, Connors E: The Ultimate Power of Resistance. Igo Publishing, 1988.
14. Burke DT, Saucier MA and Stewart G: Effects of Hydrotherapy on Pressure Ulcer Healing. Am J Phys Med Rehabil 77:394–398, 1988.
15. Campion MR: Adult Hydrotherapy: A Practical Approach. Oxford, England: Heinemann Medical Books, 1990, pp 199–239.
16. Centers for Disease Control: Microbiologic Control Branch, Bacterial Disease Division, and Bureau of Epidemiology. Atlanta, CDC, 1977.
17. Cole A, Becker B: Introduction to aquatic rehabilitation. J Back Musculoskel Rehabil 4:7, 1994.
18. Cole AJ, Eagleston RE, Moschetti M, et al: Spine pain: Aquatic rehabilitation strategies. J Back Musculoskel Rehabil 4:273, 1994.
19. Cunningham J: Halliwick method. Aquatic Rehabil 16:305-331. 1977.
20. Dadswell JV: Managing swimming, spas and other pools to prevent infection. Communicable Dis Rep 2:R37–40, 1996.
21. Basford J: Physical agents. In DeLisa J, Gans BM (eds): Rehabilitation Medicine Principles and Practice, 3rd ed. Philadelphia, Lippincott-Raven, 1998, pp 483–504.
22. De Vierville J: Aquatic rehabilitation: An historical perspective. In Becker B, Cole A (eds): Textbook of Comprehensive Aquatic Therapy. Newton, MA, Butterworth-Heinemann, 1997, pp 1–16.
23. Dressendorfer RH, Morlock JF, Baker DG, Hong SK: Effects of head out of water immersion on cardiorespiratory responses to maximal cycling exercise. Undersea Biomed Res 3:183, 1976.
24. Droegemueller W: Cold sitz baths for relief of postpartum perineal pain. Clin Obstet Gynecol 23:1039–1043, 1980.
25. Dull Harold: Watsu. Aquatic Rehabil 17:333–352, 1997.
26. Dull Harold: Watsu: Freeing the Body in Water, 2nd ed. Harbin Hot Springs, CA, Harbin Hot Springs Publishing, 1993.
27. Epstein M: Renal effects of head out immersion in humans: A 15 year update. Physiol Rev 72:563, 1992.
28. Evans BW, Cureton KJ, Purvis JW: Metabolic and circulatory responses to walking and jogging in water. Res Q 49:442–449, 1978.
29. Frantz R: Adjunctive therapy for ulcer care. Clin Geriatr Med 13:553–562, 1997.
30. Garrett G: Bad Ragaz ring method. Aquatic Rehabil 15:289–304, 1997.
31. Gatti CJ, Young RJ, Glad HL: Effect of water-training in the maintenance of cardiorespiratory endurance of athletes. Br J Sports Med 13:162, 1979.

32. Genaurio SE, Vesgo JJ: The use of a swimming pool in the rehabilitation and reconditioning of athletic injuries. Contemp Orthop 20:381–387, 1990.
33. Glass RA: Comparative biomechanical and physiological responses of suspended deep water running to hard surface running [unpublished thesis]. Auburn, AL, Auburn University, 1987.
34. Grabois M, Garrison S, et al: Therapeutic interventions. In Grabois M, et al (eds): Physical Medicine and Rehabilitation the Complete Approach. Malden, MA, Blackwell Scientific, 2000, pp 423–428.
35. Hamer TW, Morton AR: Water-running: Training effects and specificity of aerobic, anaerobic and muscular parameters following an eight-week interval training programme. Aust J Sci Med Sport 22:13, 1990.
36. Haralson K: Therapeutic pool programs. Clin Manage 5:10–13, 1986.
37. Harrison RA, Hillman M, Bulstrode S: Loading of the lower limb while partially immersed. Physiotherapy 78:165–166, 1992.
38. Konno J: Ai-chi (aquatic tai chi). In Watsu: Freeing the Body in Water. Harbin Hot Springs Publishing, 1997, pp 142–147.
39. Kowalsky L (ed): Pool-Spa Operator Handbook. San Antonio, TX, National Swimming Pool Foundation, 1990.
40. Krizek V: History of balneotherapy. In Licht S (ed): Textbook of Medical Hydrology. Baltimore, MD: Waverly Press, 1963, pp 132–149.
41. Lowman CL: Technique of Underwater Gymnastics: A Study in Practical Application. Los Angeles, American Publications, 1937, p 4.
42. Luedtke-Hoffman K, Schafer S: Pulsed lavage in wound cleansing. Am Phys Ther Assoc 80:292-300, 2000.
43. McGuckin M, Thorpe R, Abrutyn E: Hydrotherapy: An outbreak of *Pseudomonas aeruginosa* wound infections related to Hubbard tank treatments. Arch Phys Med Rehabil 62:283–285. 1981.
44. Meeker BJ: Whirlpool therapy, postoperative pain and surgical wound healing: An exploration. Patient Ed Counsel 33:39–48, 1998.
45. Miller JK, La Forrest NT, Hedberg M, Chapman V: Surveillance and control of Hubbard tank bacterial contaminants. Phys Ther 50:1482–1486, 1970.
46. O'Sullivan S: Physical modalities in wound management. In Physical Rehabilitation: Assessment and Treatment, 1988.
47. Prins J, Cutner D: Aquatic therapy in the rehabilitation of athletic injuries. Clin Sports Med 18: 447–461, 1999.
48. Ramler D, Roberts J: A Comparison of cold and warm sitz baths for relief of postpartum perineal pain. J Gynecol Nurs Nov/Dec:471–474, 1986.
49. Risch WD, Koubenec HJ, Beckmann U, et al: The effect of graded immersion on heart volume, central venous pressure, pulmonary blood distribution and heart rate in man. Pflugers Arch 374:117, 1978.
50. Rivers E, Fisher S: Burn rehabilitation. In O'Young B, Young MA, Stiens SA (eds): PM&R Secrets. Philadelphia, Hanley & Belfus, 1997, pp 418–428.
51. Schoedinger P: Adapting watsu for people with special needs. In Watsu: Freeing the Body in Water. Harbin Hot Springs, CA, Harbin Hot Springs Publishing, 1993, pp 111–121.
52. Simmons V, Hansen PD: Effectiveness of water exercise on postural mobility in the well elderly: An experimental study on balance enhancement. J Gerontol A Biol Sci Med Sci 51:M233-238, 1996.
53. Sova, Konno J: Ai Chi Flowing Aquatic Energy [handout].
54. Stanwood W, Pinzur M: Risk of contamination of the wound in a hydrotherapeutic tank. Foot Ankle Int 19:173–119. 1998.
55. Svendhag J, Seger J: Running on land and in water: Comparative exercise physiology. Med Sci Sports Exerc 24:1158, 1992.
56. Templeton MS, Booth BL, O'Kelly WD: Effects of aquatic therapy on joint flexibility and functional ability in subjects with rheumatic disease. J Orthop Sports Phys Ther 23: 376–381, 1996.
57. Trelstad A, Osmundsun D: Water Pik: Wound cleansing alternative. Plast Surg Nurs 9:117–119, 1998.
58. Walsh M: Hydrotherapy: The use of water as a therapeutic agent. In Thermal Agents in Rehabilitation, 2nd ed. pp 109–133, 1986.
59. Weston CFM, O'Hare JP, Evans JM, Corral RJM: Haemodynamic changes in man during immersion in water at different temperatures. Clin Sci (London) 73:613–616, 1987.
60. Zislis J: Hydrotherapy. In Handbook of Physical Medicine and Rehabilitation. 2nd ed. Philadelphia, WB Saunders, 1971.

Chapter 7

Ultraviolet Light and Laser Therapy

Kevin M. Means, MD

ULTRAVIOLET LIGHT THERAPY

Historical Background

Throughout history, the beneficial effects of sunlight have been recognized and appreciated by many. Some cultures, such as the ancient Egyptians, Chinese, East Indians, Romans, and Aztecs, actually worshipped the sun itself as a god. Many in these cultures believed the sunlight to have healthful effects, and the practice of sun bathing was common.[1]

The advent of Christianity resulted in suppression of pagan practices such as sun worship and sun bathing. However, a renewed interest in the sun and its powers resurfaced in the 18th and 19th centuries. As science and medicine continued to evolve, many physicians began to advocate the therapeutic use of sunlight for specific medical conditions. Unfortunately, the sun as a therapeutic agent was often unreliable (on cloudy days), inconvenient to use indoors, and difficult to regulate because of positional changes and seasonal variations in intensity. This fueled efforts to produce artificial illumination that could duplicate the therapeutic effects of sunlight.[1]

By the late 1800s, scientific investigation into the physical properties of sunlight and other forms of energy had advanced significantly. In 1868, Angstrom mapped out the invisible light spectrum, and ultraviolet light was a distinguishable entity. The medical use of ultraviolet light gained popularity. In 1877, Downes and Blunt proved that light could kill bacteria. Niels Finsen first used sunlight concentrated with lenses and later began using a carbon arc ultraviolet lamp to treat lupus vulgaris. Finsen's treatment of cutaneous tuberculosis with ultraviolet light won him the Nobel Prize in 1903.[1] By 1933, Frank Krusen published *Light Therapy* which included a complete list of over 150 conditions for which benefit was claimed for using ultraviolet light therapy (Table 1). Although this list included diseases for which the benefit of ultraviolet light therapy was well-established, it also included diseases such as hypertension, the common cold, and hyperacidity of the stomach.[1] Ironically, although ultraviolet light therapy was once popular in the early days of physical medicine and rehabilitation (PM&R), today relatively few physiatrists and decreasing numbers of other rehabilitation professionals actually use ultraviolet therapy. Its inclusion in this text and in standard PM&R textbooks is primarily for historical purposes. A more detailed account of the history of ultraviolet radiation use may be found elsewhere.[1]

Physics of Ultraviolet Light

Ultraviolet light is a form of radiant electromagnetic energy produced when the electrons in stable atoms are activated to move to higher, unstable orbits. As these electrons move back to their original orbit, they release energy in the form of elec-

TABLE 1. CONDITIONS FOR WHICH SUCCESSFUL TREATMENT WITH ULTRAVIOLET LIGHT WAS CLAIMED (IN 1933)

Alimentary Tract

Appendiceal abscess	Chronic colitis	Chronic constipation
Chronic cholecystitis	Liver cirrhosis	Hemorrhoids
Stomach hyperacidity	Ischiorectal abscess	Postoperative adhesions
Pyloric stenosis	Pylorospasm	Peritoneal tuberculosis
Intestinal tuberculosis		

Circulatory System

Anemia	Arteriosclerosis	Chlorosis
Hemophilia	Hypertension	Hypotension
Pericarditis	Phlebitis	Varicose veins

Respiratory System

Nervous System

Adapted from Licht S: History of ultraviolet therapy. In Stillwell GK (ed): Therapeutic Electricity and Ultraviolet Radiation, 3rd ed. Baltimore, Williams & Wilkins, 1983, pp 174–193.

tromagnetic radiation. Ultraviolet radiation is transmitted by oscillatory motion in the form of electromagnetic sine waves that travel in a straight line (Fig. 1). Wavelength is measured in nanometers (nm).[2]

Ultraviolet light also may be identified by its frequency, defined as the number of oscillations or cycles that occur within a given unit of time. Frequency is measured in cycles per second or Hertz (Hz). Wavelength and frequency have an inverse relationship. The longer a wavelength is, the fewer the number of cycles that may occur within a second. Conversely, the shorter the length of a wave, the higher the wave frequency and the higher its energy content. Like other forms of radiation, ultraviolet waves can be reflected, refracted (scattered), and absorbed.

Ultraviolet light was named for the position of its wavelength in the electromagnetic spectrum relative to the wavelength of violet light, which is on one extreme end of the visible light spectrum (Fig. 2). Visible light is actually composed of a broad spectrum of colors. Each color is defined by a different wavelength. The wavelengths of the visible light spectrum range from 400 nm to 800 nm, whereas the frequencies range from 7.5×10^{14} to 3.75×10^{14}.

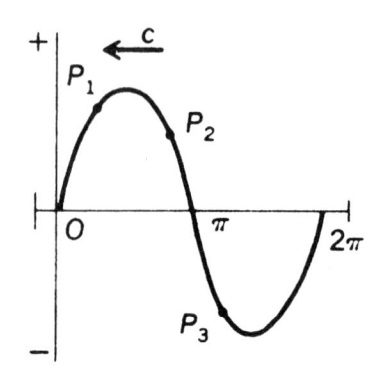

FIGURE 1. Sine wave.

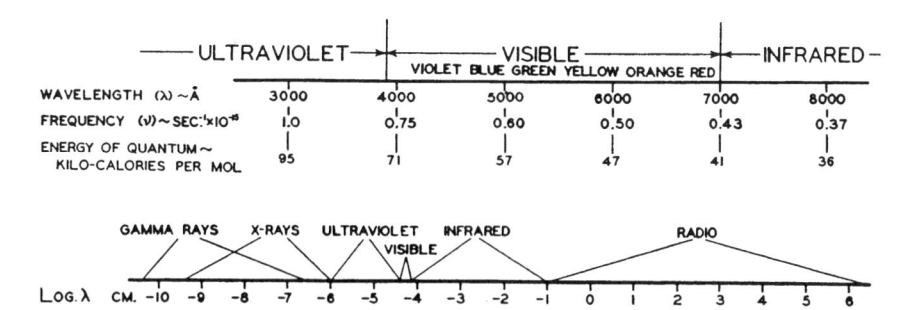

FIGURE 2. The electromagnetic spectrum. (From Blum HF: Photodynamic Action and Diseases Caused by Light. New York, Reinhold, 1941.)

The word *ultraviolet* meaning "beyond violet," is actually a misnomer because the name implies that its wavelength, which ranges from 180 nm to 400 nm, is greater than the wavelength of violet light (400nm). Some researchers have further classified ultraviolet light into three subdivisions, based on wavelength and other properties.[2] **Ultraviolet-A** (UV-A) has relatively long wavelengths, in the 320-nm to 400-nm range, closest to the visible light spectrum. UV-A also has relatively shorter frequencies. **Ultraviolet-B** (UV-B) has shorter wavelengths in the 290-nm to 320-nm range, and **ultraviolet-C** (UV-C), with the shortest range of wavelengths, at 180 nm to 290 nm, has relatively higher frequencies[2,3] (*see* Fig. 2). UV-A and UV-B are also known as *near ultraviolet* because of their proximity to the visible light spectrum, and UV-C is known as *far ultraviolet* because of its greater distance from visible light.

Photobiologic Effects

The ability of ultraviolet light to produce biologic changes in human tissue depends on several factors: (1) the wavelength of the UV radiation; (2) the amount of energy absorbed or reflected by the tissue; (3) the distance from the radiation source; (4) the angle of delivery of the radiation; and (5) the time of exposure to the radiation. Natural ultraviolet light comes from the sun's radiation, although most of the ultraviolet rays in sunlight are absorbed by the earth's atmosphere. Only 5–10% of solar energy that penetrates the atmosphere is in the ultraviolet wavelength range.[4]

Though some near ultraviolet (UV-A and UV-B) rays in sunlight penetrate the earth's atmosphere to produce biologic effects, most UV-C rays are absorbed by the upper atmosphere and never reach the earth's surface. The known biologic effects of UV-C rays are produced from exposure to artificial lamps. Ultraviolet-A radiation causes increased pigmentation or tanning of the skin and a weak erythema (sunburn) reaction.[5] Ultraviolet-B also increases skin tanning and causes a more intense (100–1000 times) erythema reaction with the possibility of blister formation. Whereas the effects of UV-A and UV-B radiation are primarily in the dermal layer of skin, the main effect of UV-C occurs in the epidermal layer. Erythema effects from a UV-C lamp peak at a wavelength of 250 nm but rarely cause an intense erythema or blistering.[6] This is because skin reflects radiation with shorter wavelength (UV-C) much more easily than radiation with longer wavelength (UV-A and UV-B).

Beneficial Effects of Ultraviolet Light

The main beneficial effects of ultraviolet light include:

Erythema. Erythema, or redness of the skin, is produced by congestion of cutaneous capillaries. If the ultraviolet dosage is sufficiently high, an inflammatory response is produced with an associated vasodilatation mediated by histamine.[7] Ultraviolet radiation wavelengths of 254 nm and 299 nm are most effective at producing erythema.

Bactericide. The bactericidal effect of ultraviolet light has been known since 1877. Ultraviolet radiation interrupts the synthesis of DNA and RNA in bacteria, and it is used to sterilize air and water. Bactericidal effects are best achieved with ultraviolet wavelengths in the 250-nm to 270-nm range.[3,4]

Wound Healing. The erythema and increased blood flow improves oxygenation to the skin and promotes wound healing by stimulation and proliferation of endothelial cells and granulation tissue. Bactericidal and virucidal effects on wound pathogenic organisms also may aid wound healing.[8,9]

Pigmentation. An increase in pigmentation (tanning) follows vascular and inflammatory changes of the erythema reaction. Previously synthesized melanin in deeper epidermal skin layers is spread by capillaries to a more superficial position within the epidermis. This produces an immediate tanning effect (within minutes). Activation of new melanin production by epidermal melanocytes and transfer of this pigment to epidermal keratinocytes results in additional delayed tanning (within days, lasts for months). Ultraviolet wavelengths of 254 nm and 297 nm are the most effective for tanning.[10]

Superficial Exfoliation. Ultraviolet light causes dead epithelial cells, eschar, and necrotic tissue to slough off. This enhances wound debridement and aids in the treatment of some cutaneous diseases.[3,8]

Application Techniques in Ultraviolet Therapy

Techniques used in the therapeutic application of ultraviolet light depend on the type and wavelength of ultraviolet radiation to be used, associated physiologic effects, and the goals of treatment (e.g., tanning, wound debridement). Protocols have been used to determine the therapeutic dosage of ultraviolet light by determining the dose (exposure time) of ultraviolet radiation required to produce desired effects.[2,3] This minimum exposure time may be different for individual patients and should be individually determined.

Normally, after skin exposure to ultraviolet light, there is a latent period of 2–6 hours. The skin then becomes red and warm from vasodilatation. This reaction peaks in intensity about 8–10 hours after exposure. Holtz reported that this reaction includes intercellular edema in the prickle cell layer of skin and a concentration of leukocytes in local blood vessels. Erythema developing after ultraviolet light exposure is divided into four levels: first, second, third, and fourth-degree erythema.[11]

First-degree erythema is a painless reddening of the skin within 4–6 hours and lasting for 24 hours. A second-degree erythema reaction also develops after 4–6 hours and involves reddening and soreness of the exposed skin area. This reaction resembles mild sunburn, lasts for 3–4 days, and is accompanied by increased pigmentation and mild superficial exfoliation. A third-degree erythema reaction starts earlier (within 2 hours) and includes more severe sunburn signs and symptoms with redness, tenderness, and edema, which may last several days. Pigmentation is more pronounced as is the exfoliation, which is typically a peeling off of superficial skin layers. Fourth-degree erythema is initially similar to third-degree erythema changes, but as severe skin edema and exudation separate the superficial skin layer from deeper layers, blister formation occurs.[4]

A device for use in determining ultraviolet radiation dosage, called an erythrometer, can be made from material that is opaque to ultraviolet such as cardboard, metal, or black paper. Some descriptions of the erythrometer and the procedure for biologic ultraviolet dosage testing differ slightly but utilize the same basic principles.[2-4,12] Four to six small (approximately 0.75 cm × 0.75 cm) openings spaced 0.75 cm apart are cut out of the opaque material and the erythmometer is then taped on the patient's volar forearm or lower abdomen. A sliding cover for the erythmometer is made from the opaque material so that one opening or all openings can be progressively covered. The patient's and the therapist's eyes should be protected, and all of the patient's skin that is in the field of the UV lamp should be draped except for the forearm.

The ultraviolet lamp is positioned 60–90 cm (2–3 feet) away from and perpendicular to the treating surface and is turned on. Initially, only the first opening is exposed. After 15 seconds of exposure, the second opening is uncovered, and the first opening remains exposed. Each of the next two to four openings is progressively uncovered at 15-second intervals, until the lamp is turned off at a total of 90 seconds of exposure. With this protocol and using an erythrometer with six openings, the first opening uncovered would have had an exposure time of 90 seconds, and the last opening uncovered would have been exposed for 15 seconds. The erythrometer is removed, but the position of each opening is marked for later reference. The patient is asked to monitor the forearm every 2 hours (while awake) for the next 48 hours and record which site becomes erythematous and when, and how long the erythema lasts. The minimal erythema dose (MED), or the minimum ultraviolet exposure time required to produce a mild (first degree), latent erythema lasting 24 hours (determined erythema reaction), can be calculated using this information.

Ultraviolet radiation dosages are in multiples of the MED exposure time for each individual patient (Table 2). For most UV lamps, 1 MED is achieved with an exposure between 5 and 15 seconds in caucasians. Exposure at 2.5 times the MED causes painful (second-degree) erythema within 6 hours, lasting 4 days. At 5–10 times the MED, painful (third-degree) erythema and blistering develops. Ultraviolet dosages in this range should be limited to small areas of exposure.[2-4]

Ultraviolet Light Administration

Procedures

Ultraviolet radiation treatment space should be private and temperature-controlled, because bare skin exposure is necessary. Absorption of ultraviolet radiation by oxygen in the air may result in ozone gas accumulation. Therefore, adequate ventilation in the treatment area is necessary. Depending on the desired effect, the physician may prescribe **generalized exposure** (mild intensity radiation for a wide-

TABLE 2. ULTRAVIOLET RADIATION DOSING PARAMETERS

- Suberythemal dose (SED) = no erythema.
- Minimal erythema dose (MED) = the dosage of UV radiation required to induce a detectable, painless (1st degree), latent erythema 2–6 hours postexposure, lasting 8–10 hours, determined with a test exposure.
- For most UV lamps, 1 MED = an exposure of 5–30 seconds at 30 inches in caucasians.
- Subsequent UV dosage (exposure) is in multiples of this 1 MED.
- 2.5 times the MED causes painful (2nd degree) erythema within 6 hours, lasting 4 days.
- 5 times the MED causes painful (3rd degree) erythema followed by intracellular edema of the prickle cell layer, then local peeling of the exposed skin.
- 10 times the MED causes superficial blister formation followed by 3rd degree erythema changes.
- Dosages of 5–10 times the MED should be limited to very small areas of the skin.

spread or generalized condition); a **regional exposure** (one or more body parts are targeted at one time while the nontreated parts are covered with a towel or drape); or a **contact exposure** (directed to a focal area, such as a wound).

Careful documentation of details of the ultraviolet treatment is required. History of past exposure to ultraviolet radiation and the erythema response is important. History of recent use or exposure to photosensitizing substances should be obtained. If more than one lamp exists in the department, the specific lamp used for the treatment should be documented as should the specific distance between the lamp and the patient. The type (generalized, regional, direct), time, and angle of exposure; response of the skin and the patient, and use of medications and topical substances after exposure should be noted.

Equipment

Early electric ultraviolet lamps were made of carbon arc electrodes. These were followed by mercury vapor lamps, and by the early twentieth century, by quartz lamps which are quartz tubes filled with argon gas and liquid mercury.[13] Some quartz lamps, known as "hot quartz lamps," are now rarely used in PM&R settings. These lamps are high pressure, high temperature, mercury-filled and air cooled. Hot quartz lamps produce ultraviolet radiation in both the near and far bands. Hot quartz lamps can be used when generalized exposure is needed or for more focused regional exposure of a body part.[3,13]

Other so-called cold quartz lamps are low-temperature, low-pressure, mercury-filled lamps. Cold quartz lamps are much more common and have the advantages of being smaller, more portable, usually hand-held devices. Cold quartz lamps emit 90% of their ultraviolet rays in the 253.7-nm (bactericidal) band, and they are typically used to treat skin ulcers and other focal cutaneous conditions.[3]

Only qualified professionals should operate ultraviolet therapy equipment. All equipment should be accurately calibrated on a regular basis and visually inspected daily. Regular servicing by qualified technicians should be performed at least every 6 months.[14]

Precautions

Because the cornea and retina are very sensitive to ultraviolet light, the eyes of the patient and the therapist or UV lamp operator should always be shielded with ultraviolet-opaque goggles.[15,16] Exposed areas of skin, particularly prominent body parts that are not intended for treatment, should be covered during ultraviolet therapy sessions.[17] Several substances are known to have photosensitizing properties, and patient consumption of these substances should be avoided prior to ultraviolet light exposure. This includes foods such as strawberries and shellfish and medicines such as insulin, quinine, sulfonamides, certain diuretics, hormones, and oral contraceptives. Exposure following intake of these substances may result in potentiation of the effects or side effects of the ultraviolet light exposure, alteration of the effect of the medication, or both. Patients should be questioned about contact with or use of these substances before ultraviolet light therapy.

Extra caution should be used in persons with very fair or atrophic skin because the relative absence of pigment or the relatively reduced skin thickness will result in decreased reflection, increased absorption, and relatively increased intensity. This effectively increases the risk of adverse effects. Because the risk of energy absorption and tissue injury could be additive, ultraviolet light therapy should be avoided immediately after application of superficial heating modalities.[3,14] In general, elderly patients, infants, and chemotherapy patients have low tolerance for ultraviolet light therapy. This physical agent should be used sparingly with these special patient populations.

Clinical Applications for Ultraviolet Light

Currently, the main clinical application in the rehabilitation setting for ultraviolet light therapy is in the treatment of pressure ulcers of the skin and other wounds. The desirable effects of ultraviolet light that aid wound healing have been studied using UV-A, UV-B, and UV-C. These effects include increasing epithelial turnover, epidermal hyperplasia, and fibroblast activity, which accelerate wound closure. The release of prostaglandin precursors, which may mediate cell proliferation, and histamine, which increases cutaneous blood flow and accelerated DNA synthesis, further assists the wound healing process.[8,18] The shorter wavelength (180–250 nm) UV-C directly applied using a hand-held cold quartz lamp is the most common method used for treatment of wounds. The bactericidal effect of UV-C inactivates bacteria to further promote healing. This property of ultraviolet light is particularly useful when treating chronically colonized or infected wounds.[8,18] In a recent in-vitro study, UV-C has been shown to inhibit growth of methicillin-resistant *Staphylococcus aureus* (MRSA) and vancomycin-resistant *Enterococcus faecalis* (VRE).[19] Despite emerging evidence supporting its effectiveness, the use of ultraviolet light for wound healing in the rehabilitation setting appears to be decreasing. This may be due to the availability of other alternative treatments, such as topical antibiotics and dressings, and the actual or perceived expense of equipment or time associated with ultraviolet therapy.

Several other conditions have been treated with ultraviolet light, though uncommonly by the physiatrist or in the rehabilitation setting.

Psoriasis. This is perhaps the skin condition most commonly treated with ultraviolet radiation. Literature support for the treatment of psoriasis is well established. Treatment is accomplished with ultraviolet radiation either alone or in combination with additive photosensitizing substances, such as tar-based topical ointments or ingested psoralen drugs. Two established anti-psoriatic treatment techniques are known by the acronyms TUVAB (Tar and UV–A and UV-B) and PUVA (Psoralen + UV-A). In the TUVAB protocol, a coal tar ointment is applied to the affected area, then removed, followed by UV-A and UV-B exposure at 4 MED, increasing daily by 2 MEDs.[3] In the PUVA protocol, the patient ingests psoralen prior to UV-A exposure. Because of some safety and side effects concerns, the PUVA protocol is indicated in only select cases.[9,20]

Acne Vulgaris. Ultraviolet radiation has been used to promote superficial desquamation in patients with acne vulgaris.

Neonatal Jaundice. Exposure to ultraviolet radiation has been used to prevent the development of jaundice in term and premature neonates.

LASER THERAPY

Laser therapy is another example of a therapeutic technology that currently is not widely used by physiatrists or in the rehabilitation setting. However, unlike ultraviolet therapy, which has been used clinically for over 100 years, laser technology is still relatively new (40 years old) and actively expanding, and the clinical use of lasers is growing. An extensive review of laser technology is beyond the scope of this chapter, but the reader is referred to a fairly recent review of this topic for further reading.[21]

The word *laser* is an acronym for light amplification by stimulated emission radiation. The use of lasers for surgical cutting and cauterization is very familiar to most clinicians. Another type of laser with more potential applications in the PM&R setting is the low-intensity laser. This type of laser is also referred to as the "cold," "low power," or "low level" laser. Laser is a form of light or radiation from another part of the same electromagnetic spectrum as ultraviolet light. Lasers characteristically produce light that is monochromatic (each laser device emits a beam of only one wavelength), coherent (waves travel in highly-ordered, parallel waves), and polarized.[22] Like other forms of radiation, laser energy can be transmitted, reflected, or absorbed by tissue. High-intensity laser radiation has output power in excess of 60–75 milliwatts (mW) which is accompanied by tissue damage and thermal effects. In contrast, low intensity laser has output power that typically is ≤0.5–1.0 mW. At such a low power, low-intensity laser beams are undetectable and not associated with any significant tissue temperature changes. Accordingly, low-intensity laser radiation works by initiating athermic photochemical reactions within cells. These reactions occur with extremely small power intensities.

The most commonly used low-intensity lasers are produced by helium-neon (HeNe), gallium arsenide (GaAs), and gallium aluminum arsenide (GaAlAs) devices. Typical wavelengths of low-intensity laser therapy using HeNe, GaAs, and GaAlAs are 632.8 nm, 904 nm, and 820 or 830 nm, respectively. A variety of delivery systems, treatment approaches, application techniques, and waveform options exist, and all of these variables may affect treatment results.[23]

The reported clinical effects of low-intensity laser radiation include marked improvements in wound healing, nerve repair, musculoskeletal pain, and various inflammatory processes.[24] A partial list of conditions that have been treated with low-intensity laser therapy appears in Table 3. Although several related studies have been conducted and literature support for low-intensity laser therapy is growing,

TABLE 3. CLINICAL CONDITIONS TREATED WITH LOW INTENSITY LASER THERAPY

Arthritic conditions	Skin/subcutaneous disorders
Rheumatoid arthritis	Pruritis
Ankylosing spondylitis	Diabetic ulcers
Sjögren syndrome	Pressure ulcers
Osteoarthritis (various sites)	Venous stasis ulcers
	Surgical wounds
Tendinitis	Radiation dermatitis
Lateral epicondylitis	Stomatitis
Medial epicondylitis	Keloids
Supraspinatus tendinitis	Hemangiomas
Bicipital tendinitis	
Achilles tendinitis	**Oral/facial pain**
	Dental surgery
Neuropathic pain	Oral dysesthesia
Carpal tunnel syndrome	Trigeminal neuralgia
Diabetic neuropathy	Temporomandibular pain
Radiculopathy	Dental hypersensitivity
Postherpetic neuralgia	
Occipital neuralgia	**Tinnitus**
Acute and chronic musculoskeletal pain	**Immune modulation**
Musculoskeletal back pain	Allergic rhinitis
Tension myalgia	Leukemia
Myofascial pain syndrome	
Cervicothoracic pain	**Peripheral and facial nerve repair**
Ankle sprain	
Muscle pull	**Pyronie's disease**
Patellofemoral pain	
Trigger point pain threshold elevation	**Headaches**

Adapted from Basford JR: Low-intensity laser therapy: Still not an established clinical tool. Lasers Surg Med 16:331–342, 1995.

many studies have been poorly controlled. More research is needed on low-intensity laser therapy, particularly well-designed controlled clinical trials to more conclusively demonstrate clinical efficacy.[21]

REFERENCES

1. Licht S: History of ultraviolet therapy. In Stillwell GK (ed): Therapeutic Electricity and Ultraviolet Radiation, 3rd ed. Baltimore, Williams & Wilkins, 1983, pp 174–193.
2. Behrens BJ: Therapeutic use of light: Ultraviolet and cold laser. In Behrens BJ, Michlovitz SL (eds): Physical Agents: Theory and Practice for the Physical Therapist Assistant. Philadelphia, F.A. Davis, 1996, pp 118–134.
3. Weisberg J: Ultraviolet irradiation. In Hecox B, Mehretaab TA, Weisberg J (eds): Physical Agents: A Comprehensive Text for Physical Therapists. Norwalk, CT, Appelton & Lange, 1994, pp 377–389.
4. Scott BO: Clinical uses of ultraviolet radiation. In Stillwell GK (ed): Therapeutic Electricity and Ultraviolet Radiation, 3rd ed. Baltimore, Williams & Wilkins, 1983, pp 228–262
5. Pathak MA: Physical units of radiation and some common terms used in photobiology. In Pathak M (ed): Sunlight and Man. Tokyo, Japan, University of Tokyo Press, 1974, pp 815–818.
6. Nussbaum E, Biemann I, Mustard B: Comparison of ultrasound/ultraviolet-C and laser treatment of pressure ulcers in patients with spinal cord injury. Phys Ther 74:812–823, 1994.

7. Greaves M, Sondergaard J: Pharmacologic agents released in ultraviolet inflammation studied by continuous skin perfusion. J Invest Dermatol 54:365–367, 1970.
8. Kloth LC: Physical modalities in wound management: UVC, therapeutic heating and electrical stimulation. Ostomy Wound Manage 41:18–20, 22–24, 26–27, 1995.
9. Kitchen SS, Partridge CJ: A review of ultraviolet radiation therapy. Physiotherapy 77:423–432, 1991.
10. Daniels F: Ultraviolet light and dermatology. In Stillwell GK (ed): Therapeutic Electricity and Ultraviolet Radiation, 3rd ed. Baltimore, Williams & Wilkins, 1983, pp 263–303.
11. Holtz F: Pharmacology of ultra-violet radiation. Br J Phys Med 15:201, 1952.
12. Leach EE, McClelland PB, Morgan P, Shelk J: Basic principles of photobiology and photochemistry for nurse phototherapists and phototechnicians. Dermatol Nurs 8:235–258, 1996.
13. Anderson WT: Instrumentation for ultraviolet therapy. In Stillwell GK (ed): Therapeutic Electricity and Ultraviolet Radiation, 3rd ed. Baltimore, Williams & Wilkins, 1983, pp 194–227.
14. Low J, Bazin S, Docker M, et al: Guidelines for the safe use of ultraviolet therapy equipment. Physiotherapy 80:89–90, 1994.
15. Morrison WL: Phototherapy and Photochemotherapy of Skin Disease, 2nd ed. New York, Raven Press, 1991.
16. Lerman S, Van Voorhees A: Cutaneous and ocular ramifications of ultraviolet radiation. Dermatol Clin 10:483–504, 1992.
17. Abel EA: Phototherapy. Dermatol Clin 13:841–849, 1995.
18. Houghton PE: Effects of therapeutic modalities on wound healing: A conservative approach to the management of chronic wounds. Phys Ther Rev 4:167–182, 1999.
19. Conner Kerr TA, Sullivan PK, Gaillard J, et al: The effects of ultraviolet radiation on antibiotic resistant bacteria in vitro. Ostomy Wound Manage 44:50–56, 1998.
20. Abel EA: Phototherapy: UVA and PUVA. Cutis 64:339–342, 1999.
21. Schindl A, Schindl M, Pernerstorfer-Schön H, Schindl L: Low-intensity laser therapy: A review. J Invest Med 48:312–326, 2000.
22. Weisberg J: Lasers. In Hecox B, Mehretaab TA, Weisberg J (eds): Physical Agents: A Comprehensive Text for Physical Therapists. Norwalk, CT, Appleton & Lange, 1994, pp 391–396.
23. Basford JR: Low-intensity laser therapy: Still not an established clinical tool. Lasers Surg Med 16:331–342, 1995.
24. Basford JR: Laser therapy: Scientific basis and clinical role. Orthopedics 16:541–547, 1993.

Chapter 8
Magnet Therapy

Sonia Williams, MD, and Butchaiah Garlapati, MD, MPH

HISTORICAL PERSPECTIVE

The term *magnet* was probably derived from Magnes, a shepherd who discovered mysterious iron deposits attracted to the nails of his sandals while walking in the area near Mount Ida, Turkey. The ancients knew magnets as Heraclen stones, lodestones, or live stones.[1]

In ancient Greece, Aristotle was the first of his time to speak about therapeutic properties of the magnets. Around 200 B.C., the Greek physician Galen found that pain from different diseases could be relieved by applying magnets. In first century a.d., the Chinese used very sensitive compasses to monitor variations in the earth's magnetic field and attributed the effects on health and disease to these variations.[2] The physician Kirches (1602–1680) used magnets to "cure" strangulated hernias.[3]

In 1762, Maximillian Hell, a Jesuit and the chief astronomer at the University of Vienna, published a treatise on the medical powers of magnets.[4,5] In 1766, Hell's younger colleague Franz Anton Mesmer (1734–1815) presented his doctoral thesis on the effects of gravitational fields and cycles on human health. Later, he proposed the theory that gravitational forces led to changes in magnetic flux, which in turn produced profound neuropsychiatric and constitutional effects, or "animal magnetism." Later, controlled, blinded experiments discredited this theory. "Animal magnetism" was determined to be self-limiting and was attributed to the power of suggestion or a psychosomatic phenomenon.[6–8]

After Mesmer was discredited, the clinical application of magnets was largely seen as quackery. By 1865, James Clerk Maxwell proposed his theory that an electric field is always accompanied by a magnetic field, and, conversely, a variable or pulsed magnetic field is always accompanied by an electric field.[9] Maxwell's theory, in part, fueled continued interest in the field of magnet therapy. Literature from the late 19th and entire 20th centuries relates growing use of magnets in clinical interventions. Despite this, there are very few scientifically sound studies supporting the efficacy or effectiveness of magnet therapy.

PHYSICS OF MAGNETS

By definition, a *magnet* is a native iron oxide (Fe3O4) that attracts iron. It is also a bar of steel or iron that attracts iron and has magnetic polarity.[10] A *magnetic field* is the region surrounding a magnet or an electric current. Pulsed magnetic fields move electrical charges or induce an electric current. Static magnetic fields do not move electrical charges or induce an electric current.

Static magnets may induce electricity when applied to arthritic joints and tender points by means of the Hall effect. In his experiments, Edwin Hall (1879) noted that when a strip of gold leaf is placed perpendicular to a magnetic field, the edges acquire different electric potentials. This suggested a small source of current.[11] This small potential may explain the useful effects of magnets in pain management. This simple concept may not apply very well to biological systems (e.g., cells, nerves, the circulatory system) because these are usually randomly oriented and likely to cancel out linear effects of magnetic fields.

Blank et al. proposed the sodium-potassium adenosine triphosphatase (Na,K-ATPase) model for electromagnetic field effects on cells and possibly various disease states. In part, this proposal asserts that electromagnetic radiation acts at the lipid membrane surface to affect the ability of ion pump enzymes to transport calcium, sodium, and potassium across the cell membrane.[12]

Of note, magnets used in the management of pain usually involve lower magnetic field strengths. These magnetic field strengths are typically less than that of a magnetic resonance imaging (MRI).

Magnetic Poles

Magnets have two kinds of poles—somewhat like two kinds of electric charges. Like poles repel each other, and unlike poles attract each other. Unlike electric charges, magnetic poles cannot be isolated. If a magnet is broken into two pieces, each piece will have two poles as shown below.[13]

Magnetic Fields

There is a magnetic field around a magnet, which looks somewhat like the electric field around a "dipole," a pair of positive and negative electric charges. A magnetic field can be shown as imaginary lines that flow out of the North Pole and into the South Pole of a magnet. The magnetic field of a bar magnet is strongest near the magnet's poles, where the lines lie closest to each other.[13]

Magnetic Fields Caused by Currents

The direction of the magnetic field is given by the **right hand rule**. Magnetism and electricity are closely related, and together they make a force called *electromagnetism*, one of the basic forces in the universe. A moving magnet near a coil of copper wire, for example, can induce (produce) an electric current flowing through a wire, creating a magnetic field around the wire. The direction of the magnetic field around a straight wire can be determined according to the right-hand rule. If you imagine that the thumb of your right hand points along the flow of the current, the fingers curl around the wire in the direction of the magnetic field.[13]

The right hand rule also applies to the magnetic field produced by a coil or a solenoid. Magnetic field lines flow through the length of a coil. If the fingers of the right hand curl around the coil in the direction of the current, the right thumb points to the coil's north pole and shows the direction of the magnetic field lines.

The right hand rule is used when the current is thought of as a flow of positive electric charges. In a simple electric circuit connected to a battery, for example, the current is defined as flowing from the battery's positive terminal to its negative terminal.

Measurement of Magnetic Fields

The strength of magnetic field is measured in units of gauss (G) or, alternatively, tesla (T). In the MKS (metric) system of units, $1\ T = 1\ 10^4\ G$. For comparison, the magnetic field of the earth at the surface is on the order of 1 G (actually $\frac{1}{2}$ G), whereas that of a neodymium magnet is on the order of 104 G. This means that neodymium magnets produce magnetic fields tens of thousands of times stronger than those of the earth. Neodymium itself is actually element, atomic number 60 on the periodic table. Neodymium magnets are made up of a compound called neodymium iron boron (NIB; $Nd_2Fe_{14}B$). This compound is one of the strongest known ferromagnetic materials.

Technically, gauss and tesla are units of magnetic induction, also known as *magnetic flux density*. Quantitatively, the force on a charged particle q moving with the velocity v is given by the vector equation: $F = qv \times B$, where B is the magnetic induction.

Another common quality of interest is the coercivity or coercive force of a magnet.[13] Also measured in gauss, the coercivity is the magnetic field required to demagnetize a material. For example, neodymium magnets typically have coercivity of about 12,000 G. Note that the coercivity is the magnetic field required for demagnetization; it is not actually a measure of the "strength" of the magnet, although the highly coercive magnets are usually quite strong.[13]

The maximum energy product is used to determine the quality of magnetic materials. The maximum energy product basically determines what materials make the best magnets.

MAGNET THERAPY DELIVERY SYSTEMS

Permanent Static Magnet Therapy

Permanent static magnets used for therapy take two forms:

1. **Unipolar**. Several discreet individual magnets are aligned with the same pole (the biomagnetic north or negative pole) facing the patient's skin. The biomagnetic south pole then faces away from the skin.[14]

2. **Bipolar**. Different shaped magnets (strips, concentric circles, squares, triangles) are aligned in alternating patterns so that both north and south poles face the patient's skin.[14]

Pulsed Electromagnetic Field Therapy

Pulsed electromagnetic field (PEMF) therapy requires an electric device in the form of a pulse generator connected to coils. The magnetic field is produced by the waveform generator that drives a current through electromagnetic coils.[15] In the "transformer" mechanism, current passes through coils adjacent to tissue, causing current flow in the tissue. This is the accepted mechanism in bone healing and the proposed mechanism with soft tissue complaints. With bone healing, the effects of PEMF therapy are likened to the natural electrical activities created within bone during movements.[16]

Unlike static magnetic fields, pulsed magnetic fields induce electric fields (Maxwell theory). Since the days of Galvani's experiments, electricity has been known to have profound effects on biological tissues. In essence, "magnetic therapy" using PEMF is based on the effects of induced electrical fields.

Commercial Products

Static magnetic field magnets come in many different designs, including pads, disks, wraps, bands, inserts, belts, necklaces, earrings, and bracelets. PEMF devices

vary by manufacturers. Features depend on available options to manipulate the different parameters of the electromagnetic field. These parameters include:
- The strength of the magnetic field in tesla or gauss
- The waveform (sine wave or pulsed)
- The frequency of the waveform (hertz, cycles/second)
- The anatomic placement and the direction of the electromagnetic field with respect to the body
- The area or volume of the body exposed to the electromagnetic field
- The time of exposure[15]

CLINICAL USES OF MAGNETS

Nerve Regeneration

In multiple sclerosis (MS), widespread axonal damage and demyelination result in loss of axonal signaling between the source and the destination. There is also loss of synchronization and coordination of neuronal signals from different parts of the brain with loss of timing and coordination. Electric and magnetic fields have effects on nerve regeneration. Borgens et al. and Kanje et al. used PEMF to pretest rats prior to crushing the sciatic nerve.[16a,16b] Regeneration of sensory nerve fibers was measured by a pinch test. Their results showed that PEMF pretreatment increased regeneration of distant fibers. They concluded that PEMF promoted sprouting and elongation of regenerated nerve fibers better than direct current fields.

Gueso studied the effects of PEMF on MS patients in a double-blinded study. Magnetic coils (Gyulin-Bordacs device, Hungary) were placed on the upper and lower spine and then on the lower extremities.[17] The magnetic waveform was 300-Hz sine waves with a 6–13 msec period of dampened oscillation. Repetition rates of 2–50 Hz were used. MS patients showed some improvement in 80% of the cases, with benefits in symptoms of pain, spasticity, and bladder incontinence. The effects were similar to those found using electrical stimulation.

Pain Reduction

Regardless of the type of pain, postpolio patients have an increased sensitivity to nociceptive stimulation, which explains their complaints about pain. Currently recommended modes of treatment are rest, physical modalities (e.g., heat, cold, ultrasound, transcutaneous electrical nerve stimulation [TENS] units), supportive braces, muscle relaxants, analgesics, and anti-inflammatory agents. Effectiveness of pharmacologic modalities is poor and often gives unwanted side effects.

A study conducted by Valbona et al. showed limited success in management of postpolio pain using static electromagnetic fields of 300–500 G.[18] The relief of pain could be from local or direct change in pain receptors. On the other hand, it could result from an indirect central response in pain perception at the cerebral cortex or subcortical areas. Pain relief could also involve change in the release of enkephalins at the reticular system.

In another human study, pain was found to be associated with a shift of T-cells into S phase.[18a] Beall and colleagues demonstrated cyclical changes in the physical state of water being organized in the S phase.[18b] Others found that water plays a major role in explaining the therapeutic effects of magnetic fields.

Localized Musculoskeletal Pain

Jesus Pujol at al. demonstrated that magnetic coil stimulators can efficiently activate neural structures without deep electrode placement and the local discomfort associated with transcutaneous electrical stimulation used for pain control.[19] In a prospective, crossover study of the effects of active versus sham repetitive magnetic stimulation of tender bony regions, active stimulation produced a 59% reduction in pain score whereas sham stimulation produced a 14% decrease in pain score. The conclusion was that powerful magnetic coil stimulation efficiently reduced pain originating from localized musculoskeletal injuries. The mechanism of this pain relief is proposed to be by interference of the abnormal neural transmission occurring in chronic pain states.

LIMITED LITERATURE REVIEW

Neurologic Disorders

Multiple Sclerosis

In 1996, Nielsen et al. conducted a double-masked study of repetitive magnetic stimulation involving 38 MS patients.[20] Both the stimulated group of 21 and the sham stimulated group of 17 were treated twice daily for 7 consecutive days. Endpoints were changes in patient's self score, clinical spasticity score, and stretch reflex threshold. Results showed statistically significant improvement of clinical spasticity and increase in stretch reflex threshold (Table 1).

In 1997, Richards et al. conducted a double-masked, placebo-controlled study in which 15 MS patients wore a PEMF device.[21] This provided a magnetic pulse in the range of 4–13 Hz, 50–100 mG to preselected sites for 10–24 hours a day over a 2-month period. Fifteen patients wore an identical but magnetically inactive device. Before and after wear, each patient was evaluated by the Expanded Disability Status Scale (EDSS), patient-reported performance scales, and quantitative electroencephalography (QEEG) during a language task. Results showed statistically significant effect of the active device on performance scales and on alpha EEG magnitude during a language task.

In the following year, these authors conducted a randomized, placebo-controlled, double-masked crossover study of PEMF therapy.[22] Using 125 MS patients from three three sites, subjects were exposed to magnetically active and inactive devices over a 10-week period. Primary outcomes were daily measures on bladder control and muscle spasticity. Secondary outcomes were symptom-rating scales on the MS Quality of Life Inventory (MSQLI). Results showed statistically significant treatment effect on the fatigue scale.

Migraines

Sherman and colleagues conducted a double-blind, placebo-controlled study of the effects of PEMF therapy on migraines.[23] Each of the 42 patients kept a 1-month log of headache activity before and after inner thigh application of PEMF therapy (active or placebo) once daily, 5 times/week for 2 weeks. Seventy-three percent of the treated group reported decreases in headaches verses 50% of the placebo group.

TABLE 1. Significant Studies of the Efficacy of Magnet Therapy

Author	Clinical Applications	Setting	Findings
Nielson et al., 1996	Multiple sclerosis	Double-blind, placebo-controlled	Changes in self score, clinical spasticity score, and stretch reflex threshold
Richard et al., 1997	Multiple sclerosis	Double-masked, placebo-controlled	Change in EDSS, patient reported performance scales, and changes in QEEG
Richards et al., 1998	Multiple sclerosis	Randomized, placebo-controlled, double-masked	Statistically significant effect on the fatigue scale
Sherman et al., 1998	Migraines	Double blind placebo controlled trial	75% decreased headache, versus 50% placebo-controlled group
Lappin, 1995	Migraines	Retrospective data analysis	2 points on a 10-point scale improvement in overall improvement. 60% reported a 5–9 point improvement on a 10-point scale
Lebet et al., 1996	Sleep	Double-blind, cross-over study	Significant improvement on sleep induction and maintenance with shorter latency, decreased onset latency, and increased duration of sleep stage B2
Weintraub et al., 1999	Diabetic neuropathy	Randomized, double-placebo, cross-over	Statistically significant decrease or resolution of numbness and tingling, compared with the 33% non-DM patients
Lin et al., 2001	Neurogenic bowel	Prospective before and after trial	Statistically significant increase in rectal pressure and decrease in CTT
Vallbona et al., 1997	Postpolio pain	Randomized, double-masked clinical trial	76% of the patients treated showed 3-point decrease in pain scale on 0–10 scale, compared to 19% patients treated with inactive device
Trock et al., 1993, 1994	Osteoarthritis	Double-masked, placebo-controlled	Six variables were measured, significant improvement noticed in treatment group.
Sharrard et al., 1990	Bone healing	Double-masked, multicenter study	92% success rate in the active group and 65% success rate in the placebo group.
Samara et al., 1997	Wounds and ulcers	Randomized, double-masked clinical trial	An 80% in ulcer volume in 33% of the PEMF and none in the standard treatment.
Lluch et al., 1996	Avascular necrosis	Prospective study	76.6% MRI success and 63.3% combined MRI and clinical successes.
Collacott et al., 2000	Low back pain	Double-blinded, placebo-controlled crossover study	No effect on outcome measure between sham and real magnets

EDSS = expanded disability status S, QEEG = quantitative electroencephalography, DM = diabetes mellitus, CTT = colonic transit time.

The 1995 retrospective data analysis of 262 migraine patients by Lappin showed that 82% reported at least a 2-point improvement on a 10-point scale of overall well-being following treatment.[24] Sixty percent reported a 5–9 point improvement on a 10-point scale.

These studies, despite encouraging results, had no control groups and therefore serve to encourage further research.

Sleep
Lebet et al. conducted a double-blind, crossover study of sleep in 52 healthy volunteers using low-energy emission therapy (LEET).[25] The electromagnetic output field was an intermittent 42.17-Hz amplitude modulation of a 27.12 MHz field. Baseline and 15-minute post-treatment EEGs were obtained. Researchers noted statistically significant effect on sleep induction and maintenance with shorter latency, decreased onset latency, and increased duration of sleep stage B2 as well as more permanently established slow waves with progression to deeper sleep stage. The conclusion was that LEET improved stage B2 sleep.

Diabetic Neuropathy
In 1999, Weintraub et al. conducted a randomized, double-placebo, crossover study of the effects of magnetized insoles on the control of neuropathic leg pain.[26] Twenty-four patients with chronic neuropathic pain (14 had diabetes mellitus [DM], and 10 had multiple myeloma, alcoholism, ischemia, or the concomitant use of simvastatin) were enrolled. Magnetized insoles (475 G) were worn in four phases over a 4-month trial period. In phase I, each patient randomly wore an active insole on one foot and an inactive one on the other. After 30 days, active and inactive sides were switched (phase II). In phases III and IV, patients wore two new active insoles (475 G) for 30 days. Using a standardized visual analog scale (VAS), patients scored their burning, numbness, and tingling pain twice a day for each foot. Nineteen patients (10 DM and 9 non-DM) completed the study. Of the 10 DM patients, 90% showed a statistically significant decrease or resolution of numbness and tingling (not burning) compared with 33% of the non-DM patients.

Neurogenic Bowel
Lin et al. conducted a prospective before- after trial of the effects of functional magnetic stimulation colonic transit time (CTT).[27] Using a PEMF device generating a 2.2 T maximum electromagnetic field, rectal pressure and CTT were measured. Results showed statistically significant increases in rectal pressure and decreases in CTT.

Musculoskeletal Disorders
Postpolio Pain
In 1997, Valbona et al. conducted a randomized, double-masked clinical trial of static magnet therapy of localized degenerative arthritis related pain in postpolio patients.[18] Fifty individuals were divided into two groups. Twenty-nine were treated with active magnet device, and 21 were treated with inactive magnet device. The device was applied to localized painful points using adhesive tape for 45 minutes. Pre-

treatment, general pain experienced was assessed by the McGill Pain Questionnaire. Post-treatment, each patient described any sensation(s) they were experiencing and used the 10-point scale to rate their pain upon palpation of the treated area by the clinician. Results showed that 76% of patients treated with an active device reported improvment (at least a 3-point decrease on the 10-point scale) of pain following treatment, whereas 19% of the patients treated with an inactive device reported improved pain post treatment. "Pain not improved" (less than a 3-point decrease on the 10-point scale) was reported by 81% of the patients treated with an inactive device and 24% of the patients treated with an active device. Exact pressures applied before and after treatment were not measured. No systematic follow-up of patients was done.

Osteoarthritis

Trock et al.28 and Miner et al.29 conducted double-masked, placebo-controlled studies that demonstrated the efficacy of PEMF therapy on osteoarthritis (OA) pain. In the Trock study, 86 patients with knee OA and 81 patients with OA of the cervical spine were subjected to 18 half-hour exposures to a 10–20 G PEMF for 1 month. Six clinical variables were measured at baseline, midpoint of therapy, end of treatment, and 1 month later. More significant changes from baseline were shown in the treated groups, and lesser significant changes were seen in the placebo group. At 1-month follow-up, these changes were maintained in the treated group, whereas loss of significance was noted in the placebo group.

Low Back Pain

Collacott and colleagues conducted a randomized, double-blind, placebo-controlled crossover pilot study of bipolar permanent static electromagnetic therapy on chronic lower back pain (LBP).[14] Twenty patients with history of LBP for a mean duration of 19 years were randomly assigned to two groups. For each patient, real or sham bipolar permanent magnets (in the form of rubberized belts) were worn 6 hours a day, 3 days a week for 1 week. After a 1-week washout period, magnets were switched and worn for 1 week. Pre- and post-treatment pain intensity on VAS, sensory, and affective components of pain on the Pain Rating Index (PRI) and lumbosacral range of motion (ROM) were measured. Results showed no effect on outcome measures between sham and real magnets.

Bone Healing

In 1990, Sharrard et al. conducted a double-masked, multicenter study of active electromagnetic stimulation of tibial shaft fractures with union delay.[30] Forty-five patients were divided into two groups. Twenty patients were plaster immobilized with active electromagnetic stimulation, and 25 patients were plaster immobilized with inactive electromagnetic stimulation for 12 weeks. Blinded and independent assessment of radiographs showed union in 9 fractures and absence of union in 11 fractures in the active group ($p = 0.002$). There was union in 3 fractures and nonunion in 22 fractures in the control group.

In the same year, Mooney et al. performed a randomized, double-masked study of the effect of therapy on lumbar interbody fusions in 195 subjects.31 Ninety-eight patients received active stimulation, and 97 had placebo stimulation. Results showed a 92% success rate in the active group and a 65% success rate in the placebo group.

In 1994, Capanna et al. conducted a double-masked, prospective, randomized study of the effect of PEMF therapy on healing of bone allograft following tumor resection.[32] Both active and control stimulation groups had a host–graft junction healing rate of 67%. In the absence of chemotherapy, the healing time of the active stimulation group was 6.7 months and 9.4 months in the control stimulation group.

In 1996, Eyres et al. performed a double-masked study of the effects of PEMF therapy on bone formation and disuse osteoporosis remodeling during limb lengthening.[33] Results showed that therapy prevented bone loss adjacent to the distraction gap but had no effect on the generating bone.

Avascular Necrosis

Lluch et al. conducted a prospective study of PEMF therapy on the progression of avascular necrosis (AVN) lesions in 21 patients with femoral head necrosis of various stages.[34] These lesions were evaluated by MRI. Results showed 76.6% MRI successes, 80% clinical successes, and 63.3% combined MRI and clinical successes.

Wounds and Ulcers

Several studies have shown that PEMF therapy is effective in the treatment of wounds and ulcers. In 1997, Sarma et al. conducted a randomized, double-masked clinical trial of the effects of PEMF therapy on plantar ulcer healing rate of leprosy patients.[35] Twenty patients received standard wound care, and 20 patients received PEMF therapy (sinusoidal form, 0.95–1.05 Hz, amplitude ±2400 nT) for 4 weeks. The volume of the ulcers was measured on day of admission and at 1 week, 2 weeks, and end of treatment. An 80% decrease in volume was observed in 33% of the PEMF group and none in the standard treatment group. A decrease in volume of more than 40% was observed in 89% of the PEMF group and 53% of the control group.

Indications and Contraindications

Based on the literature, magnet therapy is indicated for:
- Multiple sclerosis
- Postpolio syndrome pain
- Diabetes mellitus, neuropathic pain
- Osteoarthritis
- Fracture
- Peripheral vascular disease
- Wound healing
- Mood disorders
- Anxiety disorders
- Schizophrenia
- Movement disorder
- Epilepsy
- Sleep disorder

Magnet therapy is contraindicated in the presence of the following:
- Hemorrhage
- Pregnancy
- Pacemakers

TRANSCRANIAL MAGNETIC STIMULATION

Since the early 1990s, the use of magnetism in medical sciences has increased exponentially. As mentioned, electricity and magnetism are interdependent. Passing current through a coil of wire generates a magnetic field perpendicular to the current flow in the coil. If a conducting medium, such as the brain, is adjacent to the magnetic field, current will be induced in the conducting medium. The flow of the induced current will be parallel but opposite in direction to the current in the brain.

Transcranial magnetic stimulation (TMS) involves placing an electromagnetic coil on the scalp. High-intensity current is rapidly turned on and off in the coil to discharge of capacitors. This produces a time-varying magnetic field that lasts about 100–200 (sec. The magnetic field typically has strength of about 2 T (40,000 times the earth's magnetic field, or about the same intensity as the static magnetic field used in MRI). Magnetic fields are not deflected or attenuated by an intervening tissue. Other clinical applications of TMS include:

- Mood disorders
- Anxiety disorders
- Schizophrenia
- Movement disorder
- Epilepsy

CONCLUSION

The field of electromagnetic therapy continues to evolve. The exact mechanisms of action of the electromagnetic field on biological tissues remain unclear. Although well-designed studies of the effects on bone, neurologic conditions, pain, and sleep disorders are promising, further studies are necessary. Based on the available evidence, claims of therapeutic benefits should be cautiously accepted.

REFERENCES

1. Mourino MR: From Thales to Lauterbur, or from the lodestone to MR imaging: Magnetism and medicine. Radiology 180:593–612, 1991.
2. Malone KS: Magnetic healing: Applications of permanent magnets in musculoskeletal injuries. Presented at the Magnetic Healing Seminar, December 23, 1993.
3. Quinan JR: The use of magnet in medicine. Maryland Med J 14:460–465, 1885.
4. D'Occhieppo KF: Maximillian Hell. In Dictionary of Scientific Bibliography, New York, Scribner, pp 233–235.
5. Hell M: Introduction ad utilem usum magnets ex calybe. Vienna, 1762.
6. Walmsley DM: Anton Mesmer. London, Hale Press, 1967.
7. Darnton R: Mesmerism and the End of the Enlightenment in France. Cambridge, Harvard University Press, 1968.
8. Mesmer FA (G. Bloch, translator): Mesmerism [translation of the original writings of FA Mesmer]. Los Altos, CA, Kauffman, 1980.
9. Maxwell J: A dynamical theory of the electromagnetic field. Phil Trans R Soc (Lond) 155:459–512, 1865.
10. Dorland's Illustrated Medical Dictionary, 28th ed. Philadelphia, W.B. Saunders, 1994, p 979.
11. Considine D: Van Nostrand's Scientific Encyclopedia. New York, ITP, 1995, p 1534.
12. Blank M, Soo L: The Na, K-ATPase as a model for electromagnetic field effect on cells. Bioelectrochem Bioenerg 30:85–92, 1993.
13. Schawartz BB, Frankel RB: Magnetism. In Discovery Channel School, World Book Online.

http://www.discoveryschool.com/homeworkhelp/worldbook/atozscience/m338410.html. Accessed 2/1/2001.
14. Collacott EA, Zimmerman JT, White DW, Rindone JP: Bipolar permanent magnets for the treatment of chronic lower back pain. JAMA 283:1322–1325, 2000.
15. Vallbona C, Richards T: Evolution of magnetic therapy from alternative to traditional medicine. Phys Med Rehabil Clin North Am 10:729–754, 1999.
16. Bassett CAL: Bioelectromagnetics in the service of medicine. In Blank M (ed): Electromagnetic Fields: Biological Interactions and Mechanisms. Advances in Chemistry Series, 250, 1995, pp 261–275.
16a. Borgens et al.
16b. Kanje et al.
17. Gueso A: Pulsing electromagnetic field therapy of multiple sclerosis by the Gyuling-Bordacs device: Double-blind, crossover and open studies. J Bioelectr 6:23–35, 1987.
18. Vallbona C, Hazlewood CF, Gabor J: Response of pain to static magnetic fields in post-polio patients: A double-blind pilot study. Arch Phys Med Rehabil 78:1200–1203, 1997.
18a. Valbona C, et al
18b. Beall et al.
19. Pujol J, Pascual-Leone A, Dolz C, et al: The effect of repetitive magnetic stimulation on localized musculoskeletal pain. Pain 9:1745–1748, 1998.
20. Nielson JF, Sinkjaer T, Jakobsen J: Treatment of spasticity with repetitive magnetic stimulation: A double-blind, placebo-controlled study. Multiple Sclerosis 2:227–232, 1996.
21. Richards TL, Lappin MS, Acosta UJ, et al: Double-blinded study of pulsating magnetic field effects on multiple sclerosis [published erratum appears in J Altern Complement Med 3:205, 1997]. J Altern Complement Med 3:21–29, 1997.
22. Richards TL, Lappin MS, Kramer ED, et al: Evaluation of a pulsed-magnetic field device on multiple sclerosis symptoms. Presented at the Consortium of Multiple Sclerosis Centers Annual Meeting, Cleveland, October 2–4, 1998.
23. Sherman RA, Robson L, Marden LA: Initial exploration of pulsing electromagnetic fields for the treatment of migraine. Headache 38:208–213, 1998.
24. Lappin MS: Research on the Utility of Medigen Device as a Treatment for Migraines. Vancouver, BC, Energy Medicine Developments (North America) Inc, 1995.
25. Lebet JP, Barbault A, Rossel C, et al: Electroencephalographic changes following low energy emission therapy. Ann Biomed Eng 24:424–429, 1996.
26. Weintraub MI: Magnetic biostimulation in painful diabetic peripheral neuropathy: A novel intervention: A randomized, double-blind study. Am J Pain Manag 9:8–17, 1999.
27. Lin VW, Nino-Murcia M, Frost F, et al: Functional magnetic stimulation of the colon in persons with spinal cord injury. Arch Phys Med Rehabil 82:167–173, 2001.
28. Trock DH, Bollet AJ, Markoll R: The effect of pulsed electromagnetic fields in the treatment of osteoarthritis of the knee and cervical spine. Report of randomized, double bind, placebo controlled trials. J Rheumatol 21:1903–1911, 1994.
29. Miner WK, Markoll R: A double-blind trial of the clinical effects of pulsed electromagnetic fields in osteoarthritis. J Rheumatol 20:456–460, 1993.
30. Sharrad WJ: A double-blind trial of pulsed electromagnetic fields for delayed union of tibial fractures [see comments]. J Bone Joint Surg 72B:347–355, 1990.
31. Mooney V: A randomized, double-blind prospective study of the efficacy of pulsed electromagnetic fields for interbody lumbar fusions. Spine 15:708–712, 1990.
32. Campana R, Donati D, Masetti C, et al: Effect of electromagnetic fields on patients undergoing massive bone graft following bone tumor resection. A double-blind study. Clin Orthop 306:213–221, 1994.
33. Eyres KS, Saleh M, Kanis JA: Effect of pulsed electromagnetic fields on bone formation and bone loss during limb lengthening. Bone 18:505–509, 1996.
34. Lluch BC, Garcia ADG, Munoz FL, et al: Usefulness of electromagnetic fields in the treatment of hip avascular necrosis: A prospective study of 30 cases. Rev Clin Esp 196:67–74, 1996.
35. Sarma GR, Subrahmanyam S, Deenabandhu A, et al: Exposure to pulsed electromagnetic fields in the treatment of plantar ulcers in leprosy patients: A pilot, randomized, double blind, controlled clinical trial. Indian J Lepr 69:241–250, 1997.

Chapter 9

Electrical Modalities in Musculoskeletal and Pain Medicine

Viviane Ugalde, MD

The torpedo fish with electricity generating organs was used by Roman physicians to treat gout and headaches in A.D. 46.[14] In Western medicine, the first therapeutic electrical device was reported in 1744 for the treatment of finger paralysis. It was later used as a treatment of arthritis in 1747. Electrotherapy was viewed with varying degrees of acceptance by the medical establishment and was often considered a form of quackery. In the late 19th century, gynecologists used electricity through needles to treat uterine fibroids. Unfortunately, deaths were reported from peritonitis. Static electricity was used to treat a myriad of conditions through the early 20th century. Short-wave diathermy replaced most static electricity units in the 20th century. Since then, a variety of electrical applications have been developed with varying degrees of scientific confirmation. Despite of electrotherapy's illustrious past, many physicians today are skeptical of claims of its clinical improvements for a variety of ailments.[50] The best proved and most accepted use of therapeutic electricity is defibrillation in cardiac arrest. New theories on pain in the 1960s led to the development of electrical modalities to treat pain.[59] The dorsal column spinal cord stimulator and the transcutaneous electrical nerve stimulation (TENS) unit were practical applications of the theory. Electrical muscle stimulation has been used to treat musculoskeletal and neuromuscular injuries and illnesses. This modality is used by physical therapists and by athletic trainers.

At one time, electrical modalities were within the domain of physical therapists. Practice patterns in the use of electrical modalities have changed largely due to managed-care medicine. Physical therapists are no longer given the time or the authorization to see a patient for more than a few visits, making the instruction of a home exercise program the top priority. Many of the passive modalities are no longer used. However, athletic trainers commonly use muscle electrical stimulation. Electrotherapy continues to be used, particularly by pain medicine practitioners. Electrotherapy units have been designed for home use. The positive influence of managed care has been the challenge to the medical establishment to provide evidence that particular treatments are efficacious. Research with electrical modalities has been methodologically challenging, given the difficulty in designing a truly masked placebo. Many stimulation protocols call for the user to perceive a sensation or experience muscle contractions. Analysis of outcomes often involves subjective measures of pain such as the visual analog scale (VAS). The results of the VAS reported as a mean is considered an unreliable statistic, and the median is the more favored statistic.[58] Unfortunately, the mean of the VAS is a common result in much of the pain literature. A backlash of the evidence-based review of the literature is little scientific support for the modalities, lessening the potential for third-party reimbursement. However, the outcome measured in a study can be particularly important. The emphasis on reduction in opioid use is important, although likely multifactorial. The duration of the reduction of opioid use also remains an important outcome to measure, particularly in chronic pain populations. Regardless, the potential to provide patients with a non-pharmacologic alternative, particularly during work hours, is important. In employed chronic pain sufferers, opioid analgesics are not well tolerated owing to the side effect of drowsiness. If 40% of patients experience reduction in pain and medication intake from the placebo effect with electrical modalities, then there is a clinical benefit. However, cost remains a factor. An analysis would need to compare the cost savings in medication reduction and increased work productivity with the cost of the electricunit and its maintenance. This chapter reviews the research regarding the physiologic responses to electrical modalities, the medical evidence to support its use clinically, indications and contraindications, and the cost of home units.

BASIC ELECTRICAL PARAMETERS

Electrical modalities parameters were developed to stimulate motor neurons leading to muscle contraction and large–diameter afferent neurons leading to pain relief. By varying the stimulus delivery, it has been shown in isolated nerve preparations that larger A afferent nerve or motor nerve fibers can be selectively stimulated over the smaller unmyelinated nocioceptive C fibers.[49] Short-duration pulses activate large-diameter fibers, whereas longer duration pulses depolarize the smaller diameter fibers. For neuromuscular stimulation, a pulse duration of 0.1–0.5 ms should depolarize the motor fibers without activating the small nocioceptive fibers. Neuromuscular stimulation works best with intact peripheral nerves, in which the nerve depolarization can lead to full muscle contraction. Although laboratory studies of isolated nerve preparations demonstrate selective activation of large-diameter afferents over the smaller C fibers, in vivo fiber selectivity is unlikely. Stimulation through soft tissue to reach the nerve causes a nonuniform stimulation of the nerve, with more proximate fibers stimulated versus distal fibers. Electrical stimulation for pain control is rarely placed over a peripheral nerve in vivo. The large electrodes over the muscle belly can also lead to stimulation of the terminal axons as well as peripheral nerve trunks. Rectangular pulses and sine waves have also demonstrated selectivity in stimulation of different nerve fiber types. However, clinical in vivo application of the aforementioned factors has not been studied fully.[44]

Common electrical definitions are reviewed here to allow the reader to understand better descriptions of clinically applied modalities described in later sections. The amount of current is responsible for physiologic effects caused by electrical stimulation. Most units are constant current applications varying voltage to changes in impedance. Direct current (galvanic) units cause a unidirectional flow that is continuous. Alternating current causes bidirectional flow (positive and negative), which can be balanced or unbalanced or symmetric or asymmetric. Pulsed wave stimulus is neither direct current nor alternate current because there is not a continuous flow. The stimulus is delivered in a series of pulses with a pause between pulses known as the *interpulse interval*. Figures 1 and 2 depict a variety of stimulus delivery.[41]

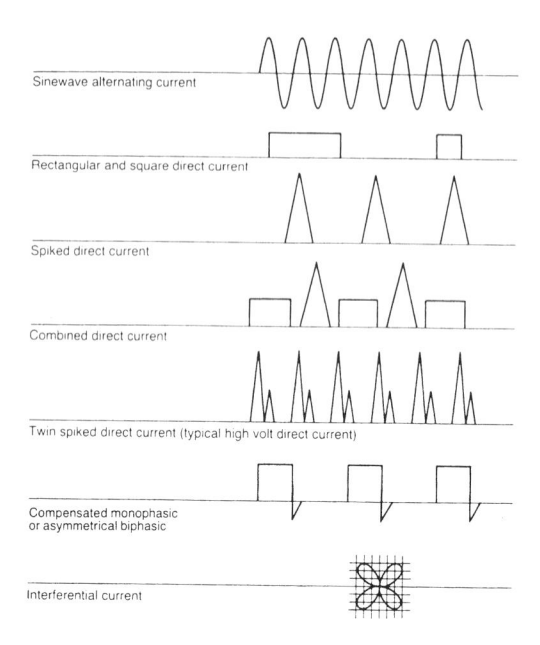

FIGURE 1. Waveforms in EMS. (From Kahn J: Electrical stimulation. In Kahn J (ed): Principles and Practice of Electrotherapy. Philadelphia, Churchill-Livingstone, 2000, pp 69–99, with permission.)

Pulsed forms can have variations in time-dependent parameters including phase duration and direction, pulse duration, interpulse interval, rise time, and decay time. Alternating current and pulse currents have frequency-dependent parameters including frequency of repetitions of the waveform or pulse and the period, which is the reciprocal of the frequency. All forms of current have the amplitude-dependent factor of peak amplitude. Pulse and alternating currents also may vary in peak amplitude of the phase, in peak-to-peak amplitude, and in phase or pulse charge, which is the area under the curve. Current modulations can also be applied and include amplitude, phase duration, pulse duration, frequency, and ramp (surge) modulations. Pulsed stimulus can be delivered in a train of repetitive, continuous pulses or in a burst fashion (interrupted train), with envelopes of stimulus separated by an interburst interval. Interferential current is a mix of alternating currents at different frequencies that are out of phase with each other.[23] Table 1 compares different electrical parameters used in medicine.

Variations in stimulus parameters have a theoretical basis in type of fiber stimulated, better patient tolerance, and variations in segmental and suprasegmental pain responses. Although electric modalities have been used for more than 200 years, systematic study of the benefits of specific electrical parameters has not been done. Available data are reviewed in each section.

NEUROMUSCULAR STIMULATION

Neuromuscular stimulation has been used in stroke and spinal cord injury rehabilitation to improve function. The bulk of the discussion focuses on the use of elec-

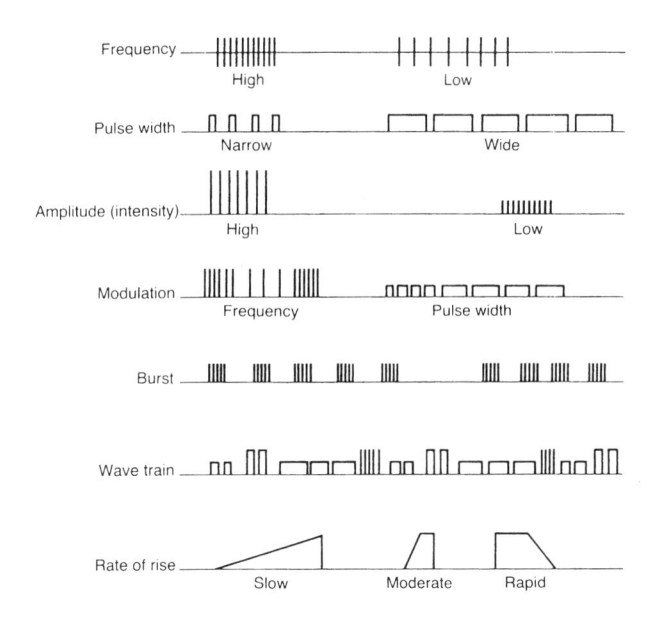

FIGURE 2. Electrical parameters used in TENS and EMS. (From Kahn J: Electrical stimulation. In Kahn J (ed): Principles and Practice of Electrotherapy. Philadelphia, Churchill-Livingstone, 2000, pp 69–99, with permission.)

trical stimulation in musculoskeletal injuries. Neuromuscular stimulation is used for overcoming reflex inhibition after an injury to allow the establishment of appropriate motor engrams. By programming appropriate engrams, the injured individual is less likely to use inappropriate muscle substitution patterns that may lead to future injury. Muscle stimulation also may be used to counteract immobilization atrophy, improve range of motion, break down adhesions in the muscle, and assist in relieving pain and muscle spasm. Athletic trainers may use muscle electrical stimulation at the end of a season to counteract fatigue and less voluntary effort during workouts.[71] It has also been marketed for improving abdominal muscle tone without having to do sit-ups. After nerve injuries such as brachial plexopathy from a football stinger, electrical stimulation has been used to maintain muscle viability.

Physiologic contraction of muscle occurs in a grade fashion, with the smaller, fatigue–resistant motor units type I, being recruited first followed by larger and larger motor units. With electrical stimulation, the larger diameter Type II fatigable fibers are recruited first. Muscle tension decreases as the fibers fatigue, unless the unit is turned up. Excessive fatigue can occur but can be limited by giving adequate rest periods between contractions and limiting the duration and frequency of the contractions.[14] Criticism of the nonphysiologic muscle contraction produced by direct muscle electrical stimulation has led to a replacement of electrical stimulation with active assisted range-of-motion exercises by the athlete.[16]

Electrical Parameters

Symmetric, biphasic square waveforms have demonstrated better patient tolerance compared with other waveforms. This waveform also allows generation of a

TABLE 1. COMPARISON OF ELECTRICAL MODALITIES SPECIFICATIONS

	Frequency	Pulse Duration (ms)	Amplitude
TENS—Low[#]	1–4 Hz	0.2–0.3 or 0.065–0.25	0-80 mA, MT
TENS—High[$]	11–150 Hz	<0.2 or 0.065–0.25	0-80 mA, PT
Brief, Intense TENS	150 Hz	> 0.3	tetany
Electrical Acupuncture*	3–10 Hz or 100 Hz	0.2–0.7	1-3 mA
PENS	4 Hz	0.1	250 µA
H-Wave	2, 16, 60, 120 Hz	0.16	35 mA, 35 V
Codetron	4 – 200 Hz		
Interferential Electro therapy	2–4 kHz	0.125	16 volts
Pulsed Electromag.	40–73 Hz	0.06-0.37	2.7 mT
E Stim—Endurance	50–200 Hz		
E Stim—Strength	2500+ Hz		0–80 mA
NMES	70 Hz	0.2–0.4	0–100 mA

*Multiple electrical protocols used.
[#]Acupuncture-like TENS
[$]Conventional TENS
Hz, Hertz; mA, milliamperes; MT, motor threshold; PT, paresthesia threshold; ms, milliseconds; V, volts; µA, microamperes.
Adapted from van Tulder MW, Cherkin DC, Berman B, et al: The effectiveness of acupuncture in the management of acute and chronic low back pain. Spine 243:1113, 1999.

larger muscle contraction compared to a monophasic waveform. Asymmetric, biphasic waveforms are used particularly with smaller muscles but have a greater incidence of burns and skin irritation owing to the accumulation of charge under one electrode. Amplitude intensity is set as tolerated by the patient up to 100 mA. The greater the intensity, the greater the force generated by the muscle contraction. Pulse duration varies from 0.2–0.4 msec and allows adjustment for patient tolerance when coupled with variable amplitude intensity. A pulse duration greater than 1.0 msec is associated with stimulation of pain afferents. Low frequencies are associated with incomplete muscle contraction. At 30 Hz, the muscle demonstrates tetanized contractions. Duty cycle is the ratio of on time (pulse train duration) to total time (on and off time) expressed as a percentage. For orthopedic problems, a 25% duty cycle has been suggested. If fatigue is a factor, then the duty cycle can be reduced. Most units have a ramp feature. Ramping is a parameter that allows a gradual increase to peak intensity that is over 2 seconds. After the peak amplitude is maintained for a specified period, the intensity is ramped down. This parameter theoretically allows an approximation of a normal muscle contraction and greater patient comfort. Indications and contraindications for neuromuscular electrical stimulation are listed in Table 2. Adverse reactions typically occur with skin allergies to the electrodes, mechanical irritation from the electrodes and occasionally itching or skin burn due to accumulation of charge under one electrode.[14]

Clinical Uses

Neuromuscular electrical stimulation use is ubiquitous with musculoskeletal injuries in athletes. After an injury, pain and joint effusion can lead to inhibition or partial inhibition of muscular contraction. This is particularly common in the initial phases of rehabilitation. Muscles near the joint are more commonly affected.

TABLE 2. NEUROMUSCULAR ELECTRICAL STIMULATION

Indications	Contraindications	Precautions
Treatment of disuse atrophy	Persons with demand cardiac pacemakers	Persons with known arrhythmia or conduction disturbances
Increase and maintenance of range of motion	During pregnancy	Near fresh incisions
Muscle re-education and facilitation	Placement along the anterior neck	Over insensate skin
Spasticity management		T6 and above spinal cord injury (autonomic dysreflexia)
Orthotic substitution		
Augmentation of motor recruitment in healthy muscle		

Adapted from DeVahl J: Neuromuscular electrical stimulation (NMES) in rehabilitation. In Gersh MR (ed): Electrotherapy In Rehabilitation. Philadelphia, FA Davis, 1992, pp 218–268.

Electrical stimulation reduces edema, likely from muscular pumping action. Once acute swelling and severe pain are controlled, neuromuscular stimulation can be an effective muscle re-education tool. Atrophy can be minimized as well. Other uses are purported to decrease muscle and tendon adhesions, and scarring. Theoretically, if a muscle or tendons are strained, scar tissue develops as a part of the healing process. The athlete may perceive a feeling of pulling or tightness. Electrical stimulation in an isometric contraction purportedly allows the most muscle stretch and break up of the adhesions and scar tissue.[71]

The effectiveness of neuromuscular stimulation in the prevention of postoperative atrophy of the quadriceps and hamstrings after anterior cruciate ligament reconstruction was studied.[64] The subjects were randomized, although the actual randomization process is not well described. All three groups underwent early postoperative exercise training. The other two groups were treated with either TENS or a neuromuscular stimulator. Outcomes were measured by a blinded examiner and included isometric and isokinetic strength testing. Although the test was described as double-blinded, there were no sham units used, thus the study was single-blinded. Each group had 14–17 subjects. The researchers found no difference in strength between any of the groups. Power analysis was not performed. Thus, the lack of difference may be due to small sample size. However, this finding is consistent with other studies in healthy subjects using combinations of electrical stimulation and exercise. There were no significant differences in strength between voluntary exercise versus voluntary exercise plus electrical stimulation even at frequencies of 2500 Hz.[14] Neuromuscular electrical stimulation has been effective in overcoming quadriceps inhibition in chondromalacia and subluxing patellae to facilitate a strength-training program.[14]

Neuromuscular electrical stimulation has also been used recently in combination with TENS for pain control in chronic back pain.[61] The combination reduced pain intensity, and subjects reported greater relief from pain compared with the use of either modality alone. All three treatment arms demonstrated reductions in pain compared with placebo. The placebo unit delivered no stimulus but had a functioning indicator light. Unfortunately, the study design was randomized repeated measures. Each subject experienced all four treatments, allowing possible unblinding of the placebo.

TRANSCUTANEOUS ELECTRICAL NERVE STIMULATION

Physiology of Action

Our understanding of the pathophysiology of pain continues to evolve. The gate control theory developed by Melzack and Wall in the 1960s led to the development of the traditional parameters of high frequency stimulation in TENS units.[23] The physiologic responses to TENS have been studied by measuring serum and spinal fluid endorphin levels,[3,35,38,75] and by observing the effects of naloxone.[1,76] In addition, the efficacy of TENS has been measured by alterations in pain threshold for various pain models.[74,78,92,94] To assist the reader, a review of pertinent studies of TENS trials is illustrated in Table 3. The optimal parameters for electrotherapy remain unknown, although recent studies have shed some light. Controversy continues regarding frequency and intensity of the stimulus and the duration of treatment. It is not surprising given the current lack of knowledge that TENS units are likely used inappropriately.

Many studies have examined the frequency of stimulation as a factor of efficacy in the treatment of pain. Lower frequency stimulation allows for greater stimulation intensity. Initially, it was believed that these electrical parameters mimicked electroacupuncture. The low frequency likely stimulates small-diameter nociocep-tive fibers and motor fibers.[92] With low frequency stimulation, muscle contraction under the electrodes is seen and is believed to be a necessary component of effectiveness.[53,76] Low frequency TENS is usually delivered at less than 10Hz and more frequently between 2 and 4 Hz. The intensity of the stimulation is 0–80 mA. In experimental design, stimulation intensity is typically set at 1.5–5 times the perception threshold. The perception threshold is the first sensation of paresthesia. Studies have focused on endorphin responses found with low-frequency TENS. An increase in cerebral spinal fluid preproenkephalins after low-frequency TENS was demonstrated in subjects with a variety of neurologic disorders.[36] Hughes measured an increase in plasma beta-endorphin levels in normal subjects after TENS.[38] An indirect measure of endorphin activity is the effect of naloxone on pain relief with TENS. Trained pulses of 2 Hz stimulation were blocked by naloxone.[77] In a rat arthritic model, analgesia was produced by 4 Hz TENS that was subsequently blocked by naloxone. The authors concluded the mu receptor at the spinal level was responsive to low-frequency TENS in rats.[79] Another measure of efficacy in pain treatment is the analgesia produce with various experimental pain models, such as ischemic, mechanical, inflamed joints, or cold-induced pain models. In an ischemic pain model, researchers found TENS modified the pain response.[94] A more specific study with the ischemic model demonstrated that low-frequency TENS at 4 Hz provided analgesia.[91] In rats, the thermal threshold remained elevated for 12 hours after the application of TENS.[78] High-frequency TENS modified pain responses to thermal pain, but not mechanical pain.[94]

High frequency described as greater than 10 Hz was formulated from the gate control theory. Stimulation of large-diameter afferents should inhibit the second order neurons from carrying pain impulses from the small-diameter afferents.[53] Thus, the small-fiber pain impulses never reach the brain. In groups of chronic pain patients or a variety of neurologic disorders, elevations of proendorphins,

Electrical Modalities in Musculoskeletal and Pain Medicine   105

TABLE 3. PHYSIOLOGY OF TENS

	Sample Size	Random	Controls	Blind	Hz	Amp	Time (min)	Tx Period	Outcome
Chapman[10]	24 Healthy vol human	No	Saline	Yes	2	44.7 mA	> 20	1 session	Naloxone blocked
Sjolund[77]	10 Chronic pain human	No	Saline	Yes	50–100	2–3x PT	> 10	3 Months	0/10 +naloxone block
	10 Chronic pain human	No	Saline	Yes	2	3–5x PT	qd—QID	3 months	6/10 +naloxone block
Abram[1]	15 Chronic pain human	No	Saline	Yes	58	12–20 mA	20	1 month	0/15 +naloxone block
Sluka[79]	122 Arthritic rats	No	No	No	100	at PT	20	1 Session	High dose +naloxone block
					4	at PT	20	1 Session	Low dose +naloxone block
Hughes[38]	10 Healthy vol human	Yes	Sham TENS	No	off	off	30	1 Session	No change endorphins
	9 Healthy vol human	Yes		No	104	32 mA	30	1 Session	Increase beta endorphins
	12 Healthy vol human	Yes		No	4	57 mA	30	1 Session	Increase beta endorphins
Salar[75]	13 no pain neuro pts	No	No	No	40–60	40–80 mA	20–90	1 Session	Incr CSF endorphins
Almay[3]	18 Chronic pain human	No	No	No	80–100	2–3x PT	15–30	1 Session	Incr CSF endorphins & subst P
Han[35]	17 Neuro pts	Yes	No	No	100	26–30 mA	30	1 Session	Incr CSF dynorphin A
	20 Neuro pts	Yes	No	No	2	26–30 mA	30	1 Session	Incr CSF enkephalin
Woolf[95]	25 Rats/thermal threshold	No	Own control	No	50–100	10–15 V	30	1 Session	40–70% relief, +Naloxone block
Woolf[94]	Ischemic	No	Yes	No	100	above PT	30	1 Session	Decr VAS, Incr Pain Tol
Roche[74]	Ischemic	No	No	No	100	4–14.2 V	> 10	1 Session	Incr Pain tol & endurance
					5	3.7 V	10	1 Session	Incr Pain tol & threshold
Walsh[91]	32 Nl Human/ischemic	Yes	No TENS/sham TENS	Yes	110	above PT	22	2 Sessions	No difference
					4	above PT	22	2 Sessions	Significant decr VAS
Sluka[78]	21 Rats/arthritic	Yes	No TENS	No	100	Below mc	20	1 Session	Incr in thermal threshold
					4	Below mc	20	1 Session	Incr in thermal threshold
Walsh[93]	50 Healthy humans	Yes	No TENS	Yes	110	above PT	45	1 Session	No difference
					4	above PT	45	1 Session	No difference

Decr, decrease; Incr, increase; mc, muscle contraction; mA, milliamperes; Neuro, neurologic; Nl, normal; PT, paresthesia threshold; Pts, patients; Subst, substance; Tol, tolerance; VAS, visual analog scale; V, volt; Vol, volunteer.

fraction 1 endorphins and substance P–like immunoractivity were found in cerebral spinal fluid.[3,35,75] In human heroin addicts, 100Hz TENS ameliorated withdrawal symptoms.[36] Hughes also found elevations of plasma endorphins in normal volunteers after 100 Hz TENS.[38] Animal studies using high-frequency TENS have demonstrated dose-dependent blockade of analgesia with naloxone.[95] However, studies in humans with chronic pain did not find reversal with naloxone.[1,77] Sluka[79] has suggested that the dose of naloxone used in the aforementioned study may not have been high enough to block the endorphin receptors involved with high-frequency TENS. With an arthritic rat model, spinal delta opioid receptors were blocked with high dose Naloxone, reversing the analgesia induced by high-frequency TENS. Interestingly, blocking of kappa opioid receptors did not reverse the analgesia in either high- or low-frequency TENS.[79] In a rat model of inflamed joints, the thermal threshold was elevated for 24 hours after TENS treatment, but there was no observable changes in joint behaviors.[78] Human studies demonstrate similar effects. A double-blind, randomized controlled trial in healthy volunteers demonstrated significant increases in the mechanical pain threshold after 10 minutes of stimulation with TENS at 110 Hz. The effect peaked at 30 minutes and lasted for 5 minutes after the unit was turned off.[56] Other studies also demonstrate that high-frequency TENS provides analgesia in mechanical pain models equivalent to 60 mg of codeine.[92]

In 13 patients with hydrocephalus, Salar found a time-dependent response to high-frequency TENS stimulation. Cerebral spinal fluid beta-endorphins were measured at time zero, 20, 45, 60 and 90 minutes of treatment with TENS. They found beta-endorphin levels peaked by 45 minutes. Interestingly, persistent treatment of 90 minutes led to a return of endorphin levels to baseline. Unfortunately, there was no control group.[75]

There are rare studies that examine parameters other than frequency of stimulation. An early study examined variations in stimulus intensity. Electroacupuncture has used high-intensity stimulation, 5–8 times the perception threshold. Sjolund[77] examined levels of analgesia produced by TENS application with burst stimuluation at 3–5 times the perception threshold. The researchers compared acupuncture like TENS with conventional high-frequency TENS delivered in a continuous fashion. Six out of the 10 with the low frequency, burst mode, and lower intensity demonstrated reductions in pain levels that were blocked by nalaxone. The high-frequency, continuous stimulation was not blocked by nalaxone. The lower intensity stimulus was better tolerated by chronic pain patients compared with higher intensity protocols.[77] Walsh found no difference in pain reduction in burst versus continuous TENS. However, high-intensity TENS was more effective with continous stimulation, whereas burst was more effective with low-intensity stimulation for an ischemic pain model.[91] Thorsteinsson and colleagues[84] found placement of the electrodes is also an important factor of efficacy. In neuropathic pain patients, stimulation directly over the involved nerve trunk provided great relief. In low-back pain, the stimulator gave significant improvement when placed over the center of the pain. This study also followed subjects for 6 months. Although subjects had an initial improvement in pain scores with TENS, 6 months later only 21/49 subjects continued to use the unit. Lack of analgesia was the most common reason for discontinuing the TENS. Thorsteinsson and associates[84] remark that perhaps the initial reduction in pain was a part of the placebo effect. Unfortunately, TENS treatment was prescribed for only 20 minutes a session. The duration of treatment may have been too short to provide maximum analgesia with TENS. Another study looked at placement of electrodes over traditional Chinese acupuncture sites on the hand versus a control point on the hand. A combination of low- and high-frequency TENS was delivered for post-operative hemorrhoidectomy pain. The group with acupoint placement had lower pain scores and required less narcotic analgesic.[11] However, 100 Hz TENS placement over auricular acupuncture points did not change electrical pain thresholds.[40]

From the available data, TENS is likely to be most efficacious if a combination of low and high frequencies are used. The duration of treatment should be at least 30–45 minutes but should not exceed an hour. The intensity of the stimulus should cause tingling or tolerable muscle contractions. Placement should be over acupuncture points, the center of maximal pain, or over involved nerve trunks (Fig. 3). Based on their study and experience with TENS, Mannheimer and Lampe[53] have recommended four stimulation modes for a variety of clinical scenarios. The conventional high-frequency TENS mode is the treatment of choice for acute, superficial pain associated with inflammation. For chronic inflammation or neurogenic pain, the acupuncture-like or low-frequency, high-intensity mode or the burst mode is recommended. When brief periods of analgesia are needed for painful procedures, the brief, intense mode can be used.[43] Clinical evidence for these protocols is lacking.

Indications for TENS are listed later with the supporting evidence. Contraindications are noted by the Food and Drug Administration (FDA) to be (1) the presence of a demand pacemaker and (2) stimulation over the carotid sinus secondary to possible vagal responses of hypotension or cardiac arrest. Precautions issued by the FDA include (1) application in the abdomen or lumbar area during pregnancy; (2) application over the eyes; (3) application internally; (4) application transcranially or cervically in persons with a history of seizures, strokes, or transient ischemic attacks; and (5) application in cognitively impaired or children without adequate supervision. Adverse reactions to TENS have been reported primarily in the integumentary system. Allergic reactions to the electrode pads are the most

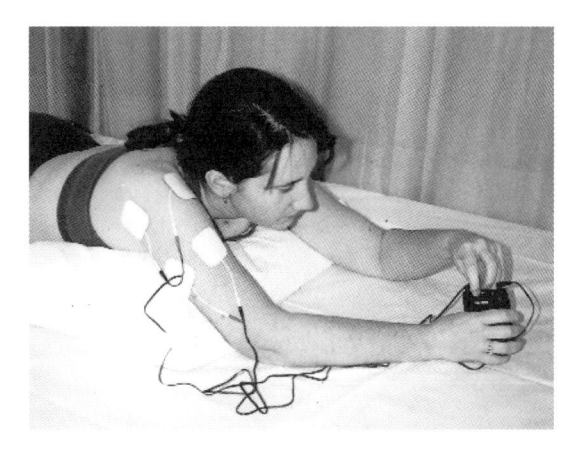

FIGURE 3. TENS unit in place over acupuncture points.

common. The carbon-silicon pads can be substituted with a karaya alternative. Mechanical irritation to the skin from pulling of the pads has also been reported. Electrical burns under the electrodes due to poor or uneven skin contact have also been reported.[23] Prevention of skin problems begins with clear instructions to the patient on proper electrode and tape use.[53]

Acute Postoperative Pain

Carroll and associates[8] published a thorough evidenced-based medicine review of the literature in 1996. They found 19 studies that provided appropriate randomization and controls. Fifteen of seventeen studies found no benefit of TENS in treating acute postoperative pain. They also comment on the lack of blinding in the studies. With lack of blinding, an exaggerated positive effect of 17% would occur. Given that the studies should have an overestimation of the treatment effect of TENS owing to lack of blinding, the negative findings in 15 studies indicate that TENS is not an effective treatment in postoperative pain for the outcomes measured.[8] Five of seven of these studies with an outcome variable of opioid consumption failed to find any significant difference with the use of TENS. Both positive and negative studies had subjects either titrate frequency or use a high-frequency setting.

In contrast, a recent double-blinded, randomized controlled report comparing low-frequency, high-frequency, and combination-frequency TENS treatment for postoperative gynecologic surgery indicated a significant 53% reduction in opioid analgesic use in the combined-frequency treatment group compared with a sham-TENS group.[34] Low or high frequency alone reduced opioid intake by only 32% and 35%. The need for rescue medication was the same in all four groups, and the number of subjects who discontinued TENS was the same in all four groups. Power analysis was performed to detect a 30% reduction in opioid use. Interestingly, pain levels as measured by the VAS were not different between the groups. Thus, the patients did not perceive reduction in pain with the TENS unit but demonstrated a 53% reduction in the need for opioid analgesia delivered through patient-administered analgesia (PCA). The difference in this more recent study and the studies reviewed by Carroll and colleagues may lie in the method of opioid analgesia delivery. With PCA, the patient has relative control of the amount of analgesia delivered. In the studies reviewed by Carroll and associates with analgesia intake as an outcome variable, analgesia was administered by nurses in amounts dictated by the physician. Also, the prior studies used only one frequency of TENS, either high frequency or a titrated level determined by the subject. Perhaps, treatment with a combination of frequencies induces the most analgesia clinically. The clinical outcome of this recent study supports the results of the proposed physiologic responses of low- and high-frequency TENS on different systems in the pathophysiology of pain (mu versus delta opioid receptors). Based on the proposed mechanism of action of low- and high-frequency TENS on alternate sites in the pain pathway, this most recent study supports the need for further exploration of the clinical use of TENS in postoperative pain control.

TENS and Spine Pain

In acute low-back pain, there is conflicting information from randomized controlled trials of limited numbers regarding outcomes of pain reduction. One trial found no improvement in function. The other found improvements in range of motion.[28] Conflicting data are also found in randomized controlled trials in chronic low-back pain. In a randomized, blind, controlled trial of exercise and TENS, 145 subjects with low-back pain of more than 3 months received treatment with sham TENS or TENS of 2 weeks of 80–100 Hz, 2 weeks of 2–4 Hz, and 2 weeks a frequency of their choice. The researchers found no difference between the TENS group and the sham TENS group but found improvements in pain and function in the exercise groups. Both the TENS and sham TENS groups had 42–47% improvement in pain indicators consistent with the placebo effect.[15] A small placebo-controlled, double-blind study focused on a combination treatment of TENS with neuromuscular electrical stimulation (NMES), which causes actual muscle contraction. Individual and combined treatment led to improvements in pain intensity and VAS of pain in sufferers of chronic low back pain.[61] The combined treatment led to the greatest improvements. However, the question of how truly blinded the sham treatments were perceived is suspect. Difficulty with blinding physical treatments remains a methodologic problem that these authors addressed as best as possible.[61] In a nonblinded trial comparing acupuncture with TENS in elderly subjects with chronic low-back pain, both groups demonstrated pain reduction and medication intake that persisted at 3-month follow-up. The authors concluded that a placebo effect could not be ruled out for both treatment interventions.[29] The Cochrane group analyzed trials of TENS and acupuncture-like TENS by evidenced-based methodology. They concluded that there is evidence from limited data that both TENS and acupuncture-like TENS are able to reduce pain and improve range of motion.[21] However, other evidenced-based reviews have found no difference in pain, functional status, or mobility.[28] In a nonrandomized, placebo-controlled trial in chronic low-back pain, high-frequency, low-intensity TENS provided pain relief in both the sensory-discriminative and motivational-affective components in the short term. Evaluation at 3 and 6 months did not show any benefit. The authors concluded that TENS may be a useful adjunct early in pain management but not over the long term.[54]

Data regarding the use of TENS for cervical pain is even more limited. The Cochrane group evaluated the literature for the use of physical medicine modalities for mechanical neck disorders. There was not evidence to support electrotherapy in this population.[31] However, they did cite two studies using pulsed electromagnetic fields that were proven effective. A miniaturized short-wave diathermy unit was built into a neck collar that the patient wore 8 hours per day for 12 weeks.[19]

TENS and Obstetrics and Gynecology

A systematic review of the literature found TENS to be of little use in relieving labor pain.[9] Randomized trials were hampered by poor blinding techniques. They report that only three of eight studies demonstrated a positive result. The only study with appropriate blinding methods and with a positive result used a post-labor recall of pain score. The pain score was lower in the TENS group versus the sham TENS groups. However, in the pain scores taken during the labor were no different between the groups.[83] A study using TENS to treat low-back pain specifically during labor found no difference between TENS and the standard treatment of massage and mobilization.[48] Comparison of TENS to sham TENS yielded no difference in first-stage labor pain as judged by the amount of reduction in self-administered analgesia.[88] All of these studies used a variety of frequencies, pulse durations, placement of electrodes, and duration of treatment, making comparison difficult. There is a suggestion that electrical stimulation can improve circulation. A recent Cochrane Review of the literature found no supporting studies for the use of TENS to improve blood flow in placental insufficiency.[32]

In a cross-over design, women with dysmenorrhea were treated with 100 Hz TENS, Ibuprofen, both TENS and ibuprofen, or sham TENS (no electricity delivered). The subjects were not adequately blinded given a cross-over design. For the active TENS unit, subjects were asked to adjust the amplitude of stimulation to a comfortable tingling sensation. Thus, the subjects would be aware of a sham TENS that did not deliver electricity. Regardless, there were no significant differences in pain and symptom relief with TENS. Ibuprofen consistently improved pain measures.[13] In a small study comparing intrauterine pressure, contractions and pain with dysmenorrhea, 12 women experienced significant relief with either naproxen or 70–100 Hz TENS with high amplitude (40–50 mA). Only the naproxen group experienced reductions in intrauterine pressure and contractions.[60] Unfortunately, the study was not blinded.

A comparison trial of TENS alone, lignocaine injection alone, and TENS combined with lignocaine was performed for the treatment of pain related to cervical laser treament. TENS alone or in combination did not provide any analgesic effects compared with lignocaine.[12] In a double-blinded randomized, controlled trial using a wrist-adapted TENS unit for the treatment of chemotherapy-related nausea, no difference was found in the intensity of the nausea or the percentage of persons with nausea.[66] However, all subjects were treated with antiemetics, diluting the possible effects of TENS. Overall, further study needs to be conducted to determine whether certain stimulus parameters might benefit obstetric and gynecologic patients.

TENS and Urologic Uses

Application of TENS in the sacral region for detrusor instability led to a reduction in maximum detrusor pressure and an increase in the pressure at which the subject felt the first desire to void. Maximum cystometric capacity was unchanged compared with control subjects with sham TENS.[7] A study with retrospective controls found pain reduced by 40% during lithotripsy with a TENS unit.[70] Well-designed clinical trials are needed to determine the efficacy of TENS for this application.

In a study of subjects with classic and nonulcerative interstitial cystitis, TENS was helpful in reducing pain. Classic interstitial cystitis had a better pain response with TENS. In addition, many with ulcers present for greater than 10 years had healing of the lesion.[17] For urologic patients, the optimal electrotherapy perscription has not been determined. However, it appears that sacral stimulation has effects on the detrusor muscle as well as an analgesic response.

Neuropathic Pain

Systematic study of electrical treatment of neuropathic pain is particularly sparse. Anecdotal reports have claimed benefit or lack of success.[81] A double–blind trial in subjects with neuropathies demonstrated significant pain relief if the TENS unit was placed over the nerve trunk.[84] There are some randomized studies using H-wave that demonstrate effectiveness in treating peripheral neuropathic pain (see later).[45,46] A pilot study looking at pulsed electrical stimulation delivered through a sock electrode overnight for a month reduced subjects' 10-cm VAS. The study was not blinded or controlled.[4]

In addition to reducing pain, electrical therapy may also improve peripheral circulation. A study used transcutaneous oximetry and laser Doppler flowmetry to study diabetics and controls before, during, and after electrical stimulation of the lower extremities. A transient, significant rise in tissue oxygenation was observed in the diabetics, but not the subjects without vascular disease.[67] A study to determine whether electrical stimulation has any positive clinical effects from the change in perfusion needs to be conducted.

Overall, further study needs to be done. Based on the limited data available it appears that electrical treatment of neuropathic pain may be a helpful adjunct for pain treatment. Possible perfusion effects may provide reduction or prevention of ischemic pain, but this needs rigorous study.

Cardiac Problems—Control of Angina and Postoperative Pain

TENS is thought to reduce angina by two methods: first, by decreasing pain, and second, by reducing ischemia by improving myocardial oxygen consumption. Lactate levels, an indicator of ischemia, were lower with the use of TENS during atrial pacing in a group with severe angina pectoris. Over a 3-week treatment period, the number of anginal episodes and nitroglycerin use were decreased. A concomitant increase in work capacity was found compared with controls.[52] An increase in coronary blood flow measured with intracoronary Doppler was demonstrated with TENS in fully innervated hearts.[5] Increased blood flow in nonstenotic coronary arteries was demonstrated during high-frequency TENS stimulation in cardiac catheterization patients.[39] Post–cardiac bypass surgery subjects using a pulsed form of TENS had reduced pain levels compared with controls. However, no difference was found between TENS and placebo TENS groups. No differences among the groups were found with outcomes of pulmonary function and narcotic intake.[20] Again, specific parameters need to be studied systematically. The effect on circulation is important. More clinical studies are needed once the optimal electrical parameters are established.

Pediatric Uses

In a well-designed study of TENS and sham TENS compared with a control group of usual care, children of all ages felt improvement in pain during venapuncture with the TENS.[47] Although the sham TENS group had reduction of pain compared with the control group, the TENS unit group had the greatest reduction. A case series of children with reflex sympathetic dystrophy and the use of TENS reported improvement in symptoms. The lack of controls, however, indicates that there is little definitive conclusions that can be drawn from this report.[42]

Other Musculoskeletal Pain

There is surprisingly little study of other musculoskeletal pain syndromes beyond spine pain.[28,72] In a group of subjects with frozen shoulder, a randomized controlled trial compared high- and low-frequency TENS with placebo. Both TENS groups had significantly lower pain levels postprocedure compared to controls.[62]

Gastroenterologic Uses

A study focusing on the correlation of esophogeal distension and chest pain found reduction in pain and esophogeal peristaltic velocity with the use of high-frequency TENS of moderate intensity (20–30 mA) and 0.2-msec pulse duration.[6] In a nonblinded, randomized, controlled trial in subjects undergoing hemorrhoindectomy, TENS stimulation at a traditional Chinese acupuncture point compared with TENS stimulation on a control point yielded pain reduction when stimulated at the acupuncture point only.[11]

ELECTRICAL ACUPUNCTURE

Researchers in China have demonstrated in rats and humans that electroacupuncture at the 100-Hz level blocked morphine withdrawal. A high dose of naloxone was able to block the electroacupuncture response in rats, implicating the kappa opioid receptor. In addition, spinal levels of dynorphin A, an endogenous opioid peptide, returned to normal levels after stimulation with electroacupuncture.[96]

Out of five studies reviewed with evidenced-based medicine principles by the Cochrane collaboration, only one generated a positive result. This study used a combination of low- and high-frequency stimulation. Improvements were demonstrated in pain description, global improvement scale, and a VAS for function. The improvements seen compared with wait list controls were maintained 6 months later.[82] The other four were neutral owing to methodologic problems.[89] There were no standard electrical parameters, and studies varied in choices of intensity, frequency, and placement. There are interesting effects with spinal opioid levels demonstrated with electroacupuncture. Future research likely will focus on optimal electrical parameters for maximal analgesia in the clinical setting.

Percutaneous Electrical Nerve Stimulation

In percutaneous electrical nerve stimulation (PENS), needles are placed through the skin into soft tissue or muscle at various sites and electricity is applied through the needles. It is believed to be a combination of TENS and electrical acupuncture.[25] With standard electrical parameters, research with PENS has been beneficial owing to the ability to compare responses in multiple studies.

In a randomized, single-blinded, cross-over study in patients with chronic low-back pain from degenerative disk disease, PENS reduced pain, improved function, and led to a reduction in opioid analgesia compared with the use of needles alone (sham PENS), TENS, or an exercise program (of questionable merit-seated flexion and extension exercise).[24] Reduction on VAS of 82% was demonstrated in the PENS group, whereas the sham PENS, TENS and exercise reduced pain by only 4–26%. Their randomization procedures were not described. Bias was likely, with subjects acting as their own controls. In a single blind study, observer bias is likely as well. The same design was applied to a group with sciatica from a herniated disk lasting more than than 6 months. Similar results were found as in the degenerative disk group.[26]

Another randomized single-blinded study with PENS and sham PENS in persons with chronic low-back pain, treatment with PENS for more than 30 minutes improved short-term VAS pain scores, oral analgesic use, physical activity, and sleep.[33] Again, how well the subjects were blinded is questionable, and a cross-over study is not the ideal design to minimize this methodologic error. Further study by this group of researchers, using cross-over design found 15–30 Hz to be the frequency of PENS leading to the greatest improvements in decreasing pain, and increasing physical activity and sleep.[25]

A single-blind, randomized study of PENS in postherpetic neuralgia demonstrated reductions in pain at 3 and 6 months but not 9 months.[2] Unfortunately, statistical analysis was not reported in the long-term component of the study. Better-designed clinical studies need to be performed for both electroacupuncture and PENS.

H-WAVE

The FDA has approved the H-wave muscle stimulator for relaxation of muscle spasm, prevention of retardation of disuse atrophy, edema control, muscle re-education, prevention of postoperative venous thrombosis, and in maintaining or improving range of motion. Low-frequency settings are used for muscle contractions, whereas the high frequency is used for pain relief (Electronic Waveform Lab, Inc). A larger unit is used in clinical practice, whereas a smaller home unit can be obtained for the patient. The unit is not designed for full portability.

In a double-blind, randomized controlled trial measuring the effect of H-wave stimulation on the mechanical pain threshold (MPT), H-wave caused significant increases in the MPT after 10 minutes of stimulation and peaked at 30 minutes. The increased MPT lasted up to 5 minutes after the H-wave stimulation was completed. These effects were similar to the analgesia provided by a comparison group using TENS.[56] Another study demonstrated similar improvements in MPT with 2-, 16-, and 60-Hz H-wave stimulation (McDowell[57]). However, ischemic pain models did not demonstrate an analgesic effect of H-wave.[57,55] This finding contradicts an earlier study demonstrating the effectiveness of H-wave therapy with 60-Hz stimulation in relieving ischemic pain.[90] However, this study was only single-blinded compared with the later study. Thus, H-wave is not likely beneficial in ischemic pain.[55]

Two randomized and controlled trials in diabetics with peripheral neuropathy demonstrated reduction in overall pain scores (0–5) and analog scores for symptoms.[45,46] Patients used a home unit 30 minutes a day for 4 weeks. In the later study, a group was chosen that was refractory to amitriptyline. In both studies, a small subgroup demonstrated 100% relief in pain. Conflicting data and poorly designed studies indicate that further study is needed.

CODETRON

Codetron delivers electrical stimulation similar to traditional a TENS unit but randomly switches stimulation between the six electrode sites every 10 seconds. The theory is by frequent changes in stimulation sites, habituation from repetitive signals is avoided. In a blinded, randomized, controlled trial of 58 subjects with acute occupational low-back injuries without objective spine pathology, Codetron offered no improvement over placebo in functional status, perceived pain, or return to work.[37] In 36 osteoarthritis subjects randomized to either codetron or sham Codetron, no improvements in 50 feet walking time, joint line tenderness, range of motion or knee circumference were found. Pain measures using the 10-cm VAS and the West Haven Yale Multidimension Pain Inventory did demonstrate significant improvements in the Codetron group.[18] However, randomization and blinding procedures were not well described. No other randomized, controlled trials were found by Medline search from 1966 to present.

INFERENTIAL CURRENT THERAPY

Inferential current is medium frequency (4000 Hz) amplitude modulated at a low frequency of 0–250 Hz. It is produced by mixing two out- of -phase currents (2000 Hz and 4000 Hz). It was developed to reduce skin resistance and allow amplification in the tissue. The current that reaches the tissue should be an average of the two frequencies, and the amplitude-modulated frequency is the difference between these two delivered frequencies The medium frequency is viewed as a "carrier" frequency for the lower frequency generating clinical analgesic effects.[65] A study focusing on the analgesic effects of inferential therapy found that the amplitude modulation did not change the response compared with nonamplitude modulation.[65] The purported benefit of interferential current therapy over TENS is a more rapid onset of analgesia within 15 minutes. The effects are likely similar to low-amplitude, burst-mode TENS.[43]

Although interferential current electrotherapy has been used in several countries,[27,51,68,73] clinical trials are rare. The reader is referred to several reviews regarding various electrotherapies.[30,85-87] A randomized, controlled trial in the Netherlands compared interferential therapy with ultrasound in the treatment of shoulder pain. A control group allowed exercise therapy alone without adjuvant treatments. Each electrotherapy group had a subgroup of sham therapy. In the interferential therapy group, the sham therapy group received a few minutes of electrical stimulation, three times over a 15-minute period. The treatment group received continuous interferential current for 15 minutes. Patient perception of recovery and physical therapy evaluation translated into VASs were the measured outcomes. No differences were found among any of the five groups. The authors concluded that ultrasound and interferential current therapy are not efficacious for the treatment of shoulder pain.[85] Other reports of interferential therapy describe benefits in the treatments of urinary stress incontinence,[30] osteoarthritis,[69,63] jaw pain,[80] and to promote fracture healing.[22] Randomized, controlled trials supporting the use of interferential therapy are lacking.

Interferential current therapy uses a novel approach to allow greater stimulation to bypass skin impedance. The relative benefits have not been proven by well-designed, randomized, controlled trials. Initially, the units were bulky and limited to physical therapy practices. Now small units are available for home use. The reimbursement rates are similar to a TENS unit (data from TENSPEDE). More randomized, controlled trials are needed to understand better the role interferential therapy plays in physical medicine and rehabilitation practice.

SUMMARY

Although clinical claims of efficacy have outpaced our understanding of the underlying physiologic mechanisms of electrotherapy, new evidence indicates that electrotherapy has effects on spinal cord opioid systems. The optimal parameters for application of electrotherapies remain to be determined. The potential benefit of a nonpharmacologic treatment for patients with pain demands rigorous pursuit of increasing our understanding of electrotherapy.

The cost of TENS units in Northern California range from $300–640 for purchase or $30–85 per month as a rental if they are obtained from medical supply companies. Units advertised on the internet range from $69-200. Interferential current stimulators are the same cost as TENS units from supply companies. From the internet, the cost is $200. Neuromuscular electrical stimulators are more expensive. From medical suppliers, the cost is $870–950 for purchase and form $73–120 per month rental. From the internet, units can cost from $99–130. The cost of supplies increases the expense. As stated in the introduction, the cost may be justified if work productivity increases with the nonsedating effects of TENS pain relief and there is a concomitant reduction in oral medications. Much work needs to be done on the basic clinical efficacy of various electrotherapy units before a meaningful cost analysis can be performed.

REFERENCES

1. Abram S, Reynold A, Cusick J: Failure of naloxone to reverse analgesia from transcutaneous electrical stimulation in patients with chronic pain. Anesth Analg 60:81, 1981.
2. Ahmed HE, Craig WF, White PF, et al: Percutaneous electrical nerve stimulation: An alternative to antiviral drugs for acute herpes zoster. Anesth Analg 87:911, 1998.
3. Almay BGL, Johansson F, Knorring L, et al: Long-term high frequency transcutaneous electrical nerve stimulation (hi-TNS) in chronic pain. Clinical response and effects on CSF-endorphins, monoamine metaboites, substance P-like immunoreactivity (SPLI) and pain measures. J Psychosom Res 29:247, 1985.
4. Armstrong DG, Lavery LA, Fleischli JG, Gilham KA: Is electrical stimulation effective in reducing neuropathic pain in patients with diabetes? J Foot Ankle Surg 36:260, 1997.
5. Borjessson M: Visceral chest pain in unstable angina pectoris and effects of transcutaneous electrical nerve stimulation (TENS): A review. Herz 24:114, 1999.
6. Borjesson M, Pilhall M, Eliasson T, et al: Esophageal visceral pain sensitivity: Effects of TENS and correlation with manometric findings. Dig Dis Sci 43:1621, 1998.
7. Bower WF, Moore KH, Adams RD, Sheperd R: A urodynamic study of surface neuromodulation versus sham in detrusor instability and sensory urgency. J Urol 160:2133, 1998.
8. Carroll D, Tramer M, McQuay H, et al: Randomization is important in studies with pain outcomes: Systematic review of transcutaneous electrical nerve stimulation in acute postoperative pain. Br J Anaesth 77:798, 1996.
9. Carroll D, Tramer M, McQuay H, et al: Transcutaneous electrical nerve stimulation in labour pain: A systematic review. Br J Obstet Gynaecol 104:169, 1997.
10. Chapman CR, Benedetti C: Analgesia following transcutaneous electrical stimulation and its partial reversal by a narcotic antagonist. Life Sci 21:1645–1648, 1977.
11. Chiu J, Chen W, Chen C, et al: Effect of transcutaneous electrical nerve stimulation for pain relief on patients undergoing hemorrhoidectomy. Dis Colon Rectum 42:180, 1999.
12. Crompton AC, Johnson N, Dudek U, et al: Is transcutaneous electrical nerve stimulation of any value during cervical laser treatment? Br J Obstet Gynaecol 99:492, 1992.
13. Dawood MY, Ramos J: Transcutaneous electrical nerve stimulation (TENS) for the treatment of

primary dysmenorrhea: A randomized crossover comparison with placebo TENS and Ibuprofen. Obstet Gynecol 75:656, 1990.
14. DeVahl J: Neuromuscular electrical stimulation (NMES) in rehabilitation. In Gersh MR (ed): Electrotherapy in Rehabilitation. Philadelphia, FA Davis, 1992, pp 218–268.
15. Deyo RA, Walsh NE, Martin DC, et al: A controlled trial of transcutaneous electrical nerve stimulation (TENS) and exercise for chronic low back pain. N Engl J Med 322 1627, 1990.
16. Ellenbecker T: Modalities in issues in rehabilitation. Advanced Team Physician Course Syllabus, Indianapolis, American College of Sports Medicine, 1999, pp 123–127.
17. Fall M, Lindstrom S: Transcutaneous electrical nerve stimulation in classic and nonulcer interstitial cystitis. Urol Clin N Am 21:131, 1994.
18. Fargas-Babjak AM, Pomeranz B, Rooney PJ, et al: Acupuncture-like stimulation with CODETRON for rehabilitation of patients with chronic pain syndrome and osteoarthritis. Acupunct Electrothera Res 17:95, 1992.
19. Foley-Nolan D, Moor K, Codd M, et al: Low energy high frequency pulsed electromagnetic therapy for acute whiplash injuries—a double blind randomized controlled study. Scand J Rehab Med 24:51, 1992.
20. Forster EL, Kramer JF, Lucy DL, et al: Effect of TENS on pain, medications, and pulmonary function following coronary artery bypass graft surgery. Chest 106:1343, 1994.
21. Gadsby JG, Flowerdew MW: Transcutaneous electrical nerve stimulation and acupuncture-like transcutaneous electrical nerve stimulation for chronic low back pain. (Cochrane Review). In The Cochrane Library, Issue 2. Oxford, Update Software, 2000.
22. Ganne JM, Speculund B, Mayne LH, Goss AN: Intereferntial therapy to promote union of mandibular fractures. Aust N Z J Surg 49:81, 1979.
23. Gersh MR: Transcutaneous electrical nerve stimulation for management of pain. In Gersh MR (ed): Electrotherapy in Rehabilitation. Philadelphia, FA Davis, 1992, pp 149–196.
24. Ghoname EA, Craig WF, White PF, et al: Percutaneous electrical nerve stimulation for low back pain—a randomized crossover study. JAMA 281:818, 1999.
25. Ghoname EA, Craig WF, White PF, et al: The effect of stimulus frequency on the analgesic response to percutaneous electrical nerve stimulation in patients with chronic low back pain. Anesth Analg 88:841, 1999.
26. Ghoname EA, White PF, Ahmed HE, et al: Percutaneous electrical nerve stimulation: An alternative to TENS in the management of sciatica. Pain 83:193, 1999.
27. Goats GC: Interferential current therapy. Br J Sports Med 24:87, 1990.
28. Godlee F (ed): Clinical Evidence. London, British Medical Journal Publishing Group, 2000, pp 486–572.
29. Grant DJ, Bishop-Miller J, Winchester DM, et al: A randomized comparative trial of acupuncture versus transcutaneous electrical nerve stimulation for chronic back pain in the elderly. Pain 82:9, 1999.
30. Green S, Buchbinder R, Glazier R, Forbes A: Systematic review of randomized controlled trials of interventions of painful shoulder: Selection criteria, outcome assessment, and eficacy. BMJ 316:354, 1998.
31. Gross AR, Aker PD, Goldsmith CH, Peloso P: Physical medicine modalities for mechanical neck disorders (Cochrane Review). In The Cochrane Library, Issue 3. Oxford: Update Software, 2000.
32. Gulmezoglu AM, Hofmeyr GJ: Transcutaneous electrostimulaiton for suspected placental insufficiency (diagnosed by Doppler studies) (Cochrane Review). In The Cochrane Library, Issue 3. Oxford, Update Software, 2000.
33. Hamza MA, Ghoname EA, White PF, et al: Effect of the duration of electrical stimulation on the analgesic respone in patients with low back pain. Anesthesiology 91:1622, 1999.
34. Hamza MA, White PF, Ahmed HE, Ghoname EA: Effect of the frequency of transcutaneous electrical stimulation on the postoperative opioid analgesic requirement and recovery profile. Anesthesiology 91: 1232, 1999.
35. Han JS, Chen XH, Sun SL, et al: Effect of low- and high-frequency TENS on Met-enkephalin-Arg-Phe and dynorphoin A immunoreactivity in human lumbar CSF. Pain 47:295, 1991.
36. Han JS, Wu LZ, Cui CL: Heroin addicts treated with transcutaneous electrical nerve stimulation of identified frquencies. Regul Pept 54:115, 1994.
37. Herman E, Williams R, Stratford P, et al: A randomized controlled trial of transcutaneous electrical nerve stimulation (CODETRON) to determine its benefits in a rehabilitation program for acute occupational low back pain. Spine 19:261, 1994.

38. Hughes G, Lichstein P, Whitlock D, Harker C: Response of plasma beta-endorphins to transcutaneous electrical nerve stimulation in healthy subjects. Phys Ther 64:1062, 1984.
39. Jessurun GAJ, Tio RA, De Jongste MJL, et al: Coronary blood flow dynamics during transcutaneous electrical nerve stimulation for stable angina pectoris associated with severe narrowing of one major coronary artery. Am J Cariol 82:921, 1998.
40. Johnson MI, Hajela VK, Ashton CH, Thompson JW: The effects of auricular trancutaneous electrical nerve stimulation (TENS) on experimental pain threshold and autonomic function in healthy subjects. Pain 46:337, 1991.
41. Kahn, J: Electrical Stimulation. In Kahn J (ed): Princliples and Practice of Electrotherapy. Philadelphia, Churchill-Livingstone, 2000, pp 69-99.
42. Kesler RW, Saulsbury FT, Miller LT, Rowlingson JC: Reflex sympathetic dystrophy in children: Treatment with transcutaneous electric nerve stimulation. Pediatrics 83:728, 1988.
43. Kloth LC: Electrotherapeutic alternatives for the treatment of pain. In Gersh MR (ed): Electrotherpy in Rehabilitation. Philadelphia, FA Davis, 1992, pp 197–217.
44. Kukulka CG: Principles of neuromuscular excitation. In Gersh MR (ed): Electrotherapy In Rehabilitation. Philadelphia, FA Davis, 1992, pp 3–25.
45. Kumar D, Alvaro MS, Julka IS, Marshall HJ: Diabetic peripheral neuropahy. Effectiveness of electrotherapy and amitriptyline for symptomatic relief. Diabetes Care 21:1322, 1998.
46. Kumar D, Marshall HJ: Diabetic peripheral neuropathy: amelioration of pain with transcutaneous electrostimulation. Diabetes Care 20:1702, 1997.
47. Lander J, Fowler-Kerry S: TENS for children's procedural pain. Pain 52:209, 1993.
48. Labrecque M, Nouwen A, Bergeron M, et al: A randomized controlled trial of nonpharmacologic approaches for relief of low back pain during labor. J Fam Pract 48:259, 1999.
49. Li CL, Bak A: Excitability characteristics of the A and C fibers in a peripheral nerve. Exp Neurol 50:67, 1976.
50. Licht S: History of electotherapy. In Stillwell GK (ed): Therapeutic Electricity and Ultraviolet Radiation, 3rd ed. Baltimore, Williams & Wilkins, 1983, pp 1–64.
51. Lindsay DM, Dearness J, McGinley CC: Electrotherapy usage trend in private practice in Alberta. Physiother Can 47:30, 1995.
52. Mannheimer C, Carlsson CA, Emanuelsson H, et al: The effects of transcutaneous electrical nerve stimulation in patients with severe angina pectoris. Circulation 71:308, 1985.
53. Mannheimer JS, Lampe GN: Clinical Transcutaneous Electrical Nerve Stimulation. Philadelphia, FA Davis, 1984.
54. Marchand S, Charest J, Li J, et al: Is TENS purely a placebo effect? A controlled study on chronic low back pain. Pain 54:99, 1993.
55. McDowell BC, Lowe AS, Walsh DM, et al: The lack of hypoalgesic effect of H-wave therapy on experimental ischemic pain. Pain 61:27, 1995.
56. McDowell BC, McCormack K, Walsh DM, et al: Comparative analgesic effects of H-Wave therapy and transcutaneous electrical nerve stimulation on pain threshold in humans. Arch Phys Med Rehabil 80:1001, 1999.
57. McDowell BC, Robinson JI, Cherry HR, et al: The comparative hypoalgesic efficacy of H-wave therapy (HWT) and oral analgesics on experimental ischaemic pain in humans. Pain Clinic 9:93, 1996.
58. McQuay H, Carroll D, Moore A: Variation in the placebo effect in randomized controlled trials of analgesics: all is as blind as it seems. Pain 64:331, 1995.
59. Melzack R, Wall PD: Pain mechanisms: A new theory. Science 150:971, 1965.
60. Milsom I, Hedner N, Mannheimer C: A comparative study of the effect of high-intensity transcutaneous nerve stimulation and oral naproxen on intrauterine pressure and menstrual pain in patients with primary dysmenorrhea. Am J Obstet Gynecol 170: 123, 1994.
61. Moore SR, Shurman J: Combined neuromuscular electrical stimulation and transcutaneous electrical nerve stimulation for treatment of chronic back pain: a double—blind, repeated measures comparison. Arch Phys Med Rehabil 78:55, 1997.
62. Nash TP, William JD, Machin D: TENS: Does the type of stimulus really matter? Pain Clinic 3:161, 1990.
63. Ni Chiosoig F, Hendirks O, Malone J: A pilot study of the therapeutic effects of bipolar and quadripolar interferential therapy, using bilateral osteoarthosis as a model. Physiother Ire 15:3, 1994.

64. Paternostro-Sluga R, Fialka Ch, Alacamliogliu Y, et al: Neuromuscular electrical stimualtion after anterior cruciate ligament surgery. Clin Orthop Relat Res 368:166, 1999.
65. Palmer ST, Martin DJ, Steedman WM, Ravey J: Alteration of Interferential current and transcutaneous electrical nerve stimulation frequency: effects on nerve excitation. Arch Phys Med Rehabil 80:1065, 1999,
66. Pearl ML, Fischer M, McCauley DL, et al: Transcutaneous electrical nerve stimulation as an adjunct for controlling chemotherapy-induced nausea and vomiting in gynecologic oncology patients. Cancer Nursing 22:307, 1999.
67. Peters EJ, Armstrong DG, Wunderlich RP, et al: The benefit of electrical stimualtion to enhance perfusion in persons with diabetes mellitus. J Foot Ankle Surg 37:396, 1998.
68. Pope GD, Mocket SP, Wright JP: A survey of electrotherapeutic modalities: Ownership and use in the NHS in England. Physiotherapy 81:82, 1995.
69. Quirk A, Newman R, Newman K: An evaluation of interferential therapy, shortwave diathermy and exercise in the treatment of osteoarthrosis of the knee. Physiotherapy 71:55, 1985.
70. Reichelt O, Zermann DH, Wunderlich H, et al: Effective analgesia for extracorporeal shock wave lithotripsy: Transcutaneous electrical nerve stimulation. Urology 54:433–436, 1999.
71. Reid DC: Physical modalities. In Sport Injury: Assessment and Rehabilitation. New York, Churchill Livingstone, 1992, pp 31–64.
72. Rey B, Gerber NJ: Shoulder pain trials. In Slapbach P, Berber NJ (eds). Physiotherapy: Controlled Trials and Facts. Basel, Karger, 1991, pp 91–98.
73. Robinson A, Snyder-Mackler L: Clinical application of electrotherapeutic modalities. Phys Ther 68:1235, 1988.
74. Roche PA, Gijsbers K, Belch JJF, Forbes CD: Modification of induced ischaemic pain by transcutaneous electrical nerve stimulation. Pain 20:45, 1984.
75. Salar G, Job I, Minigrino S, et al: Effect of transcutaneous electrotherapy on CSF beta-endorphin content in patients without pain problems. Pain 10:169, 1981.
76. Sjolund, GH: Peripheral nerve stimulation suppression of c-fiber–evoked flexion reflex in rats. Part 2. Parameters of low rate train stimulation of skin and muscle afferent nerves. J Neurosurg 68:279, 1988.
77. Sjolund B, Eriksson M: The influence of naloxone on analgesia produced by peripheral conditioning stimulation. Brain Res 173: 295, 1979.
78. Sluka KA, Bailey K, Bogush J, et al: Treatment with either high or low frequency TENS reduces the secondary hyperalgesia observed after injection of kaolin and carrageenan into the knee joint. Pain 77:97, 1998.
79. Sluka KA, Deacon M, Stibal A, et al: Spinal blockade of opioid receptors prevents the analgesia produced by TENS in arthritic rats. J Pharmacology Exp Ther 289:840, 1999.
80. Taylor K, Newton R, Personius W, Bush F: Effects of interferetial current stimulation for treatment of subjects with recurrent jaw pain. Phys Ther 67:346, 1987.
81. Thomas PK, Eliasson SG: Diabetic neuropathy. In Dyck PJ (ed): Diseases of the Peripheral Nervous System. Philadelphia, WB Saunders, 1987, pp 1773–1810.
82. Thomas M, Lundberg T: Importance of modes of acupuncture in the treatment of chronic nociceptive low back pain. Acta Anaesthesiol Scand 38:83, 1994.
83. Thomas IL, Yle V, Webster J, Neilson A: An evaluation of transcutaneous electrical nerve stimulation for pain relief in labour. Aust N Z J Obstet Gynaecol 28:182, 1988.
84. Thorsteinsson G, Stonnington HH, Stillwell GK, et al: Transcutaneous electrical stimulation: A double-blind trial of its efficacy for pain. Arch Phys Med Rehabil 58:8, 1977.
85. van der Heijden GJMG, Leffers P, Wolters PJMC, et al: No effect of bipolar interferential electrotherapy and pulsed ultrasound for soft tissue disorders: A randomized controlled trial. Ann Rheum Dis 58:530, 1999.
86. van der Heijden GJMG, Torenbeek M, van der Windt DAWM, et al: Transcutaneous electrotherapy for musculoskeletal disorders: A systematic review. Final report for the Health Council of the Netherlands. Hoensbroek, Institute for Rehabilitaiton Research, 1999.
87. van der Heijden GJMG, van der Windt DAWM, De Winter AF: Physiotherapy for soft-tissue shoulder disorders. A systematic review of randomized clinical trials. BMJ 315:25, 1997.
88. van der Ploeg JM, Vervest HAM, Liem AL, Schagen van Leeuwen JH: Transcutaneous nerve stimulation (TENS) during the first stage of labour: A randomized clinical trial. Pain 68:75, 1996.

89. van Tulder MW, Cherkin DC, Berman B, et al: The effectiveness of acupuncture in the management of acute and chronic low back pain. Spine 243:1113, 1999.
90. Walsh DM, Baxter GD, Allen JM, Bell AJ: An investigation f the hypoalgesic effects of H-wave therapy upon experimentally induced ischaemic pain. Ir J Med Sci 161:472, 1992.
91. Walsh DM, Foster NE, Baxter GD, Allen JM: Transcutaneous electrical nerve stimulation: Relevance of stimulation parameters to neurophysiological and hypoalgesic effects. Am J Phys Med Rehabil 74:199, 1995.
92. Walsh DM, Liggett C, Baxter D, Allen JM: A double-blind investigation of the hypoalgesic effects of transcutaneous electrical nerve stimulation upon experimentally induced ischaemic pain. Pain 61:39, 1995.
93. Walsh DM, Noble G, Baxter GD, Allen JM: Study of the effects of various transcutaneous electrical nerve stimulation (TENS) parameters upon the RIII nociceptive and H-reflexes in humans. Clin Physiol 20:191–199, 2000.
94. Woolf CJ: Transcutaneous electrical nerve stimulation and the reaction to experimental pain in human subjects. Pain 7:115–27, 1979.
95. Woolf CJ, Barett D, Mitchell D, Myres R: Naloxone-reversible peripheral electroanalgesia in intact and spinal rats. Eur J Pharmacol 45:311, 1977.
96. Wu LZ, Cui CL, Tian JB, et al: Suppression of morphine withdrawal by electroacupuncture in rats: Dynorphin and kappa–opioid receptor implicated. Brain Res 851:290, 1999.

Chapter 10
Therapeutic Exercise

Rajeswari Kumar, MD, and Michelle Voss, DPT

Exercise is the most commonly applied therapeutic modality. Exercises are prescribed to improve strength, endurance, and range of motion (ROM). *Absolute muscle strength* is the maximal force that the muscle may develop and is directly proportional to its size or physiologic cross-sectional area.[1] *Endurance* is the ability to continue a specific task for a prolonged period of time and is related to both the cardiovascular system and muscle strength. *Range of motion* of a specific joint depends on the flexibility of tendons and ligaments and the integrity of the joint. In addition to improving strength and endurance, exercise has been shown to affect various organ systems in the body.[1]

PHYSIOLOGY OF EXERCISE

Energy for muscle contraction is obtained from adenosine triphosphate (ATP), which is hydrolyzed to adenosine diphosphate (ADP). ADP is regenerated to ATP with the available phosphocreatine (PC), another high-energy compound.[1] The sources of ATP are glucose, glycogen, fatty acids, and amino acids, which enter the Krebs cycle and yield ATP. During glycolysis, glucose is broken down to pyruvate and ATP. In the presence of oxygen (O_2), the pyruvate is converted to acetyl coenzyme A and transported to mitochondria, which then enter the Krebs cycle. In the absence of O_2, pyruvate is reduced to lactate, which enters the venous blood and subsequently is reoxidized in the liver when oxygen supply is available. There are three phase of energy production during exercise. During the **lactic phase**, energy is produced from the stored high-energy phosphates. During the **glycolytic phase**, high-energy phosphates are produced from anaerobic metabolism of glucose and glycogen. In the **aerobic phase**, there is an increase in ventilation, and oxygen becomes available. Subsequently, ATP is generated aerobically through oxidation of glucose, fat, and protein.[1]

Historically, the presence of lactate during high-intensity exercise was thought to stimulate respiration.[2] Lactate accumulation in blood was thought to reflect a point at which oxygen supply to the muscle was inadequate to meet the oxygen demand. In the 1960s, Hollman and colleagues linked lactate production in the blood to endurance performance, which challenged the previous belief that lactate accumulation occurs in short strenuous exercise. In 1964, Wasserman and McIlroy developed the concept of the *critical threshold* that exists during prolonged exercise. At the critical threshold, metabolic need for oxygen in the muscle exceeds the cardiopulmonary system's supply, after which there is a sudden increase in anaerobic metabolism causing lactate production in the muscle.[2]

In recent years, isotopic tracer technology has revealed that muscles could produce lactate even in the presence of adequate supply of oxygen.[2] It is now recognized that lactate production and removal is a continuous process. Change in rate of the production or removal of lactate determines blood lactate level. The concept that a threshold exists after which there is a sudden onset of anaerobic metabolism currently is being challenged.[2] Recent studies have shown that blood lactate accumulation is due to beta-adrenergic stimulation of muscle glyconeogenesis. Lactate also acts as a substrate and may be the predominant fuel for heart and slow-twitch muscle fibers during exercise. There is also a misconception that accumulation of lactate causes muscle fatigue and soreness. Studies have shown that accumulation of lactate occurs after a bout of strenuous exercise, and in these instances, people experience very little fatigue. Moreover, direct infusion of lactate does not seem to cause fatigue or muscle soreness.[2]

Physiologic Response to Exercise

Muscle

Strengthening exercises cause muscle fiber hypertrophy in all fiber types, as evidenced by an increase in cross-sectional area of the muscle.[3] Muscle hypertrophy is a result of increase in the number of myofibrils resulting from an increase in protein synthesis. There is an increase in the density of actin and myosin, which may explain fiber hypertrophy, although such changes are seen even in fibers that do not show any hypertrophy. Muscle fiber hypertrophy is commonly recognizable after 6 weeks of training. There is controversy regarding conversion of slow-twitch muscle fibers to fast-twitch muscle fibers with strengthening exercise. It is also questionable whether there is muscle fiber splitting and increase in the number of muscle fibers with strengthening program. With endurance exercise, the aerobic capacity in both type I and II fibers increases. In addition, oxidative enzymes, myoglobin, mitochondrial density, and number of capillaries increase. An increase in aerobic capacity is evidenced by an increase in the difference in arteriovenous oxygen saturation. Fiber type conversion is not well documented with endurance exercise programs. There is also an increase in glycolytic capacity in the muscle fibers with endurance exercise.[1,3]

Nervous System

Even before a person begins to exercise, there are changes in the central neural activity called *central command*. This phenomenon withdraws cardiac parasympathetic activity and causes reduced vagal tone. There is an increase in sympathetic activity that results in increased heart rate, increased cardiac output, increased sympathetic vasoconstrictor tone, and reduced cutaneous blood flow.[4,5]

During exercise, ischemic metabolites (lactic acid, diprotonated phosphates, and adenosine) accumulate in the exercising muscle bed. These metabolites activate chemosensitive afferent nerve fibers called *muscle metaboreceptors*. This activation increases the sympathetic activity in the exercising and the nonexercising muscles. In the nonexercising muscles, the result is vasoconstriction. In the exercising muscle, these effects compete with the direct vasodilator effect of local ischemic metabolites on the vascular smooth muscles, eventually causing vasodilatation. This sympathetically mediated activity is called *metaboreflex*.[6]

Exercise causes synchronization of motor unit recruitment, especially in the prime movers. Strength and performance depend not only on the quality of the involved muscles but also on the ability of the nervous system to activate appropriately the changes within the nervous system that cause activation of agonist muscle groups and inactivation of antagonist muscles. These changes allow the activation of prime movers in specific movements and better coordination and activation of all relevant muscles, thereby affecting a greater net force in the intended direction of movement.[7]

Gastrointestinal System

Exercise reduces splanchnic blood flow, which results in the reduction in absorption of food from the intestine. A study was done in 10 healthy, well-trained subjects to determine the various effects of exercise on gastrointestinal function.[8] These subjects underwent rest–cycling–rest protocol, and a rest–rest–rest protocol. Esophageal motility, gastroesophageal reflux, intragastric pH, and gastric motility were measured using a transnasal catheter. A sugar absorption test was performed to determine intestinal permeability and glucose absorption. The result of this study showed that neither gastric emptying nor transit time was different between rest and cycling periods. There was no difference between gastric pH and the number of gastroesophageal reflux among pre-exercise, exercise, and postexercise.[8] Gastric absorption of glucose was significantly lower during the period of exercise. Thus, gastric emptying depends on a number of other factors including meal osmolality, meal temperature, and exercise conditions. It is commonly known that light exercise enhances liquid gastric emptying, and vigorous exercise delays solid emptying.[9,10]

Gastrointestinal symptoms are very common among athletes, particularly women runners. Foods rich in fat, protein, dietary fiber, and hypertonic drinks decrease gastrointestinal symptoms of diarrhea, abdominal pain, and urge to defecate.[9] Symptoms of gastric acid reflex or heartburn are of particular concern because these symptoms may mimic cardiac symptoms. The gut adapts to increases in exercise-induced physiologic stress. Adequate training leads to a less dramatic decrease in gastrointestinal blood flow at submaximal exercise intensities and is important in the prevention of gastrointestinal symptoms.[10]

Cardiovascular System

Beneficial effects of exercise on the cardiovascular system include increases in exercise tolerance, cardiac output, and maximum oxygen consumption. A regular exercise program, at least 3 days a week, increases the exercise tolerance level. An 8-week exercise program at 60% or more of the maximal heart rate achieved at baseline testing increased the subjects' exercise tolerance on the treadmill by 30% and increased the maximum oxygen consumption by 15–20%.[11] The beneficial effects are more prominent in sedentary individuals.[11] Higher intensity exercises are shown to have a better short-term improvement but no statistically significant difference after 1 year. Older individuals may require a prolonged period of training compared with younger individuals.[3,11]

Regular exercises have been shown to reduce the severity of anginal symptoms and increase anginal threshold in subjects with chronic stable angina[11] and have been shown to improve cardiac function among patients with chronic heart failure and cardiomyopathy. Dipyridamole-thallium tests in these patients have shown increased uptake of thallium suggesting increased coronary perfusion.[11] The clinical improvement in patients with heart disease is also due to peripheral adaptation such as increased oxidative enzyme capacity and improved peripheral oxygen uptake.[11]

The effect of exercise programs on the reduction of blood pressure (BP) is controversial. Some studies have shown that exercises reduce average BP by 10–13 points, but others have not found similar results. Progressive increase in blood pressure is a normal phenomenon during endurance and strengthening exercise.[11,12] Strengthening exercises cause a slightly higher elevation of BP compared with endurance exercise. Short bouts of strengthening exercises are commonly associated with the Valsalva maneuver, which sometime causes dangerously high levels of BP. Meta-analysis was conducted on 15 studies in which subjects were involved in a 4-week progressive resistive exercise program. Analysis showed that progressive resistive exercise had beneficial effects in reducing systolic and diastolic blood pressure in hypertensive individuals.[13] However, a well-controlled study to determine the efficacy of progressive resistive exercise as a measure to control high blood pressure is lacking.

An increase in heart rate after exercise is due to reduction in vagal tone. Similarly, recovery of heart rate is due to vagal reactivation. Cole et al. showed that the recovery of heart rate might be a powerful predictor of overall mortality due to cardiovascular disease.[14] In this study, 2428 subjects without coronary revascularization or heart failure were followed for 5 years. Recovery of heat rate was defined as decrease in heart rate by 12 beats in 1 minute after stopping the exercise. The mortality rate showed that a delayed decrease in heart rate during the first minute after exercise might be a powerful predictor of overall mortality (95% confidence interval of 1.5–2.7; $p < 0.001$).[14]

Pulmonary

During exercise, the minute ventilation increases linearly to a point, and then the increase become steeper. There are no measurable changes in pO_2 and pCO_2, even with moderate intensity of exercise.[1,15] pH decreases with an increase in workload, and there is a slight decrease in pO_2 with a very high workload. These changes in pH and pO_2 are not proportional to the metabolic demand and suggest a neural reflex mechanism.[1] The stimulus or the pathway of this reflex is not clear. In healthy, fit subjects, there are few changes in airway caliber during or after exercise. In young healthy subjects with average fitness, little ventilatory constraint exists during exercise. In older subjects, there is a decline in ventilatory capacity due to reduced elastic recoil. Flow limitations occur at a lower level of ventilation in older patients than in younger patients.[16]

Renal

Renal circulation receives more blood flow per tissue weight at rest than any other organ. With exercise, there is a reduction in renal cortical blood flow and an increase in renal vascular resistance.[1,17] An immediate decrease in blood flow after exercise is due to central command and metaboreflex.[4] Further decrease in renal blood flow during exercise is thought to be due to increased metabolic demand during exercise and shunting of the blood to the exercising muscles.[17] Radionuclide angiographic studies in healthy volunteers showed that renal blood flow was decreased by 53.4% immediately after exhausting exercise. Renal blood flow remained decreased by 17% 30 minutes after exercise and by 21.1% 60 minutes after exercise.[17,18] Similar studies on renal blood flow on healthy volunteers with static handgrip exercise showed that renal cortical blood flow decreases and renal cortical vasculature resistance increases after exercise.[17,18] Renal vascular constriction during exercise is not an autoregulatory mechanism because renal blood flow falls below the basal value. Normally, autoregulation helps the blood flow to remain at control levels. There are no relationships between renal blood flow and plasma angiotensin, plasma rennin, or noradrenalin. As a result of the reduced blood flow, the urine output is reduced and urine is concentrated.

Renal blood flow changes during exercise are influenced by age of the individual. One study found that there was less reduction in blood flow to the kidney during exercise in an older population (mean age 67 years) when compared with a younger population (mean age 24 years). During the recovery period, the renal blood flow fell below the resting value in older subjects compared with younger subjects.[19] Renal blood flow is also influenced by nonsteroidal anti-inflammatory medications (NSAIDs). Indomethacin (Indocin) produces no change in renal blood flow or renal vascular resistance at rest compared to control values, but significant reduction in renal blood flow was noticed ($p < 0.027$) after exercise. Patients who routinely take NSAIDs should be warned about the effects of NSAIDs during exercise. Adequate fluid supplementation is very important in these patients and in older subjects.[20]

Reproductive System

The female reproductive system is influenced by exercise. A wide spectrum of menstrual dysfunction has been found in athletes and some women involved in a vigorous exercise program.[21] Ovarian function and menstrual regularity depend on normal pituitary gonadotropic stimulation. Gonadotropin levels were found to be too low or below normal in women long-distance runners, reflecting central suppression of the reproductive axis. Hypothalamic hypofunction has been shown to be the cause of pituitary hypofunction; however, the cause of hypothalamus dysfunction in athletes has not been investigated. Delayed menarche, oligomenorrhea, anovulation, and amenorrhea are the most common documented menstrual dysfunctions in female athletes.[21,22] Exercise-induced menstrual irregularity is multifactorial in origin and is a diagnosis of exclusion. Reduction of exercise levels and dietary modification can produce dramatic changes in menstrual function.

There is an association between body fat composition and initiation and maintenance of menstrual periods. Seventeen percent body fat is required for initiation of menstruation, and 22% body fat is required for maintenance of menstrual periods. Athletes who have amenorrhea are shown to have a lower percentage of body fat or a lower body weight.[22]

Vascular

Nitrous oxide (NO) has been identified as a potential mediator for the vascular benefit of exercise. Elevation of shear stress on vascular endothelium causes NO production. Previous studies have postulated that NO derived from endothelium is responsible for vasodilatation of feed arteries in the muscles, which therefore permits increased vascular flow to the muscle without a decrease in perfusion pressure.[23] This vasodilatation is also presumed to be responsible for reduction in blood pressure with regular exercise. A brisk walk for 30 minutes five to seven times per week was found to improve endothelial function in normotensive and hypertensive individuals. This may help to contribute to cardiovascular protective effects of exercise training. The important effect was on coronary arteries. Exercise training improved endothelial-dependent vasodilatation both in the epicardial coronary vessels and in resistance vessels in patients with coronary artery disease.[24]

Psychological

Meta-analyses on the effect of regular exercise have shown that physical activity enhances self-esteem, improves mood state, reduces anxiety, and improves physical self-perception. Both aerobic and resistance exercises enhance mood state.[25,26] Serum levels of norepinephrine were found to be low in depressed individuals, and mood state is thought to be improved by the high levels of norepinephrine that are present after exercise.[26] In addition, aerobic exercise increases beta-endorphin levels in plasma, which may result in mild euphoria.[26]

Improvement in depression has been documented by significant improvement in Beck Depression Inventory scale. Improvement was more rapid in subjects who exercised in addition to taking antidepressant medication compared with those who were treated with medication alone. Weaker evidence also suggests that exercise improves cognitive function in patients with chronic fatigue syndrome.[27]

Hematologic

Exercise enhances thrombin-induced platelet fibrinogen binding and platelet aggregability.[28] These changes were reversible with recovery 60 minutes after completion of exercise. Various intensities of exercise affect platelet function differently. For example, moderate exercise desensitizes and strenuous exercise potentiates platelet aggregability.[29,30] Severe exercise may potentiate platelet activity by elevating the norepinephrine level, which is a potent platelet-activating agent.[30] These factors may explain exercise-induced acute myocardial infarction and cardiac arrest. Other hematologic effects of exercise include increased neutrophil migration from the marginated pools into circulation. This mainly occurs after exhaustive exercise.[31]

Endocrine

During exercise, the whole body consumption of O_2 increases as much as 20-fold. To meet the increase in energy demand during exercise, skeletal muscle uses its own stores of glycogen, triglyceride, and free fatty acids derived from breakdown of adipose tissue from the muscle and uses glucose derived from the liver.[32]

Blood glucose level is well maintained during exercise in order to preserve central nervous system function and muscle function. The metabolic adjustment that preserves normoglycemia during exercise is hormonally mediated. There is a decrease in plasma insulin and increase in glucagon during early part of exercise. This helps mobilize glucose from the liver.[33] During prolonged exercise, there is increase in catecholamines, which plays an important role in mobilization of glucose. The central command and withdrawal of vagal tone are responsible for increase in catecholamine levels in blood.[33]

COMPONENTS OF THERAPEUTIC EXERCISE

There are several types of therapeutic exercise, and the clinician must weigh the advantages and disadvantages of each when formulating an exercise prescription to achieve maximum benefit. Components of exercise regimens include flexibility, ROM, strengthening, and endurance. Most often, a combination of these exercise regimens leads to the most optimal results.

Flexibility Training

Muscles produce their maximal amount of tension when fibers are at their optimal resting length.[34] The resting length of a muscle may become shortened as a result of immobility from factors such as prolonged casting, soft tissue injury, restricted joint mobility, and neurologic disorders. Stretching is a key component of most exercise regimens and serves to maintain muscles at their optimal resting length to enhance muscle function. The American College of Sports Medicine (ACSM) has established guidelines for stretching prescription, which include (1) a minimum of three days per week, (2) stretch to a position of mild discomfort, (3) hold the stretch for 15–30 seconds, (4) complete three to five repetitions for each stretch, and (5) perform static stretching, that is, avoid ballistic, bouncing movements, with emphasis on the lower back and thigh area.[35]

Many methods for stretching include manual passive stretching, mechanical stretching, and the contract-relax technique. During manual passive stretching, the body segment is passively moved to a position just beyond the resting length of the involved tissues[36] and may be held in this position from 15 to 30 seconds.[36] Mechanical stretching may be accomplished by use of serial casting or a dynamic splinting device, which provide a low-intensity stretch for a prolonged period of time and are typically used to reduce joint contractures. Dynamic splinting devices may be worn 8–10 hours per day.[37] The contract-relax technique is commonly used by therapists to improve muscle length.[38] In this technique, the person isometrically contracts the tight muscle and then relaxes. After the relaxation is complete, the therapist passively lengthens the muscle. The type of stretching procedure that is prescribed ultimately will be based on individual ability and need.

Stretching exercise performed for lower body segments has beneficial effects for proximal body segments.[39] For example, a 3-week program of daily hamstring muscle stretching, performed for 10 repetitions with 15-second hold, resulted in increased straight-leg raise range and hip motion during forward bending.[40] Thus, increased flexibility of the hip may reduce the amount of lumbar spine motion necessary to complete an activity.

Stretching is commonly recommended before exercise with the belief that injuries will be prevented.[35] However, some studies have found that static stretching performed exclusively before exercise had no significant difference in delayed onset of muscle soreness[41,42] or preventing injury[43] when compared with exercise without a stretching component. Therefore, to maintain optimal flexibility, stretching exercise should be done on a regular basis rather than only before exercise.

Studies have shown that stretching exercise, if not done properly, has potential to cause injury.[41,44] Injury may be avoided through active warm-up before stretching,[35] use of heat prior to stretching,[36,44] and avoidance of bouncing, ballistic movements.[35,36] Stretching must be prescribed individually because stretching exercises may be contraindicated for certain musculoskeletal disorders with active joint pathology, and some people may not have adequate flexibility to properly perform certain stretches.

Range-of-Motion Exercises

Each joint has an optimal ROM for performance of daily activities. Many orthopedic and neurologic conditions, such as contracture after prolonged casting or spasticity resulting from a stroke, may negatively affect joint ROM. ROM may be increased by several different methods including passive, active-assisted, and active ROM. Passive range of motion (PROM) is exercise in which there is no voluntary muscle contraction of the involved body segment as the joint is moved through its available range. PROM may be used to maintain joint ROM when active exercise is contraindicated. These exercises are helpful after recent tendon or muscle repair surgery or active inflammatory process of a joint. PROM is prescribed when a person is incapable of active muscle contraction such as in the case of paralysis or severe pain. PROM may be accomplished using gravity, another person, another body segment, or mechanical devices. A continuous passive motion (CPM) machine is commonly used to maintain knee joint ROM passively after total knee replacement.[45] Similarly, Codman's pendulum exercises use gravity to maintain flexibility in shoulder joints after surgical repair of a tendon or joint replacement.[46]

Active-assisted range of motion (AAROM) is a type of exercise in which the involved limb is assisted through the ROM when a person is unable to move his or her limb actively through the full available range because of pain, weakness, or poor motor control.[37] It is important that as little assistance as possible is rendered so that the weaker muscles are allowed to generate their maximum force throughout the range. The involved limb may be assisted by many sources such as the uninvolved limb, use of mechanical devices, or the buoyancy of water.[36]

Active range of motion (AROM) is defined as the movement of a body segment through its available ROM with the person's own effort. AROM may be performed through a limited range, in the presence of recent surgery or pain, or through full available range. The exercise program progresses to include moving the extremity through full range against resistance when indicated. The time it takes to advance a person from PROM exercise to AROM exercise depends on the nature of the disease, injury, or surgery performed.

Strength Training

Muscle strength has been defined as "the maximum force a muscle can produce during a single exertion to create joint torque."[46] Several types of muscle contractions lead to increases in muscle strength including isometric,[47,48] isotonic,[36,46] concentric,[49,50] eccentric,[41,50] isokinetic,[50,51] and plyometric.[52] Human movement is composed of concentric, eccentric, and isometric contractions. Isotonic and isokinetic contractions are dependent on a fixed load or fixed velocity, respectively, that are controlled external to the body and do not often occur outside of a controlled evaluation or treatment situation.

Isometric

An isometric contraction is elicited when the external force placed on the muscle equals the force generated by the muscle and yields no net change in muscle length. For example, isometric contractions are elicited in the trunk musculature to maintain upright posture.

Isotonic Contractions

An isotonic contraction is elicited when a constant load is placed on the muscle and the length of the muscle is not fixed. The load remains the same, but the velocity of muscle shortening changes. For example, concentric or eccentric isotonic contractions may be elicited using free weights in a typical strengthening program.

Concentric Contractions

A concentric contraction results in a net shortening of the muscle as force generated from the muscle fibers exceeds the external force applied to the muscle. Concentric contractions may be isotonic or isokinetic.

Eccentric Contractions

An eccentric contraction results in a net lengthening of the muscle as the external force applied to the muscle exceeds the force generated from muscle fibers. The potential for skeletal muscle soreness is greatest during training that emphasizes eccentric contractions as compared to isometric or concentric contractions.[35,53] Eccentric contractions may be isotonic or isokinetic.

Isokinetic Contractions

An isokinetic contraction occurs under constant velocity with varying torque. Isokinetic contractions may be elicited for purposes of training or evaluation of strength, and may be concentric or eccentric in nature. This type of contraction is performed with an isokinetic dynamometer, which is set at a velocity between 0 and 400°/second.[54] Maximal tension is maintained throughout the ROM as the force applied by the muscle is translated to resistance.[54] Bast and colleagues found that the eccentric isokinetic training group showed a greater increase in peak force and peak torque compared with the combined concentric and eccentric isokinetic training group for training of shoulder abduction in the scapular plane with the humerus internally rotated.[51] This study involved 28 healthy male and female subjects who completed a protocol of 12 sets of 10 repetitions at maximum weight, three times per week for 4 weeks with 30 seconds rest between repetitions.

Plyometric Contractions

A plyometric contraction is elicited when the muscle is placed on stretch before a concentric or shortening contraction.[52] For example, a person may crouch down, placing his or her gastrocnemius and soleus muscles on stretch, before bounding up to a step.

Open-Chain versus Closed-Chain Exercises

Resistance exercises may be performed in either an open-chain or closed-chain[55] environment. An open-chain environment is one in which the distal end of the exercising limb is not in contact with another surface. A closed-chain environment is one in which the distal end of the exercising limb is in contact with another surface, resulting in weight bearing through the limb. Examples of open-chain exercises of the knee are hamstring curls and knee extensions, whereas examples of closed-chain exercises are standing squats or leg presses. Open-chain exercises tend to elicit contraction of a single muscle group and may or may not elicit contraction of the antagonist muscle. Closed-chain exercises tend to elicit cocontraction of agonist and antagonist muscle groups.[56]

Strengthening protocols. The "overload principle," in which the resistance to movement or the frequency or duration of the activity is increased to levels above those normally experienced,[35,46] guides increases in strength and endurance. Strength training may result in physiologic benefits including an increase in bone mass, an increase in connective tissue strength, improvement in cardiorespiratory fitness, reduction in body fat, a reduction in blood pressure, improvement in glucose tolerance, and improvement in blood lipid and lipoprotein profiles.[35] Exercise intensity may be increased or decreased by varying the amount of weight used, the number of repetitions, the number of sets and the length of rest periods. Several authors have proposed protocols for increasing strength.[35,57,58] The ACSM recommends that a minimum of 8–10 separate exercises be performed to target major muscle groups. They recommend a duration of less than 1 hour per session to increase compliance and one set of 8–12 repetitions performed through full ROM to the point of fatigue at least twice per week. Exercises should be performed both eccentrically and concentrically in a slow, controlled manner, maintaining a normal breathing pattern to prevent hyperventilation or hypoventilation.[35]

In 1945, DeLorme proposed that progressive resistance exercise (PRE) be performed at a certain percentage of the 10-repetition maximum (RM).[57] The 10-RM is the amount of load that may be placed on the muscle to allow only 10 repetitions to be performed before muscle fatigue. The 10-RM should be determined for each muscle group being trained and must be re-established once each week. DeLorme also proposed that sessions should be performed daily, not less than three times per week, with the following protocol: 10 repetitions at 50% of the 10-RM, followed by 10 repetitions at 75% 10-RM, then 10 repetitions at 100% 10-RM. Often however, subjects are not able to perform 10 repetitions at 100% 10-RM due to fatigue from the previous submaximal contractions.

The Oxford technique is a training method in which a person performs 10 repetitions each at 100% 10-RM, then 75% 10-RM, and ending at 50% 10-RM.[58] This method has been shown to elicit less fatigue than the DeLorme method. The Oxford technique may be less effective than the DeLorme method, because a certain level of fatigue has been shown to be necessary to achieve training effects.[46]

Circuit weight training is a method of training in which a series of exercises are performed in succession with minimal rest between exercises For example, a series of exercises are performed to strengthen upper extremity muscles, followed by series of exercises to strengthen different muscles groups in the lower body.[35] Taafe and associates achieved training effects in male subjects ranging from 65 to 82 years old after performing a circuit of heavy resistance training three times per week for 14 weeks. The circuit included 10 exercises involving both upper and lower body muscle groups performed for a total of three sets of eight repetitions for each exercise at 75% of 1- RM, which is defined as the maximal load the subject could lift. The 1-RM was re-established every 2 weeks, and training weight was adjusted accordingly.[59]

Yarasheski and associates achieved training effects in 62- to 75-year-old men after a 16-week program of weight-lifting exercises.[60] The exercises were progressed from moderate to high-intensity, including four sets of 4–10 repetitions of each exercise, four times per week at 75–90% 1-RM. The subjects used Nautilus equipment and alternated daily between upper body (biceps curls, shoulder press, deltoid lifts, bench press, latissimus pull downs, arm crosses) and lower body (leg press, knee flexion, knee extension) exercises. Thus, many strengthening regimens have proved to be beneficial, and the most optimal regimen must be determined on an individual basis.

Endurance Training

Endurance may be defined as the ability to maintain a force or effort for a prolonged period of time. Endurance training has several beneficial effects such as improving general fitness, improving cardiovascular condition, and enabling one to sustain a particular activity for an increased period of time in order to perform daily or recreational activities. Any type of endurance training should incorporate a warm-up and a cool-down phase to prevent injury.[35,36]

Aerobic exercise is important to maintain or improve general fitness level. The ability to achieve improved aerobic capacity through endurance training is directly related to the frequency per week, duration per session, and intensity (% VO_2max) of training.[61] The ACSM recommends maintaining an exercise intensity of 60–90% maximum heart rate or 50–85% of VO_2max to achieve a training effect in healthy individuals. Exercises aimed at increasing endurance should last for a duration of 20–60 minutes and have a frequency of 3–5 sessions per week.[61] For deconditioned individuals, a training effect may be achieved with lower exercise intensities of 50–60% maximum heart rate at a minimum exercise duration starting at < 10 minutes three times per week.[35] Aerobic exercise may include use of equipment such as stationary bikes, treadmills, upper extremity ergometers, and free weights. Endurance exercise with free weights consists of lifting weights that are significantly below maximum resistance with a high number of repetitions (e.g., 8–12 repetitions).[35]

EXERCISE PRESCRIPTION

Before prescribing an exercise program, it is important to obtain a good history, including the risk factors for coronary artery disease. ACSM guidelines provide clear indications for exercise testing before starting exercise program.[35]

Intensity of exercise is based on the target heart rate (THR). THR is established usually between 70% and 90% of maximum heart rate (MHR). In patients who are deconditioned, intensity should be less than 70%, and in those who are well conditioned, the starting THR could be greater than 90%.

One method of determining maximum heart rate is 220 minus the patient's age. This method is not recommended in cardiac patients because variability of predicted heart rate is found to be very high. Another commonly used method of determining THR is the Karvonen formula.[35] This formula measures THR as maximum heart rate minus resting heart rate (RHR). The resulting value, called the *heart rate reserve*, is then multiplied by intensity of the exercise and added to the resting heart rate (THR = max HR – rest HR × [0.4 – 0.9] + rest HR). Intensity of the exercise is usually set at 50% of heart rate reserve in patients with known cardiac disease and gradually increased to 90%.[35,62]

Intensity of exercise can also be determined by perceived exertion. A common method that is used is the Borg scale of perceived exertion. In asymptomatic patients, the perceived intensity should be 12–16. In cardiac patients, it should be < 13.[62]

Frequency of exercise should be at least three to four times a week. The duration of exercise is usually 30 minutes or more if the individual is highly trained. This is preceded by 5–10 minutes of warm-up exercises, which may include light aerobic exercise such as walking or bicycling. Following the activity session, there should be cool-down period, which is similar to the warm-up, and this gradually brings the heart rate down to the resting value.[62]

The mode of exercise is often sport related for athletes. There is no best type of exercise to improve cardiovascular fitness for nonathletes. Walking, outside or on a treadmill, and bicycling are a few of the modes commonly prescribed. Addition of resistance strength training in conjunction with aerobic training has been shown to be beneficial in young patients and in patients with heart disease in the absence of congestive heart failure.[62]

The prescription for a specific musculoskeletal condition or neurologic disease needs to be individualized and is based on the specific diagnosis. Some common conditions in which exercises are prescribed are briefly described in the following paragraphs.

Cardiovascular Condition

Exercise is an important part of rehabilitation in patients after any cardiac event, including myocardial infarction, coronary revascularization, valve replacement, and unstable angina. Meta-analysis of 21 randomized, control trials showed a 25% reduction in mortality in patients with known cardiac disease after cardiac rehabilitation during a 3-year follow-up. These studies included other modalities such as dietary modification, beta-blocking agents, and thrombolytic agents. There was a positive correlation between training-induced peak exercise capacity and lower mortality rate suggesting the independent effect of exercise.[11] Supervised exercise training in cardiac patients was found to be extremely safe, with mortality rate of 1 death per 116,00 patients.[11] Exercise in cardiac patients improves exercise tolerance and quality of life. Exercise also decreases the chance of nonfatal myocardial infarction over 5 years (28.5% to 39.9%). Previous studies examining the effect of exercise training on patients with chronic stable angina have reported an increase in anginal threshold and reduction in severity of angina compared to the control group.[11] In patients with ischemic cardiomyopathy, exercise has been shown to decrease dyspnea and fatigue.[11,63]

Immediately following an acute cardiac event, the physical or occupational therapist should see the patient to plan an early exercise program. Exercises requiring 1.2–1.5 METs should be introduced. Frequent, brief sessions, rather than a longer single session, are preferable to avoid fatigue. Patients should be started on a program with 1 minute of exercise followed by a 2-minute rest period and progress as tolerated. Patients who have just had a cardiac event should be started on a phase I exercise program during their inpatient stay. The target heart rate should not exceed 20 points above the resting value (< resting HR + 20). Each session should last 5–10 minutes and should be progressed as tolerated. After discharge, patients should be started on a more intensive phase II exercise program lasting 20 minutes to a maximum of 30 minutes at 60–70% of maximum heart rate. Even though the phase II program is monitored, all patients should undergo exercise tolerance before entering this phase to determine the maximum heart rate. Patients then can advance to a supervised but unmonitored phase III program and subsequently to a community-based unsupervised program (phase IV). It is important to obtain a stress test prior to advancing to a nonmonitored exercise setting.[63a]

Chronic Obstructive Pulmonary Disease

In addition to medications, exercise plays an important part in the rehabilitation of chronic obstructive pulmonary disease (COPD). Poor exercise tolerance in COPD is due to increased flow resistance, poor gas exchange, ventilatory pump impairment, and deconditioning. Mode, frequency, and duration remain the same as for healthy individuals. An increase in resting heart rate due to inhalers is commonly seen in patients with COPD, and use of inhalers should not exclude patients from exercising to their tolerance. Despite high respiratory rate, the ventilatory response to hypoxia and hypercapnia is reduced.[15] Many of these patients are deconditioned, and an exercise program to improve the cardiovascular condition has been shown to improve their functional status and psychological well-being. Many patients attain only 60–70% of the predicted maximum heart rate. Reconditioning exercises are shown to improve pO_2, vital capacity, and FEV_1, even in patients with $FEV_1 < 2$ L. Studies have shown that presence of hypercapnia is not a contraindication to exercise and pCO_2 does not increase with an intensive exercise program.[15] The guideline for exercise is similar as for any deconditioned patients, but gradual increase in the exercise intensity is strongly recommended. Evaluation of pulmonary function test guides the physician to prescribe the exercise program tailored to the patient's needs.

Diabetes

Before prescribing an exercise program, a diabetic patient should undergo a complete physical examination including heart and lung examination, peripheral pulse, and sensation and vision testing. The physical examination and history should focus on signs and symptoms affecting the heart, blood vessels, kidneys, eyes, and nervous system. It is important to check the glucose level before and after exercise in diabetic patients until the glucose levels are stable for two or three consecutive exercise sessions. Hormonally mediated mobilization of glucose is lost in diabetic individuals. In type 1 diabetics, mobilization of glucose in the absence of insulin production may produce hyperglycemia. Exogenous administration of insulin in these patients may increase insulin availability during exercise, and hypoglycemia may ensue. Self-monitored blood glucose data and adjustment of insulin and intensity of exercise among these individuals are recommended.[33] Many studies have proved the beneficial effects of exercise in type 2 diabetes in glycemic control and prevention of cardiovascular disease, hyperlipidemia, and obesity. Improvement of hemoglobin A1C was noted in diabetic patients who were involved in a exercise program three to four times a week compared with control subjects.[33]

Diabetic patients with known coronary artery disease should undergo an exercise stress test. Any symptoms of peripheral vascular disease need to be noted. Patients should have proper footwear to prevent skin irritation in the feet during impact exercise such as treadmill walking or jogging.

It is important to remember that presence of autonomic neuropathy may limit the individual's capacity during exercise and increases the risk of adverse cardiovascular event during exercise. Resting tachycardia (> 100/min), orthostasis, or other disturbances of autonomic function involving skin, pupil, gastrointestinal system, and genitourinary system indicate presence of autonomic neuropathy.

Hypotension and hypertension after vigorous exercises are more common in patients with autonomic neuropathy. Because these individuals have difficulty with thermoregulation, they should not exercise in a hot or cold environment and should be more attentive to adequate hydration. An exercise tolerance test or thallium stress test may be performed in these patients prior to exercise prescription.[33]

Psychiatric Conditions

Many psychiatric disorders are associated with psychomotor retardation. Exercise prescription is based on age and other comorbid conditions. Aerobic conditioning exercises are commonly prescribed for this population. Many psychiatric patients are nonexercisers. The prescription should start at 40–50% of heart rate reserve and increase gradually to 60–70%. Exercise is an important aspect of treatment in chronic fatigue syndrome. Improvement in cognitive function and sleep patterns was noted in patients with chronic fatigue syndrome.[25,27]

Neurologic Disorders

Exercise is an important treatment modality for patients with various neurologic disorders including stroke, Parkinson's disease, and multiple sclerosis. During the initial recovery period of stroke, patients receive passive ROM. This is followed by strengthening exercise and incorporation of various neuromuscular facilitation techniques (e.g., Bobath, proprioceptive neuromuscular facilitation, Rood technique). The exercise prescription for Parkinson's disease patients includes strengthening, ROM exercises, and flexibility exercises. Exercises for multiple sclerosis depend on the stage of the disease. A combination of strengthening, ROM, and aerobic exercises are prescribed for these patients.[64]

Peripheral Vascular Disease

One of the nonsurgical approaches to peripheral vascular disease (PVD) involves progressive walking exercise.[65] Exercise programs that had patients walk to the near maximum tolerable claudication pain had better improvement of symptoms compared with those that had patients walk to the onset of claudication symptoms. The ischemia produced within the muscles presumably caused better metabolic and hemodynamic adaptations resulting in improvement in pain symptoms. The other important factors are the length of the program and mode of exercise. Programs that lasted 6 months and that involved walking had better improvement of symptoms compared with those that had a variety of physical activities.[65]

In a randomized study, 19 patients reported 125% increase in treadmill walking time. The initial intensity of exercise should match the onset of claudication symptoms. The client should start treadmill walking at a speed and grade that they can tolerate for 3–5 minutes. After the individual can walk at this baseline value for 10 minutes or longer, the speed and grade are gradually increased to the point of maximum or moderate pain tolerance. If he or she is able to walk at only at a speed less than 2 mph, the speed is increased before increasing the grade. Each session should last for 40–50 minutes with rest periods interspersed with periods of treadmill walking. After each exercise session, the condition of the skin should be checked.[66]

Musculoskeletal Conditions

Exercises are prescribed for many arthritic conditions. Light aerobic exercises are beneficial in patients with rheumatoid arthritis. One study of patients with rheumatoid arthritis (RA) involved a gentle dance exercise program without weight bearing or impact exercise.[67] The patients' subjective parameters showed improvement, and there was no increase in pain. Stationary bicycle and water aerobic exercises are also prescribed for these patients. Intense physical exercises and weight-bearing exercises are not commonly prescribed for patients with arthritis. In patients with RA, vigorous physical hand exercise has been shown to enhance the radiographic changes in small joints. In patients with acute joint involvement, isometric exercises are prescribed to maintain muscle strength without causing painful movement of the joint.[67]

Many orthopedic spinal conditions benefit from exercise. Williams flexion exercises help strengthen the abdominal muscles that help support the spinal column. This is a common exercise prescribed for patients with mechanical low back pain. McKenzie extension exercises help alter the forces on the disc, which helps to reduce radicular symptoms and centralize the pain. Patients with ankylosing spondylosis are prescribed spinal extension exercises and postural exercises to help maintain the correct posture as long as possible.

The contributory effect of vigorous weight-bearing exercises and heavy work as a causative factor for osteoarthritis is not well studied. A few controlled studies showed that recreational exercises within the limits of comfort do not lead to development of osteoarthritis.[68]

Obesity

Fat reduction is accomplished by prolonged aerobic exercise using as many muscle groups as possible. Examples of such exercises include walking, jogging, bicycling, and rowing. Previous studies have shown that substantial weight change did not occur until the patients exercised 60 minutes, and there was no change in weight when they exercised 30 minutes everyday. Gwinup noted that swimming in an unheated swimming pool caused slight weight gain, which is thought to be the protective effect of cold water.[68a] The study suggested that a regimen of swimming without dietary restrictions is not effective for weight reduction. The amount of fat burned depends on the intensity of exercise. Ideally the target heart rate should stay at 75% of age-predicted maximum heart rate.

Prolonged exercise at a lower intensity is more effective than shorter exercise at a higher intensity. For example, bicycling at 50 W for 60 minute is more effective than 30 minutes bicycling at 100 W. It is also recommended that the client exercise for 60 minutes, 7 days a week. Low-repetition, high-resistance exercise, which is common for strength training, is rarely associated with fat reduction. In brief bursts of exercise, carbohydrate is burned rather than fat. This increases hunger, which may cause weight gain.[69]

Exercise for the Geriatric Population

More than 12% of the United States population is 65 years old or older, representing approximately one third of patients seen by primary care physicians.[70]

Muscle mass reaches peak values by age 25–30 years and declines 25–30% by age 65 years. This decline in muscle mass is attributed to a combination of reduced physical activity and age-related changes to skeletal muscle.[52] Exercise training may be aimed at delaying or reversing this decrease in muscle mass to the point that the person may perform at a higher functional level or simply be able to perform activities of daily living.[71] For example, master athletes have been shown to maintain lean body mass well into their 70s.[72] The same training effects that are observed in young or middle-aged individuals are found in the elderly population. However, the effects may take place at a slower rate.

Several studies have outlined different exercise parameters that have proved beneficial for elderly individuals. McMurdo and Rennie found that quadriceps strength increased in elderly individuals after a 45-minute session (10-minute warm-up, 25 minutes of isometric exercises, and a 10-minute cool-down period) set to music two times per week for 6 months.[47] Rogind and colleagues found that isokinetic, isometric strength, and walking speed improved after a 3- month exercise program of general lower extremity therapeutic exercises performed two times per week in the clinic and four times per week as a home exercise program.[73] Results of a study by Sagiv and associates found that older adults should not be prescribed weight-lifting intensity greater than 30% 1-RM.[74]

Aerobic capacity in elderly individuals may fall below the level necessary for performance of daily activities, which may significantly impair their functional ability. Several studies have demonstrated gains of about 20% in VO_2max,[75,76] increased cardiac output, and increased stroke volume after 4–6 months of low- to moderate-endurance exercise programs.[52] Another benefit of regular exercise is the significant role exercise plays in the prevention of osteoporosis.[77,78]

When prescribing exercise for the elderly, exercise stress testing is helpful if the person has any cardiac history or if the person is considered to be at a high risk for complications. ACSM recommends that cardiac screening be completed before the initiation of high-intensity exercise; this is not necessary for moderate-intensity exercise such as brisk walking.[35] Swimming and walking are commonly prescribed exercise modes. The target heart rate is best determined by exercise stress testing because of the potential confounding illnesses, medication effects, or impairments with which the person may present; however, use of relative perceived exertion scales may be more appropriate. Exercise prescription for the elderly population often proves challenging owing to the common medical problems of arthritis, cardiac involvement, osteoporosis, impaired vision, impaired balance, and diabetes. In general, exercise prescription for the elderly population should include slow progression of intensity and duration, slow and careful warm-ups, slow cool-down before showering until heart rate is below 100, and static stretching to maintain adequate flexibility.[79]

Exercises for Pediatric Clients

Obesity is a common problem among children in United States. Obesity is directly correlated with lack of exercise and physical activities. There are no special guidelines for exercise prescription other than encouragement for daily exercise participation. Exercise has been shown to reduce levels of low-density lipoprotein even in preadolescent children. Risk prevention of coronary heart disease, high blood pressure, and hyperlipidemia should start from childhood with the incorporation of a routine exercise program in their daily life.[80]

NEGATIVE EFFECTS OF EXERCISE

The negative psychological effects of exercise are seen in habitual exercisers. Mood disturbances, restlessness, anxiety, irritability and increased sleep disturbance can occur 24–48 hours after exercise deprivation. A correlation has been established between compulsive running and anorexia nervosa.[81]

Exercise-related transient abdominal pain (ETAP), commonly referred to as a "stitch," causes sharp cramping abdominal pain mainly in the right or left lumbar region. The suggested etiology for this include diaphragmatic ischemia, stress on the visceral ligaments, and irritation of parietal peritoneum. This is usually a self-limiting disease and improves after stopping the exercise.[82]

Exercise-induced urticaria and anaphylaxis have been recognized in the past two decades. Mast cell activation during exercise is thought to be the etiology of these conditions. Use of antihistamine before exercise is recommended in these patients.[83]

All health care personnel should be aware of the occurrence of sudden death after vigorous physical activity. Exercise-related cardiac death has been reported to be 5.4 deaths per 100,000 individuals. Possible causes of death include atherosclerotic plaque rupture, coronary artery spasm in the disease segments of the coronary arteries, and catecholamine-induced platelet aggregation. Graded exercise testing before starting a vigorous exercise program in high-risk individuals (men > 40 years and women > 50 years, individuals with more than one coronary risk factors, and those with known coronary artery disease) helps prevent such untoward outcomes.[35]

REIMBURSEMENT

Physicians, physical therapists, and occupational therapists may prescribe therapeutic exercise. A physician's referral is required for a client to gain access to physical or occupational therapists in most states; however, some states permit direct access to physical therapists (i.e., without a physician referral), which offsets the cost of physicians' fees. Cost of services provided may be reflective of the overhead cost, but most physicians and therapists base their fees on the Medicare resource-based relative value scale (RBRVS). The RBRVS uses geographic location, practice and malpractice costs, nationally uniform relative value units, and a nationally uniform conversion factor to calculate an allowed amount for each **current procedural terminology** (CPT) code.[84] Reimbursement may be obtained through health-care plans such as managed care, fee-for-service, Medicare, or MediCal. Most physicians and therapists in outpatient settings, including rehabilitation agencies, CORFs, outpatient services to residents in skilled nursing facilities, hospital outpatient services, and outpatient services to non–home-bound care clients, bill using CPT codes based on the RBRVS. Documentation must be present in the client's chart to justify the procedural code that is billed. Specific payors may have different requirements for coding and billing procedures.

Treatment is billed in units of time with each unit averaging 15 minutes in length. As of April 1, 2000, the Health Care Financing Administration defined one unit as at least 8 minutes but not greater than 23 minutes with each additional unit representing another 15-minute interval. If more than one client is seen by one therapist within the same unit of time, a group therapy code must be used. For example, a physical therapist who supervised or instructed a client in a therapeutic exercise regimen for 30 minutes would bill the following: 2 units of therapeutic exercises (CPT code: 97110). In Los Angeles, during April, 2000, this therapist would be reimbursed at a rate of $25.46 per unit for a total of $50.92 for the treatment session. If two clients were seen during the same unit of time, the physical therapist would bill for 2 units of group therapeutic procedures (CPT code: 97150). This physical therapist would be reimbursed at a rate of $21.15 per unit for a total of $42.30 for the treatment session. In Alabama, during the year 2000, the physical therapist would be reimbursed $22.18 per unit of therapeutic exercise. Therefore, each provider of therapeutic exercise should be mindful that CPT codes and cost of services are constantly changing and differ regionally. In addition, different payors often have different coding systems for services rendered. Contact the appropriate intermediary or carrier for specific questions.

REFERENCES

1. Moldavar JR, Borg-Stein: Exercise and fatigue. In Downey J (ed): The Physiological Basis of Rehabilitation Medicine. Boston, Butterworth-Heinemann, 1994, pp 393–409.
2. Myers J, Ashley E: Dangerous curves: A perspective on exercise, lactate and anaerobic threshold. Chest 111:787–795, 1997.
3. Joynt RL: Therapeutic exercise. In DeLisa JA (ed): Rehabilitation Medicine: Principles and Practice. Philadelphia, J.B. Lippincott, 1988, pp 346–371.
4. Vissing SF, Scherer U, Victor RG: Stimulation of skin sympathetic nerve discharge by central command: Differential control of sympathetic flow. Circulation 69:228–238, 1991.
5. Mark AL, Victor RG, Nerhed G, Wallin BG: Microneurographic studies of the mechanism of sympathetic nerve responses to static exercise in humans. Circulation 57:461–469, 1985.
6. Sinoway LI, Smith MB, Enders B, et al: Role of diprotonated phosphate in evoking muscle reflex response in cats and humans. Am J Physiol 267:H770–H778, 1994.
7. DeLateur JB: Strength and local muscle endurance. Phys Med Rehabil Clin North Am 5:269–289, 1994.
8. van Nieuwenhoven MA, Brouns F, Brummer RJ: The effect of physical exercise on parameters of gastrointestinal function. Neurogastroenterol Motil 11:431–439, 1999.
9. Moses FM: The effect of exercise on the gastrointestinal tract. Sports Med 9:159–72, 1990.
10. Brouns F, Beckers E: Is the gut an athletic organ? Digestion, absorption and exercise. Sports Med 15:242–257, 1993.
11. Ades P, Coello CE: Effects of exercise and cardiac rehabilitation on cardiovascular outcomes: Risk factor modification for cardiac disease. Med Clin North Am 84:245–261, 2000.
12. Higashi Y, Sasaki S, Kurisu S, at al: Regular aerobic exercise augments endothelium-dependent vascular relaxation in normotensive as well as hypertensive subjects: Role of endothelium derived nitric oxide. Circulation 100:194–202, 1999
13. Kelley GA, Kelley KS: Progressive resistance exercise and resting blood pressure: A meta-analysis of randomized controlled trials. Hypertension 35:838–843, 2000.
14. Cole CR, Blackstone EH, Pashkow FJ, et al: Heart rate recovery immediately after exercise as a predictor of mortality. N Engl J Med 341:1351–1371, 1999.
15. Rondinelli RD, Hill NS: Rehabilitation of the patient with pulmonary disease. In DeLisa JA (ed): Rehabilitation Medicine: Principles and Practice. Philadelphia, J.B. Lippincott, 1988, pp 688–707.
16. Johnson BD, Weisman IM, Zeballos RJ: Emerging concepts in the evaluation of ventilatory limitation: The exercise tidal volume loop. Chest 11:488–503, 1999.
17. Middlekauff HR, Nitzche FU, Alison H, et al: Modulation of renal cortical blood flow during static exercise in humans. Circ Res 80:62–68, 1997.

18. Middlekauff HR, Nitzche FU, Hoh C, et al: Exaggerated renal vasoconstriction during exercise in heart failure patients. Circulation 101:784–795, 2000.
19. Kenny WL, Zappe DH: Effect of age on renal blood flow during exercise. Aging 6:293–302, 1994.
20. Walker RJ, Fawcett JP, Flannery FM, Gerrard DF: Indomethacin potentiates exercise-induced reduction in renal hemodynamics in athletes. Med Sci Sports Exerc 26:1302–1306, 1994.
21. Chen EC, Brzyski RG: Exercise and reproductive dysfunction. Fertil Steril 71:1–6, 1999.
22. Warren MP, Steihl AL: Exercise and female adolescent. JAMA 54:115–120, 1999.
23. Lewis TV, Dart AM, Chin-Dusting JPF, Kingwell BA: Exercise training increases basal nitric oxide production from the forearm of hypercholesterolemic patients. Arterioscler Thromb Vasc Biol 19:2782–2787, 1999.
24. Hambrecht R, Wolf A, Gielen S, et al: Effect of exercise on coronary endothelial function in patients with coronary artery disease. N Engl J Med 342:454–460, 2000.
25. Blumenthal JA, Babyak MA, Moore KA, et al: Effects of exercise on older patients with major depression. Arch Intern Med 159:2349–2356, 1999.
26. Perrig-Chiello P, Perrig WJ, Ehrsam R, et al: The effects of resistance training on well-being and memory in elderly volunteers. Age Ageing 27:469–475, 1998.
27. Lane, RJM, Burgess AP, Flint J, et al: Exercise responsiveness and psychiatric disorder in chronic fatigue syndrome. BMJ 311:544–546, 1995.
28. Lund T, Kvernmo HD, Osterud B: Cellular activation in response to physical exercise: The effect of platelets and granulocytes on monocyte activity. Blood Coagul Fibrinolysis 9:63–69, 1998.
29. Wallen NH, Goodall AH, Li N, Hjemdahl P: Activation of haemostasis by exercise, mental stress and adrenaline: Effects on platelet sensitivity to thrombin and thrombin generation. Clin Sci 97:27–35, 1999.
30. Wang JS, Jen CJ, Kung HC, et al: Different effects of strenuous exercise and moderate exercise on platelet function in men. Circulation 90:2877–2885, 1994.
31. Yamada M, Suzuki K, Kudo S, et al: Effect of exhaustive exercise on human neutrophils in athletes. Luminescence 15:15–20, 2000.
32. Hargreaves M: Interaction between muscle glycogen and blood glucose during exercise. Exerc Sports Sci Rev 25:21–39, 1997.
33. Zinman B, Ruderman N, Campaigne BC, et al: Diabetes melllitus and exercise. Diabetic Care 20:1908–1912, 1997.
34. Crawford GNC, James NT: The design of muscles. In Owen R, Goodfellow J, Bullough P (eds): Scientific Foundations of Orthopedics and Traumatology. London, William Heinemann, 1980, pp 67–74.
35. ACSM's Guidelines for Exercise Testing and Prescription, 6th ed. Baltimore, Lippincott Williams & Wilkins, 2000.
36. Kisner CK, Colby LA: Therapeutic Exercise: Foundations and Techniques, 2nd ed. Philadelphia, F.A. Davis, 1990, pp 19–22, 49–50, 56–58, 68–72, 120–124.
37. Hepburn G, Crivelli, K: Use of elbow Dynasplint for reduction of elbow flexion contracture: A case study. J Orthop Sports Phys Ther 5:269, 1984.
38. Condon SN, Hutton RS: Soleus muscle electromyographic activity and ankle dorsiflexion range of motion during four stretching procedures. Phys Ther 67:24, 1987.
39. Bridger RS, Orkin D, Henneberg M: A quantitative investigation of lumbar and pelvic postures in standing and sitting: Interrelationships with body position and hip muscle length. Int J Industr Ergonom 9:235–244, 1992.
40. Li Y, McClure PW, Pratt N: The effect of hamstring muscle stretching on standing posture and on lumbar and hip motions during forward bending. Phys Ther 76:836–849, 1996.
41. Johansson PH, Lindstrom L, Sundelin G, Lindstrom B: The effects of pre-exercise stretching on muscular soreness, tenderness and force loss following heavy eccentric exercise. Scand J Med Sci Sports 9:219–225, 1999.
42. Lund H, Vestergaard-Poulsen P, Kanstrup IL, Sejrsen P: The effect of passive stretching on delayed onset muscle soreness and other detrimental effects following eccentric exercise. Scand J Med Sci Sports 8:216–221, 1998.
43. Pope RP, Herbert RD, Kirwan JD, Graham BJ: A randomized trial of pre-exercise stretching for prevention of lower-limb injury. Med Sci Sports Exerc 32:271–277, 2000.
44. Halbertsma JPK, Goeken LNH: Stretching exercises: Effect on passive extensibility and stiffness in short hamstrings of healthy subjects. Arch Phys Med Rehabil 75:976–981, 1994.

45. Gose J: Continuous passive motion in the postoperative treatment of patients with total knee replacement. Phys Ther 67:39, 1987.
46. de Lateur BJ: Strength and local muscle endurance. Phys Med Rehabil Clin North Am 5:284, 304–306, 1994.
47. McMurdo MET, Rennie LM: Improvements in quadriceps strength with regular seated exercise in the institutionalized elderly. Arch Phys Med Rehabil 75:600–603, 1994.
48. Carroll TJ, Abernathy PJ, Logan PA, et al: Resistance training frequency: Strength and myosin heavy chain responses to two and three bouts per week. Eur J Appl Physiol 78:270–275, 1998.
49. Neder JA, Nery LE, Shinzato GT, et al: Reference values for concentric knee isokinetic strength and power in nonathletic men and women from 20–80 years old. J Orthop Sports Phys Ther 29:116–126, 1999.
50. Wu Y, Li RCT, Maffulli N, et al: Relationship between isokinetic concentric and eccentric contraction modes in the knee flexor and extensor muscle groups. J Orthop Sports Phys Ther 26:143–149, 1997.
51. Bast SC, Vangsness CT, Takemura J, et al: The effects of concentric versus eccentric isokinetic strength training of the rotator cuff in the plane of the scapula at various speeds. Bull Hosp Jt Dis 57:139–144, 1998.
52. Brooks GA, Fahey TD, White TP: Exercise physiology: Human bioenergetics and its applications, 2nd ed. Mountain View, CA, Mayfield Publishing Company, 1996.
53. Evans WJ: Exercise induced skeletal muscle damage. Phys Sport Med 15:89, 1987.
54. Esselman PC, Lacerte M: Principles of isokinetic exercise. Phys Med Rehabil Clin North Am 5:256, 1994.
55. Davies GJ, Heiderscheit BC: Reliability of the Lido Linea closed kinetic chain dynamometer. J Orthop Sports Phys Ther 25:133–136, 1997.
56. Ohkoshi Y, Kazunori K, Kaneda K, et al: Biomechanical analysis of rehabilitation in the standing position. Am J Sports Med 19:605, 1991.
57. DeLorme TL: Restoration of muscle power by heavy-resistance exercise. J Bone Joint Surg 27:645, 1945.
58. Zinovieff AN: Heavy resistance exercises. The Oxford technique. Br J Phys Med 14:129–132, 1951.
59. Taafe DR, Pruitt L, Reim J, et al: Effect of recombinant human growth hormone on the muscle strength to resistance exercise in elderly men. J Clin Endocrinol Metab 79:1361–1366, 1994.
60. Yarahevski KE, Zachwieja JJ, Campell JA, Bier DM: Effect of growth hormone and resistance exercise on muscle growth and strength in older men. Am J Physiol 268:E268–E276, 1995.
61. American College of Sports Medicine: The recommended quantity and quality of exercise for developing and maintaining cardio respiratory and muscular fitness in healthy adults. Med Sci Sports Exerc 22:265, 1990.
62. Fardy P, Yanowitz FG: Exercise prescription. In Pine JW (ed): Cardiac Rehabilitation, Adult Fitness and Testing. Baltimore, Williams & Wilkins, 1993, pp 245–260.
63. McGowan GA, Murali S, Loftus S, Uretsky B: Comparison of metabolic, ventilatory, and neurohormonal responses during light forearm isometric exercises and isotonic exercise in congestive heart failure. Am J Cardiol 77:391–396, 1996.
63a. Brammel HL: Rehabilitation of the cardiac patients. In DeLisa JA (ed): Rehabilitation Medicine Principles and practice. Philadelphia, JB Lippincott Publishing, 1988, pp 671–687.
64. Kumar R, Broadbent S: Therapeutic exercise in neurological disorders. In Shankar K (ed): Exercise Prescription. Philadelphia, Hanley & Belfus, 1998, pp 677–689.
65. Gardner AW, Poehlman ET: Exercise rehabilitation programs for the treatment of claudication pain: Meta-analysis. JAMA 274:975–980, 1995.
66. Hiatt WR, Regensteiner JG: Nonsurgical management of peripheral arterial disease. Hosp Pract 28:59–81, 1993.
67. van den Ende CH, Hazes JM, Le Cessie S, et al: Comparison of high and low intensity training in well controlled rheumatoid arthritis. Results of a randomized clinical trial. Ann Rheum Dis 55:798–805, 1996.
68. Panush S: Does exercise cause arthritis? Long term consequences of exercise on musculoskeletal system. Rheum Dis Clin North Am 16:389–395, 1990.
69. de Lateur BJ: Application of exercise to fat reduction. Phys Med Rehabil Clin North Am 5:309–316, 1994.

70. Kane RL, Ouslander JG, Abrass IB: Essentials of Clinical Geriatrics, 3rd ed. New York, McGraw-Hill, 1994, p 21.
71. Wagner EH, LaCroix AZ, Buchner DM: Effects of physical activity on health status in older adults: Observational studies. Annu Rev Public Health 13:451, 1992.
72. Kavanagh T, Shepard RJ: Can regular sports participation slow the aging process? Data on masters athletes. Phys Sports Med 18:94–104, 1990.
73. Rogind H, Bibow-Nielsen B, Jensen B, et al: The effects of a physical training program on patients with osteoarthritis of the knees. Arch Phys Med Rehabil 79:1421–1427, 1998.
74. Sagiv M, Fisher N, Yaniv A, et al: Effect of running versus isometric training programs on healthy elderly at rest. Gerontology 35:72, 1989.
75. Belman MJ, Gaesser GA: Exercise training below and above the lactate threshold in the elderly. Med Sci Sports Exerc 23:562, 1991.
76. Posner JD, Gorman DK, Windsor-Landsberg L, et al: Low to moderate intensity endurance training in healthy older adults: Physiological responses after 4 months. J Am Geriatr Soc 40:1, 1992.
77. US Preventive Services Task Force: Exercise Counseling. Guide to Clinical Preventive Services. An Assessment of the Effectiveness of 169 Interventions. Baltimore, Williams & Wilkins, 1989, p 297.
78. Smith EL, Reddan W, Smith PE: Physical activity and calcium modalities for bone mineral increase in aged women. Med Sci Sports Exerc 12:60, 1981.
79. DeVries H: Tips on prescribing exercise regimens for your older patients. Geriatrics 35:75–81, 1979.
80. Craig SB, Bandini LG, Lichtenstein AH, et al: Impact of physical activity on lipids, lipoproteins and blood pressure in preadolescent girls. Pediatrics 98:389–395, 1996.
81. Mondin GW, Morgan WP, Piering PN, et al: Psychological consequences of exercise deprivation in habitual exercisers. Med Sci Sports Exerc 28:199–203, 1996.
82. Morton DP, Callister R: Characteristics and etiology of exercise related transient abdominal pain. Med Sci Sports Exerc 32:432–438, 2000.
83. Volcheck GW, Li JT: Exercise induced urticaria and anaphylaxis. Mayo Clin Proc 72:140–147, 1999.
84. Coding and Payment Guide for the Physical Therapist: An Essential Coding, Billing, and Reimbursement Resource for the Physical Therapist. Reston, VA, Ingenix Publishing, 1999.

Chapter 11
Massage Therapy

Sanjiv Jain, MD

Massage has been used as a therapeutic intervention for thousands of years. There are specific references in various texts written in different languages in different countries and at different times. References in the literature from China and India appear to be the oldest.[1] The *Yellow Emperor's Classic of Internal Medicine*, which dates back to 2500 B.C., discussed the use of therapeutic massage.[2,3] The *Ayurveda*, the oldest known medical writing in India, dates to around 1500–1200 B.C. and references the use of massage.[4,5] Ancient Greek and Roman writings by Hippocrates, Plato, Socrates, and Aschepiades also reference massage, or "rubbing," as an important therapeutic intervention (500–300 B.C.).[5] In the last 200 years, one of the most influential people in the development of massage is Per Henrick Ling (1776–1839) a Swedish teacher of physical education. He adapted French terms (*effleurage, petrissage*, and *tapotement*) to describe various common massage strokes. He developed a system of "medical gymnastics" that has become known as Swedish massage.[4] The Royal Institute of Gymnastics was established in Stockholm, Sweden, in 1813 with additional centers following in Europe and subsequently in New York in 1916. Other notables include Lucas-Championniere (1843–1913), who advocated the use of massage in the management of fractures as an adjunctive treatment.[2] Elizabeth Dicke found that deep massage over one part of the body had observable effects on distal body parts and called this approach "reflex zone massage," or *Bindegeswebmassages*. In England, Cyriax and Menell used friction massage in very specific areas of acute and chronic injury to promote healing.[1]

Massage as an intervention can be defined broadly, and, depending on your definition, it can encompass a variety of interventions, some of which are covered elsewhere in this text. Massage is typically understood as a treatment that involves a practitioner physically "laying hands on" (touching) a patient and moving his or her hands to move or manipulate the patient's soft tissues. Several different factors can further classify this intervention, including the amount of pressure administered, the rate and rhythm of the movement, the direction the stroke travels, the part of the practitioner's body that is used, whether the patient's limb or joint is moved through space, and the duration of the massage. Different combinations of these factors can describe different types of strokes within a type of massage as well as altogether different types of massages. As broad as this definition is, it is still incomplete because it includes only treatment administered by direct human touch. Devices can be used to mimic or enhance treatment delivered by the hands that may be considered massage therapy. Examples include pneumatic compression devices used in deep venous thrombosis prevention, vibratory tools, and ultrasound. This chapter will focus only on "hands on" treatment interventions.

In the rush to embrace all things scientific (modern medicine), many less serious ailments of the human body and mind often are not adequately addressed or are overlooked altogether. The understanding that "alternative" treatments such as massage and acupuncture have a track record of use spanning centuries (or even millennia) is now beginning to emerge. Most treatments that do not have a basis in modern science are associated in some way with claims that they can treat virtually any illness, regardless of how serious. However, these dubious claims should not be used to rule out all the benefits a modality such as massage does have. This is where our skeptical, scientific mind is useful in differentiating likely benefits from the highly improbable or impossible.

Using the scientific method, controlled and uncontrolled studies are now helping to support and define the utility of massage therapy. These studies attempt to find likely benefits of massage, although inadequacies in outcome measurement can make it difficult to find and prove benefit where some actually exists. Similarly, overinterpreting results by assigning benefits to massage when they may be due to confounding factors also poses a potential problem. Limitations of many studies on massage therapy include small sample size, lack of a control group, selection bias concerns, poorly defined massage technique and duration, and lack of rigorous statistical analysis. Confounding factors that are difficult to control include the attention and time of the therapist (being the important factor rather than the actual massage itself), the patient's expectation of benefit, the difficulty in performing true double-blind studies (in active hands-on treatment), and the potential differences in the therapist's skill that may lead to different outcomes. Nonetheless some general beneficial effects of massage therapy can be put forth.

Massage therapy has been used throughout history to reduce pain and discomfort. The benefits of decreasing anxiety, promoting relaxation, and decreasing stress are also well supported. Numerous other uses have been advocated including increasing flexibility, decreasing muscle tension, improving circulation, improving immune function, enhancing growth and development, decreasing swelling, and enhancing overall function and health.[1,2,6]

MECHANISM OF ACTION

The mechanisms by which massage therapy achieves its effects are still unknown, although different theories exist and the mechanism of action is likely to be multifactorial. Mechanical effects produced by massage are related to the physical pressure on the specific area massaged. This includes stretching and mobilizing muscle fibers, which may physically release adhesions by shear force and thus increase flexibility. The compression of soft tissues and blood vessels may lead to pushing fluid out of the massaged area, thereby decreasing edema and promoting improved circulation. Vibration of soft tissues may lead to loosening mucus in congested airways, improving flow of thick secretions. Activation of peripheral sensory receptors may modulate the perception of pain through the gate control theory of Melzack and Wall.[7] The activation of deep mechanoreceptors in deep tissue or muscle may diminish the H-reflex and contribute to decreasing tone and spasticity in muscle.[8] Other potential mechanical effects include physically stimulating cells. For example, mast cells may be physically stimulated to release histamine, causing the triple response of redness, flare, and wheal formation.

Reflexive responses are related to obtaining an effect at a site distant to the site of massage as well as causing central effects such as increased relaxation that have been clearly noted but are difficult to explain. Manipulation of the parasympathetic and autonomic nervous systems, the release of neurohumeral factors, and the stimulation of Golgi tendon organs are just some possibilities, none of which have been clearly supported. The theory behind Eastern massage holds that the application of pressure along certain paths of energy flow is beneficial and that manipulating that flow of energy will return the body to a state of energy balance and, thus, normal health. Obviously, the physical presence and contact between therapist and patient also create potentially powerful effects by way of the mind–body connection. The patient may feel increased attention, closeness, security, trust, and caring from the therapist that, in turn, affects the physical response to massage therapy.

Although some research has attempted to delineate the physiologic mechanism by which massage elicits its effect, the primary focus in this review of the literature is the use of massage in clinical situations. Massage, especially in more recent literature, has been examined in clinical settings with attempts made to provide for controls, consistency in massage techniques, and more comparable outcome analysis. This chapter focuses on areas of research that include massage in growth and development (of infants), massage in pain and palliative care, massage in pulmonary and critical care, massage in lymphedema management, massage in pregnancy, and massage in various other clinical conditions.

RESEARCH AND MASSAGE THERAPY

The amount of research conducted in the area of massage is steadily increasing and becoming more sophisticated. Evaluating and documenting effectiveness in terms of parameters that are difficult to quantify (though important), such as relaxation, anxiety, and stress, as well as in more objective terms, such as hormone levels, weight gain, and blood pressure, are being pursued. Research concerning massage therapy typically has limitations, as noted earlier, however significant effort has been made to address some of these potential problems in this literature.

Infant Massage

There is considerable literature concerning the benefit of massage in preterm and full-term infant development. In a study of preterm infants treated in a neonatal intensive care unit, the effect of massage therapy can be seen clearly.[6] The infants were massaged through portholes in incubators for 14 minutes three times per day for 10 days. Treated (massaged) infants gained 47% more weight than control (unmassaged) infants, and norepinephrine and epinephrine levels increased. Massaged infants were also hospitalized for an average of 6 days less, resulting in a significant savings in cost per infant. Relative gains were noted on the Brazelton Neonatal Behavioral Assessment Scale. Persistent gains in weight and on motor and mental functioning scales (Bayley Scales of Infant Development) were noted after 1 year. The early improvements may have allowed more early and active stimulation from caregivers that lead to the sustained gains. Similar results have been obtained in various studies with surprisingly consistent amounts of weight gain (31–47%).[9–13]

Studies of infants exposed to cocaine and HIV have also demonstrated significant improvements in weight gain for massaged infants. Moreover, the additional benefits of decreasing anxiety in parents and perhaps improving parent–infant bonding are noted as well.[14] Expanding this concept to full term infants without concomitant medical problems continues to demonstrate relative benefits of massage. The results in this group are less dramatic, but the ability to quantify subjective improvement also makes it difficult to demonstrate benefits. In one study, full-term infants were either massaged or rocked for 15 minutes an average of 12 times over a 6-week period. During sessions, infants seemed to be more alert, cry less, and have lower salivary cortisol levels. Longer term effects after the 6-week study were also suggested (including more weight gain, improved "soothability," decreased stress hormones), although more research is needed to support and verify these results.[15]

Pain and Cancer Treatment

The use of massage in the settings of pain management and palliative care is quite common. Decreased anxiety and stress are cited as benefits of massage in these groups of patients. Studies attempting to support this benefit are becoming more commonplace. A study by Wilkinson of 103 patients receiving palliative care demonstrated decreased anxiety, improved quality of life, and improved psychological measures with massage therapy and with massage coupled with aromatherapy.[16]

Ashles et al. examined the effects of massage therapy on patients undergoing autologous bone marrow transplants.[17] Patients receiving 20-minute massages of the shoulder, head, and neck were compared to standard (no massage) treatment. Immediate effects of the treated group included significantly decreased distress, fatigue, nausea, and anxiety, with persistent improvement only in the amount of fatigue by the predischarge session.

An evaluation of the effect of massage and exercise combined with and without ultrasound was examined (compared with a control group) in the treatment of myofascial trigger points.[18] The massage and exercise groups demonstrated a decrease in the number and intensity of trigger points compared with the control group. Of note, however, was that the patients' complaints of neck and shoulder pain remained similar to the control group.

The use of massage in back pain is a common practice. However, as with many treatments for back pain, demonstrating efficacy is difficult. Ernst performed a systematic review of the literature on massage therapy for back pain and concluded that too few trials existed for a reliable evaluation of its efficacy, although he noted after his review that massage may have some potential as a therapy for low back pain.[19]

Pulmonary and Critical Care

An interesting study by Hayes took advantage of the intensive monitoring already in place of critically ill patients in intensive care units (ICUs).[20] Twenty-five ICU patients (68 sessions) received 5-minute foot massages. Significant reductions in heart rate, blood pressure, and respiratory rate were noted during the massage.

A study of the effects of back massage on promoting sleep was conducted with 69 patients in a hospital critical care unit.[21] The results suggested that back massage was useful in promoting sleep in critically ill older men.

Another study examined the effect of manual vibratory massage in 8 patients (3 were status post heart transplant, 3 were status post lung transplant, and 2 were status post coronary artery bypass grafting) in the intensive care unit.[22] In the 10-minute period following the massage, a 30% increase in tidal volume ($p = 0.008$), an increase in PO_2 (percutaneous oxygen saturation), an 11% decrease in central venous pressure ($p = 0.04$), and an 18% decrease in pulmonary vessel resistance ($p = 0.001$) were found.

Researchers examined the effect of neuromuscular release massage therapy in 5 patients with chronic obstructive lung disease.[23] Twenty-four weekly massage sessions were performed, and the results suggested improvements in several pulmonary function tests including heart rate, oxygenation saturation, and time of breath hold.

Massage therapy was performed in a group of 20 pediatric patients with cystic fibrosis.[24] Parents in the massage group, who were instructed in massage technique, performed massage for 20 minutes per day at bedtime, whereas the control group parents instead read to their children for those 20 minutes. Children and parents in the massage group reported reduced anxiety. Improved peak air flow in the treated group suggesting that massage may facilitate breathing by decreasing anxiety and improving mood.

Another study by Field examined the effect of massage on children with asthma.[25] Two age groups of children (age 4–8 years old and age 9–14 years old) were examined. Again, parents were taught how to administer the massage in one session and then performed the massage for 20 minutes each night at bedtime for 30 days. In both age groups, reduced anxiety and improved attitude toward asthma were found. In younger children, a decrease in cortisol levels and improvement in peak air flow and other pulmonary functions were noted, whereas in older children pulmonary forced expiratory flow was the only parameter noted to improve.

The use of traditional Chinese massage in treating and preventing recurrent respiratory tract infections in children was examined in a study published in the *Journal of Traditional Chinese Medicine*.[26] This study suggested that the treatment group faired significantly better than the control at 3 and 6 months following the massage sessions.

Gastrointestinal System

A German study examined 130 patients undergoing abdominal surgery for various gynecologic conditions who were placed in three groups: foot reflexology, simple foot massage, and simple conversation (no massage).[27] Simple massage was noted to be relaxing and a positive experience. However, foot reflexology was associated with various effects, some of which were negative, including increased abdominal pain. Secondary to this, the study did not recommend foot reflexology on patients following recent abdominal surgery for gynecologic reasons.

Abdominal massage is also used to treat or decrease constipation. Ernst performed a systematic review of four articles.[28] He concluded that although further research and better studies were needed, massage could be a promising treatment for chronic constipation (Fig. 1).

Pregnancy

The relative benefit of massage during pregnancy has also been examined. In a study by Field, 26 pregnant women received either massage or relaxation therapy

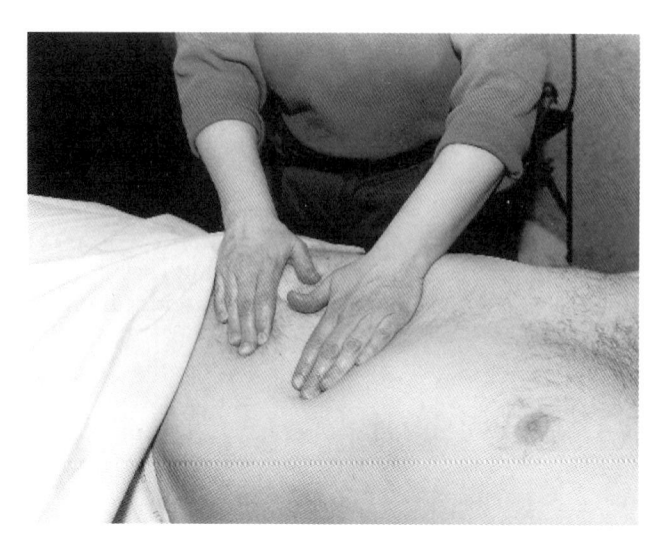

FIGURE 1. Abdominal effleurage (in right to left direction for constipation).

(each for 20 minutes 2 times per day).[29] The massage group reported less anxiety and back pain and improved mood compared with the relaxation group. The results also suggested that the massage therapy group had fewer complications during labor and less prematurity. Further and larger studies are needed to prove significant differences.

In another study, partners of pregnant women learned how to administer massage during labor.[30] Compared with a control group coached only in traditional breathing techniques, results suggested that the massaged mothers experienced less anxiety, shorter labor, shorter hospital stays, and less postpartum depression.

Soft Tissue Mobilization

More research is beginning to emerge on soft tissue mobilization therapy. The theorized mechanism in one type of soft tissue mobilization, augmented soft tissue mobilization (ASTM), in successfully treating chronic tendinitis is that it promotes healing through a controlled application of microtrauma. In a study of 30 (enzyme-induced) injured rat Achilles tendons, different levels of pressure of ASTM were compared.[31] In the heavy-pressure ASTM group, a statistically greater number of fibroblasts were noted, which theoretically implies more healing potential. Another study of rat Achilles tendons with induced tendinitis showed an increase in fibroblast proliferation after ASTM.[32]

A case report on ASTM describes its effectiveness in treating one athlete's chronic ankle pain, fibrosis, and diminished range of motion with 6 weeks of directed ASTM.[33]

Smoking Cessation

A study of 20 adult smokers examined the effect of self-hand or self-ear massage performed during three cravings per month compared with a control group that was not taught the massage techniques.[34] The massage group reported that they experienced less anxiety, improved mood, and fewer withdrawal symptoms and smoked fewer cigarettes per day by the end of the month-long study.

General Hospital Patients

A study of 113 hospitalized patients was performed to evaluate qualitative benefits of massage to patients.[35] Patients received between 1 and 4 massages and filled out surveys or provided narrative reports of their experiences. Of the range of comments and perceived benefits that was obtained, the most common were increased relaxation (98%), improved feeling of well-being (93%), and positive mood change (88%).

Bulimia

In a study of 24 bulimic adolescent girls, the patients were assigned either to massage or to control (no massage) groups.[36] Improvement in depression and in some psychological and behavioral measures and lower cortisol and higher dopamine levels were suggested by the results.

Dermatologic Conditions

A study of young children with atopic dermatitis and the use of massage therapy (administered by parents) was performed.[37] One group received traditional topical therapy coupled with parent-performed massage therapy for 20 minutes per day for 1 month. The control group received the traditional topical therapy only. The children in the massage group improved on all clinical measures including alleviation of redness, scaling, lichenification, excoriation, and pruritus, whereas the control group improved on the scaling measure only. Decreased anxiety in parents and children was noted as well in the massage group. The study concluded that massage may be a cost-effective adjunct treatment for atopic dermatitis because only a one-time expense of about $30 was incurred for the initial massage training session for the child and parent.

Sports Massage/Exercise

In a review of the literature, the effectiveness of massage after exercise to decrease delayed-onset muscle soreness (DOMS) was examined.[38] Significant methodologic flaws were noted in all studies; nonetheless, the authors concluded that massage may be helpful in alleviating DOMS and that further studies were warranted.

Controversy exists surrounding the role of massage following exercise. A review of the literature by Tiidus covering the scientific evidence of benefits of massage on specific parameters after exercise prompted their conclusion that a demonstrated beneficial effect was not shown.[39] In another study, a combination of different massage techniques in muscles of small (forearm) and large (quadriceps) muscle mass were performed.[40] Massage did not increase Doppler-measured muscle blood flow. The results did indicate that light exercise increases blood flow and would be beneficial if that is the desired therapeutic effect.

Lymphedema

Manual lymph drainage (a light massage technique directed at improving lymphatic flow) significantly decreases edema in affected extremities, and coupled with appropriate compression, it can lead to sustained edema reduction. This technique is largely replacing automated mechanical compression devices because of improved outcomes and fewer complications.

Large and prospective studies have been performed showing ≥ 50% reduction in limb size. A comprehensive program involving skin care, manual lymph drainage, exercises, and compression bandaging resulted in sustained reduction in size on follow-up after 9 months.[41,42] A case study by Weiss demonstrated significant reduction in leg edema (by 80%) 1 year after injury with multiple fractures and persistent nonhealing wounds using manual lymph drainage, compression bandages, and exercise.[43]

Tone and Spasticity

As evidenced by a reduction in H-reflex amplitude after massage performed to the triceps surae, massage decreases spinal reflex arc excitability.[44] This modulation appears likely secondary to deep mechanoreceptors rather than stimulation of cutaneous mechanoreceptors.[45] This supports the theory that patients with muscle spasm and cramps (increased muscle tone) will likely benefit from massage.

Caregivers and Miscellaneous Disorders

Massage performed on primary caregivers of hospice patients as a form of respite intervention was examined and found to be of benefit in stress reduction, among other areas of benefit.[46]

A study of massage administered by parents to children with juvenile rheumatoid arthritis was performed with a control group using relaxation techniques alone. The massages were performed 15 minutes per day for 30 days, resulting in a decrease in children's anxiety, cortisol level, and pain as assessed by self-reports, patient reports, and physician reports.[47]

Wounds and Burns

Bass et al. reviewed the literature to evaluate the effectiveness of massage on preventing pressure sores.[48] The authors concluded that sufficient evidence was not available to support the use of massage in preventing pressure sores and that its use for this problem was not recommended.

Friction massage to decrease hypertrophic scar formation or to improve pliability and decrease scar banding is commonly incorporated but still not clearly shown to be beneficial. In one study of 30 pediatric patients, massage sessions of 10 minutes per day over 3 months did not demonstrate significant improvement in vascularity, pliability, or height of the scar.[49] However, in a study of 28 patients assigned to either a massage or control group during the active debridement of a wound, benefits were noted in patient comfort.[50] The massage group did have decreased anxiety, pain, and depression.

Chair Massage

The use of massage in Western culture has now progressed to utilizing the modality in the workplace. Further research is needed to help define the benefit of chair massage in a working environment, but decreased stress, anxiety, and improved attention, concentration, and worker satisfaction are proposed benefits (Fig. 2). One study of 52 individuals receiving a 15-minute chair massage found a significant decline in systolic and diastolic blood pressure; however, no control group was used.[51]

Aromatherapy

Using aromatic agents in the massage oil is proposed to be more beneficial than massage without aromatic agents. In one study, the addition of aromatherapy massage (in this case using Roman chamomile essential oil) compared with massage with a carrier oil alone suggested a greater relative decrease in anxiety level and relative benefits in psychological well-being in patients with cancers undergoing palliative care.[52]

TYPES OF MASSAGE

Because of massage's long history in many countries, many different types of massage have evolved. Within each type of massage, different techniques can be used to treat different types of problems, although certain types of massage may be

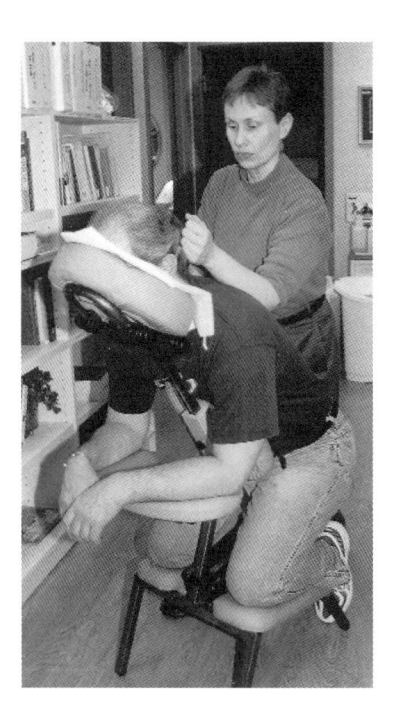

FIGURE 2. Chair massage. Compression is applied to the rhomboid and trapezius area.

better suited to achieve certain goals in specific situations. For example, manual lymph drainage would be a good choice to reduce edema in a postmastectomy patient, whereas friction massage or myofascial release is not a good choice for achieving a general state of relaxation for stress reduction.

Classic Western Massage

Classic Western massage has much in common with Swedish massage and is the most common type of massage practiced in the United States. The basic types of strokes can be categorized in different ways, but the most common are petrissage, effleurage, friction, and tapotement. Each category contains many distinct, specific strokes that are similar to the basic stroke in that category.

Petrissage involves compression of a body's tissues, typically between the therapist's hands or between therapist's hand and bony structures of the patient. Specific strokes include kneading, picking up, rolling, and wringing (Figs. 3–5). These techniques can be used to mobilize fluids in tissues, and mobilize adhesions.

Effleurage describes stroking or gliding movements over the body and can be either superficial or deep (Figs. 6–8). These slow rhythmic hand movements can begin with light pressure to induce a general state of relaxation and accelerate both in speed and pressure to improve muscle tone and tissue fluid movement respectively.

Friction massage is directed circular or transverse motions applied through the fingertips, thumb, or palm of the hand to a small area of tissue. The movement initially involves light pressure and progressively becomes more firm and deeper as adhesions, contractions, tendinitis, and other localized areas of tissue damage are targeted (Fig. 9).

Tapotement is a percussion massage usually produced by rapid, rhythmic, vigorous movements of the hands on the patient. Types of strokes include clapping, cupping, hacking, vibration, and tapping (Fig. 10). Increasing muscle tone, mobilizing tissue fluid and in the case of more vigorous vibration, loosening impacted

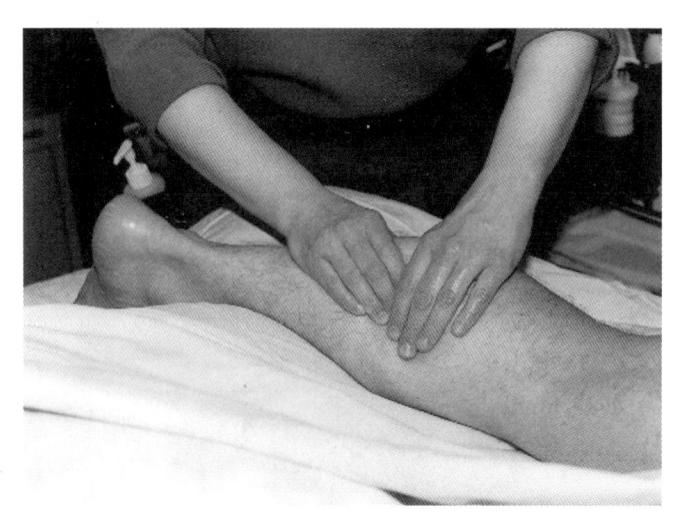

FIGURE 3. Petrissage to calf muscles.

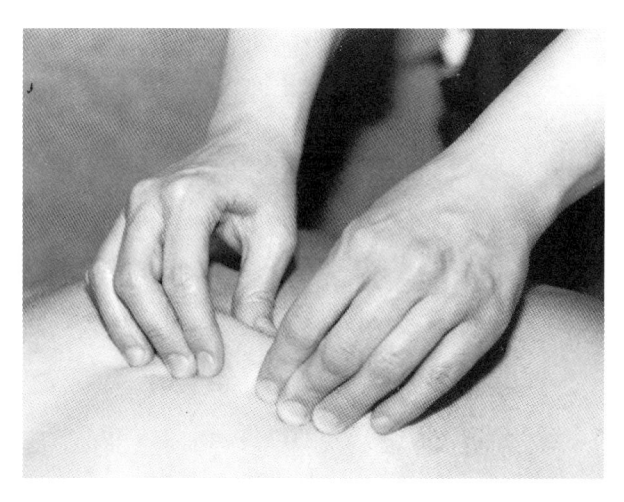

FIGURE 4. Rolfing, a type of myofascial release, to the back.

secretions in the respiratory tree (for use with chest physiotherapy) are some potential uses for these strokes.

Myofascial Release and Neuromuscular Massage

These techniques, although largely different, are similar in that they work toward removing fascial restrictions or myofascial trigger points or nodules (with the stripping technique defined by Travell). Myofascial release involves gentle pressure and passive stretching in the direction of muscle fibers followed by a hold, until a release is felt (Fig. 11). With Rolfing, the focus is on deep friction massage

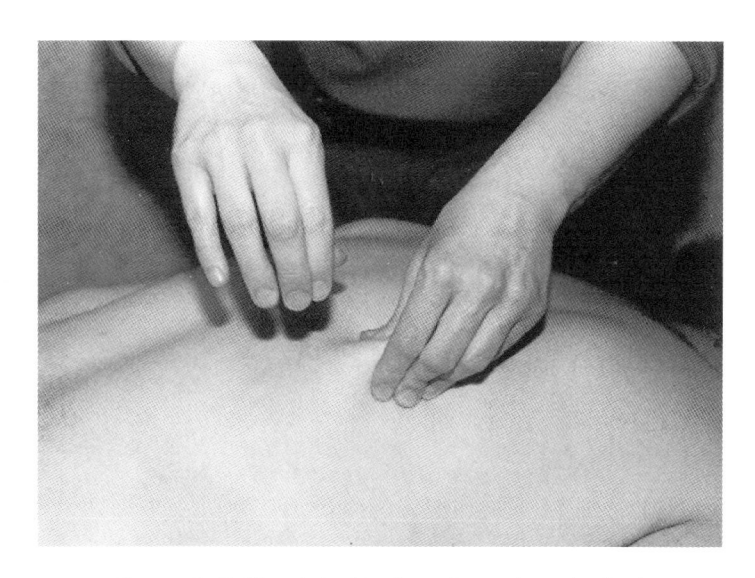

FIGURE 5. Fulling (plucking) performed on the back.

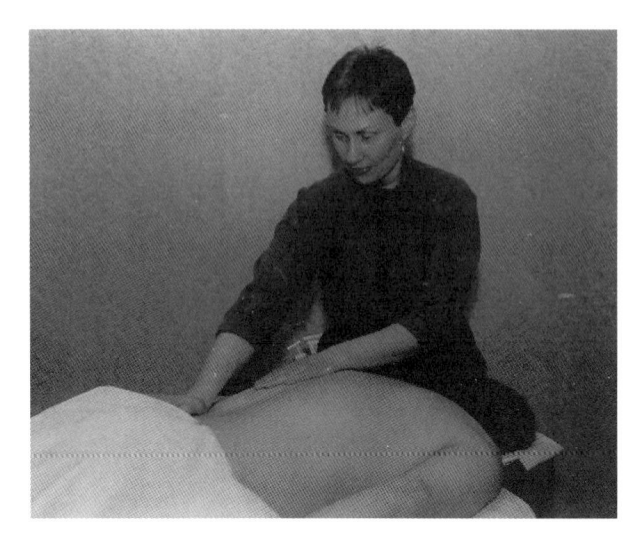

FIGURE 6. Effleurage (gliding) to back.

to realign deep fascial planes in the body. Stripping massage is a stroking technique applied slowly and deeply to a relaxed (not taut) muscle. A sliding and milking movement is performed along the length of the muscle up to and then over and past the trigger point or nodule that is encountered.

Cross-Fiber Friction Massage and Deep Transverse Friction Massage

In this technique as described by Cyriax, the therapist's fingertip is placed on the exact site of the lesion and rubbed hard *across* the direction of the fibers of the affected muscle fiber, tendon, or ligament. The key here is that the therapeutic movement is confined to a very small spot. The proposed effect is to break down

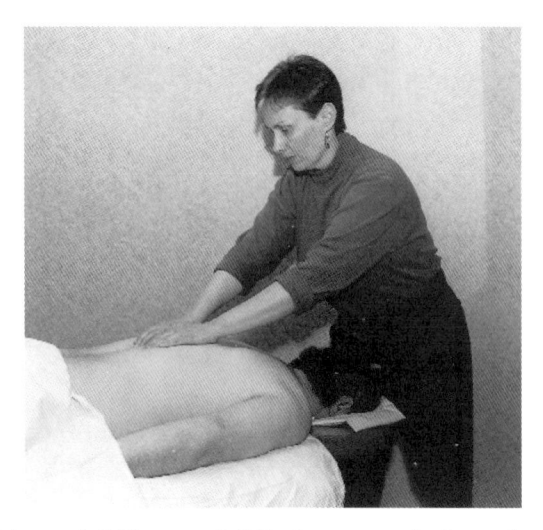

FIGURE 7. Effleurage (gliding) on paraspinal muscles.

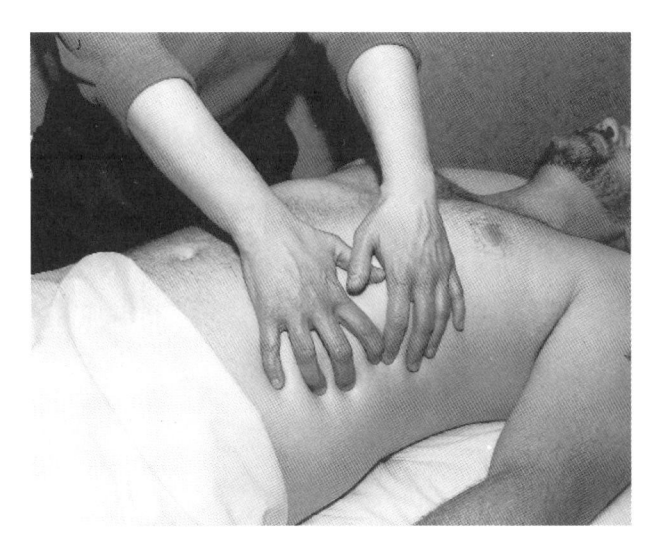

FIGURE 8. Deep effleurage (raking) to the intercostals.

adhesions in muscles, tendons and ligaments. With tenosynovitis, it is proposed to smooth rough edges of the tendon.[53]

Manual Lymph Drainage and Complete Decongestive Physiotherapy

This technique consists of slow, light, and repetitive strokes that help move lymph fluid through the system of vessels and nodes. The massage is carried out in a systematic way to move the fluid to the intact parts of the lymphatic system and thus to return it into circulation. This technique is also known as complex physical therapy (CPT) and complete decongestive physiotherapy (CDT). The technique

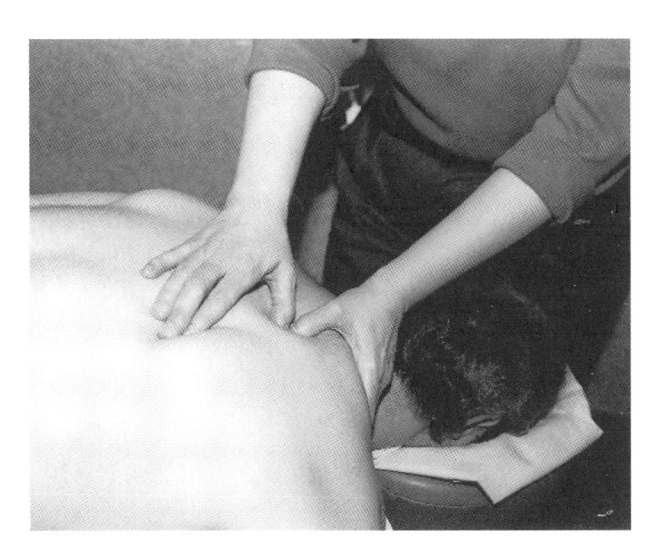

FIGURE 9. Ischemic compression with thumbs.

156   Massage Therapy

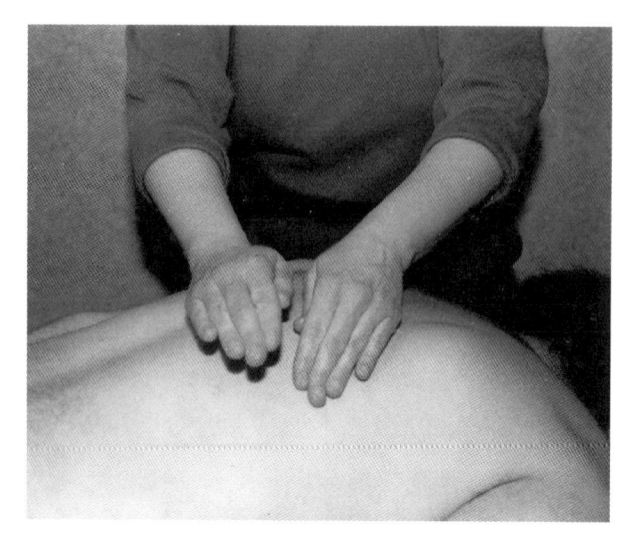

FIGURE 10. Tapotement to the back.

first begins proximally to clear the lymph from the proximal lymph channels, lymph nodes, and thoracic duct. Then it proceeds down the distal involved extremity, thus making room proximally for the fluid coming from the more distal site as you work your way down.

Connective Tissue Massage (Bindegewebsmassage)

This technique is primarily used in Europe. The intent is to affect underlying organs whose innervation theoretically corresponds to cutaneous dermatomes. This supposed influence over the nervous system is similar to that in Eastern massage, although obviously with a different underlying philosophy and a much shorter history.

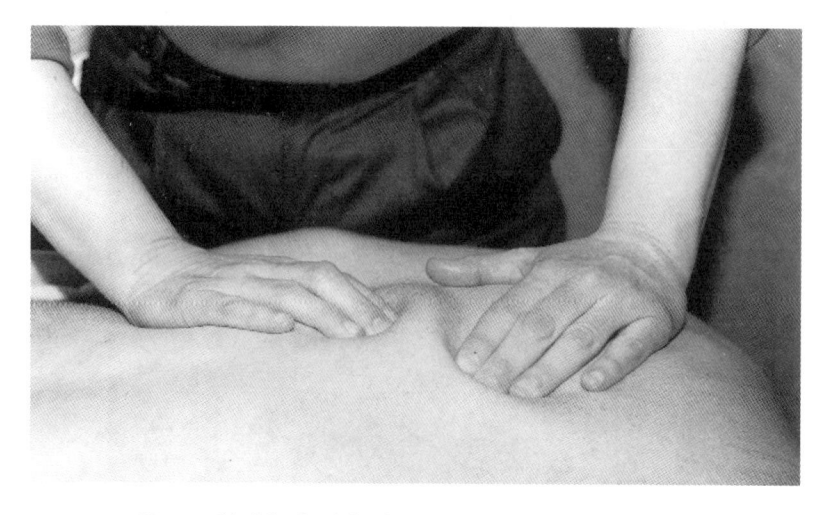

FIGURE 11. Myofascial release technique to the back.

Acupuncture, Shiatsu, and Reflexology

In these techniques, the fingers apply pressure over specific points determined by Chinese meridian theory. Acupressure points are situated along channels or meridians of the body along which energy (*chi*) circulates. Manipulation of these points affects this flow of energy and consequently the balance of this energy in one's body. Shiatsu (*shi* meaning "finger" and *atsu* meaning "pressure"), which dates back over a thousand years, is the Japanese equivalent of this treatment. Reflexology involves deep finger pressure applied to specific points over the sole of the foot (Fig. 12). These similarly are supposed to correspond to specific organs and parts of the body and are also based in part on meridian theory.

Sports Massage

Sports massage can entail a full body massage, but more typically it focuses on the main muscles used in the athletic activity. A pre-event massage may be used to relax and ready the muscles for exercise as well as to decrease anxiety in the participant. The postexercise massage attempts to mobilize waste products accumulated during the exercise, while stretching and decreasing tension and stiffness in those muscles.

CONTRAINDICATIONS

Contraindications to massage are largely empirically derived and based on common sense. Massage over infected tissues, cellulitis, or more deep-seated infections is contraindicated to avoid dissemination of the infection. Massage in a systemic febrile illness may also lead to an increased rate of dissemination of bacteria through increased lymphatic flow. Massage of deep venous thrombosis (DVT) or arterial thrombi is contraindicated to prevent dislodging the clot. Massage over an open wound exposes the therapist to the risk of contracting blood-borne

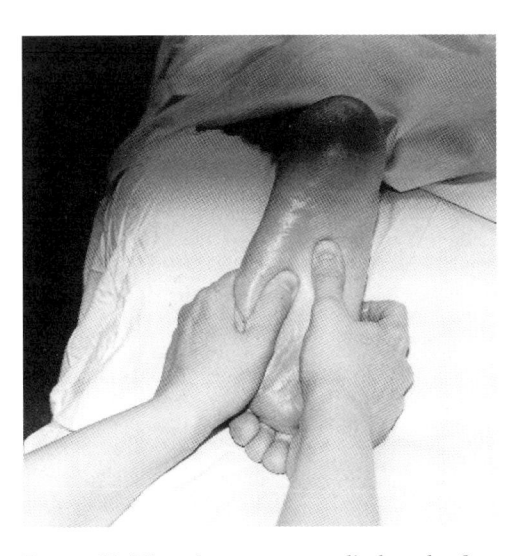

FIGURE 12. Thumb pressure applied to the foot.

pathogens. Too vigorous massage over or near a wound that has not completely healed may lead to that surgical wound reopening.

Massage is relatively contraindicated over malignancies, secondary to the perceived risk of further disseminating the tumor by physical manipulation or by increasing circulation to the tumor and promoting dissemination in that way. Relative contraindications and special precautions should also be taken with fragile skin (to avoid breakdown), with patients with active cardiac problems (secondary to increased venous return and increased demands placed on the heart), in pregnant patients (positioning issues and other unique factors must be evaluated), and in the anticoagulated patient.

During a deep massage (e.g., Rolfing technique), a 51-year-old woman with a history of ureteral stenosis and calculi developed severe left flank pain.[54] Displacement of her left ureteral double-J stent was noted in her evaluation in the emergency department, with resolution of her pain when the stent was replaced. Other complications noted in the literature, although rare, include nerve injury, hematoma formation after massage in a patient taking anticoagulation medication, induction of thyrotoxicosis, and massage-related sigmoid colon perforation.[2,55–58]

CONCLUSION

The use of massage has a history spanning well over 2000 years. Massage in different forms is used throughout the world and is becoming more and more popular in Western countries. Research efforts are beginning to bear out some of the beneficial effects that massage is purported to have. In some cases, third-party carriers are providing coverage for massage therapy, and massage is becoming more prevalent in hospital settings, office settings, with athletic training, and in stress reduction, as well as for specific ailments described here. Further controlled studies will help provide evidence of its effectiveness. As an adjunctive treatment, massage may be of considerable benefit to patients in various clinical conditions.

I would like to thank Julie Pendzialek, a registered nurse and licensed massage therapist at Carle Foundation Hospital, for her review of this manuscript as well as her and her husband Walter's volunteering to model for the photographs.

REFERENCES

1. Geringer S, Kincaid C, Rechtien J: Traction, manipulation, and massage. In DeLisa J (ed): Rehabilitation Medicine: Principles and Practice, 2nd ed. Philadelphia, Lippincott, Williams & Wilkins, 1993.
2. Braverman D, Schulman R: Massage techniques in rehabilitation medicine. Phys Med Rehabil Clin North Am 10:631, 1999.
3. Monte T: World Medicine: The East West Guide to Healing Your Body. 1993.
4. Atchinson J, Stoll S, Gilliar W: Manipulation, traction, and massage. In Braddon RL (ed): Physical Medicine and Rehabilitation. Philadelphia, W.B. Saunders, 1996.
5. Kanemetz H: History of massage. In Basmajian J (ed): Manipulation, Traction, and Massage. 1985, pp 211–255.
6. Field T: Massage therapy effects. Am Psychologist 53:1270–1280, 1998.
7. Melzack A, Wall P: Pain mechanisms: A new theory. Science 50:971–979, 1965.
8. Morelli M, Sullivan SJ, Chapman CE: Inhibitory influence of soleus massage onto the medial gastrocnemius H-reflex: Electromyogr Clin Neurophysiol 38:87–93, 1998.

9. Goldstein-Ferber S: Massage in preterm infants. Presented at the 11th Annual International Conference on Infant Studies, Atlanta, Georgia, 1998.
10. Jinon S: The effect of infant massage on growth of the preterm infant. In Yarbes-Almirante C, De Luma M (eds): Increasing Safe and Successful Pregnancy. 1996, pp 265–269.
11. Field T, et al: Tactile/kinesthetic stimulation effects on preterm neonates. Pediatrics 77:654–658, 1986.
12. Scafidi F, et al: Massage stimulates growth in preterm infants: A replication: Infant Behav Devel 13:167–188.
13. Dieter J, et al: Weight gain can increase in preterm infants following only one week of massage. Presented at the 12th Annual International Conference on Infant Studies, Atlanta Georgia, 1998.
14. Wheedon A, et al: Massage effects on cocaine-exposed preterm neonates. J Dev Behav Pediatr 14:318–322, 1993.
15. Field T, et al: Massage therapy for infants of depressed mothers. Infant Behav Dev 19:109–114, 1996.
16. Wilkinson S: An evaluation of aromatherapy massage in palliative care. Palliative Med 13:409–417, 1999.
17. Ashles TA, et al: Massage therapy for patients undergoing autologous bone marrow transplantation. J Pain Sympt Manag 18:157–163, 1999.
18. Gam AN, et al: Treatment of myofascial trigger points with ultrasound combined with massage and exercise a randomized controlled trial. Pain 77:73–79, 1998.
19. Ernst E: Massage therapy for low back pain: A systematic review. J Pain Symptom Manag 17:65–69, 1999.
20. Hayes J, Cox C: Immediate effects of a five-minute foot massage on patients in critical care. Intens Crit Care Nurs 15:77–82, 1999.
21. Richards KC: Effects of a back massage and relaxation intervention on sleep in critically ill patients. Am J Crit Care 7:288–299, 1999.
22. Doering TJ, et al: External stimuli in the form of vibratory massage after heart or lung transplantation. Am J Phys Med Rehabil 78:108–110, 1998.
23. Beeken JE, et al: The effectiveness of neuromuscular release massage therapy in five individuals with chronic obstructive lung disease. Clin Nurs Res 7:309–325, 1998.
24. Hernandez-Reif M, et al: Children with cystic fibrosis benefit from massage therapy. J Pediatr Psychol 24:175–181, 1999.
25. Field T, et al: Children with asthma have improved pulmonary function after massage therapy. J Pediatr 132:854–858, 1998.
26. Zhu S, et al: A clinical investigation on massage for prevention and treatment of recurrent respiratory tract infection in children. J Trad Chin Med 18:285–291, 1998.
27. Kesselring A: Foot reflexology massage: A clinical study [German]. Forschende Komplementarmedizen 6(suppl 1):38–40, 1999.
28. Ernst E: Abdominal massage therapy for chronic constipation. A systematic review of controlled clinical trials: Forschende Komplementarmedizin 6:149–151, 1999.
29. Field T, et al: Pregnant women benefit from massage therapy. J Psychosomat Obstet Gynecol 18:31–38, 1999.
30. Field T, et al: Labor pain is reduced by massage therapy. J Psychosomat Obstet Gynecol 18:281–291, 1997.
31. Gehlsen GM, Ganion LR, Helfst R: Fibroblast responses to variation in soft tissue mobilization pressure. Med Sci Sports Exerc 34:531–535, 1999.
32. Davidson CJ, et al: Rat tendon morphologic and functional changes resulting from soft tissue mobilization pressure. Med Sci Sports Exerc 29:313–319, 1997.
33. Melham TJ, et al: Chronic ankle pain and fibrosis successfully treated with a new noninvasive augmented soft tissue mobilization technique (ASTM): A case report. Med Sci Sports Exerc 30:801–804, 1998.
34. Hernandez-Reif M, Field T, Hart S: Smoking cravings and reduced by self-massage. Prevent Med 28:28–32, 1999.
35. Smith MC, et al: Benefits of massage therapy for hospitalized patients: A descriptive and qualitative evaluation. Altern Ther Health Med 5:64–71, 1999.
36. Field T, et al: Bulimic adolescents benefit from massage therapy: Adolescence 33:555–563, 1998.
37. Schachner L, et al: Atopic dermatitis symptoms decreased in children following massage therapy: Pediatr Dermatol 15:390–395, 1998.

38. Ernst E: Does post-exercise massage treatment reduce delayed onset muscle soreness? A systematic review. Br J Sports Med 32:212–214, 1998.
39. Tiidus PM: Manual massage and recovery of muscle function following exercise: A literature review. J Orthop Sports Phys Ther 25:107–112, 1997.
40. Shoemaker JK, Tiidus PM, Mader R: Failure of manual massage to alter limb blood flow: Measures by Doppler ultrasound. Med Sci Sports Exercise 29:610–614, 1997.
41. Foldi M: Treatment of lymphadema [editorial]. Lymphology 27:1–5, 1994.
42. Ko DSC, Lerner R, Klose G, et al: Effective treatment of lymphadema of the extremities. Arch Surg 133:452–457, 1998.
43. Weiss JM: Treatment of leg edema and wounds in a patient with severe musculoskeletal injuries. Phys Ther 78:1104–1113, 1998.
44. Morelli M, Sullivan SJ, Chapman CE: Inhibitory influence of soleus massage onto the medial gastrocnemius H-reflex. Electromyogr Clin Neurophysiol 38:87–93, 1998.
45. Morelli M, Chapman CE, Sullivan SJ: Do cutaneous receptors contribute to the changes in the amplitude of the H-reflex during massage? Electromyograph 39:441–447, 1999.
46. MacDonald G: Massage as a respite intervention for primary caregivers. Am J Hospice Palliative Care 15:43–47, 1998.
47. Field T, et al: Juvenile rheumatoid arthritis: Benefits from massage therapy. J Pediatr Psychology 22:607–617, 1997.
48. Bass IC, Halfens RJ, Abu-Saab HH: The effectiveness of massage in preventing pressure sores: A literature review. Rehabil Nurs 22:229–234, 1997.
49. Patino O, et al: Massage in hypertrophic scars. J Burn Care Rehabil 20:268–271, 1999.
50. See reference 49.
51. Cady SH, Jones GE: Massage therapy as a workplace intervention for reduction of stress. Perceptual Motor Skills 84:157–158, 1997.
52. Wilkinson S, et al: An evaluation of aromatherapy in palliative care. Palliative Med 13:409–417, 1999.
53. Cyriax JH, Cyriax PJ: Cyriax's Illustrated Manual of Orthopedic Medicine, 2nd ed. 1993, pp 20–22.
54. Kerr HD: Ureteral stent displacement associated with deep massage: WMJ 96:57–58, 1997.
55. Herskovitz S, Strauch B, Gordon MJV: Shiatsu induced injury of the median recurrent motor branch [letter]. Muscle Nerve 15:12–15, 1992.
56. Yeo TC, Choo MH, Tay MB: Massive haematoma from digital massage in an anticoagulated patient: A case report. Singapore Med J 35:319–320, 1994.
57. Tachi J, Amino N, Miyai K: Massage therapy on the neck: A contributing factor for destructive thyotoxicosis? Thyroidology 2:25–27, 1990.
58. Rahman MN, McAll G, Chai KG: Massage-related perforation of the sigmoid colon in Kelantan. Med J Malasia 42:56–57, 1987.

Chapter 12
Spinal Traction

Ernest H. Winkenwerder, MPT, and Kamala Shankar, MD

Traction is a drawing force, specifically defined by *Merriam Webster's New Collegiate Dictionary* as a "state of tension created by a pulling force exerted on a skeletal structure by means of a special device."[67] In spinal traction, this force could best be described as axial distraction drawing spinal segments apart to achieve a desired physiological end. Applying traction also causes some amount of gliding, especially at the facet joints. Although some recent reviews and studies have called the utility of traction into question,[6,64] spinal traction is still a widely used and touted modality in the treatment choices for physicians and physical therapists.[1,12,19]

This chapter focuses on the methodology of applying effective traction after discussing the indications and contraindications for various conditions. The latest literature and current controversies is reviewed, followed by some personal reflections based on clinical experience.

This critical look is needed because traction varies widely in usage. If five therapists or physiatrists were asked about the use of ultrasound for subacute low back strain, each may reach a general agreement on dosage (1.5 w/cm^2 × 8–10 minutes for six sessions) with comments on the utility or uselessness of the treatment. Each practitioner would probably have a much wider variation in opinion on traction, which Caillet states varies often due to "personal preference and patient response which dictates method, force, duration and frequency of treatment."[8]

HISTORY

Traction has a long history, with the oldest known reference found in Hindu mythology (3500–1800 B.C.), in which Krishna is found using a stretching technique to correct a hunchback deformity of one of his devotees.[38] Traction was described and illustrated by Hippocrates (460–355 B.C.) for conditions of scoliosis and khyphosis.[25] In his treatise *On Setting Joints by Leverage*, he described an extension force that was exerted on a prone patient pulled by ropes attached to levers, coupled with a manipulative hand maneuver.[47] Galen, (A.D. 131–201), a follower of Hippocrates, used axial traction with direct pressure for spinal conditions.[38] In 1692, Nuchen used continuous traction with body weight as countertraction to treat wry neck syndrome.[24]

Modern literature was scanty through the first part of the 20th century. Traction did receive renewed interest after the 1920s as intervertebral disk pathology began to be seen as an etiology of treatable low back pain.[24] In the 1950s in his *Textbook of Orthopedic Medicine*, James Cyriax popularized the use of traction for lumbar disk protrusion.[13,15] Since then, a number of researchers have investigated the methods and utility of spinal traction. A study of treatment modalities in the Netherlands in 1995 found that traction was used in 7% of the 21 million annual physical therapy treatments in that country.[64]

Continuous bed traction was used for years with very poor results noted by therapists, physicians, and patients. This may be one reason why only 28% of physicians surveyed would recommend traction in the case of radicular pain.[9]

Currently mechanical traction is often used in conjunction with other conservative treatments,[10,45,59,71] but evidence for certain efficacy of traction is scanty.[6,64] Also, new techniques in positioning[17] and equipment[48,59] have appeared over the last 10 years, making assessment of traction more complicated.

INDICATIONS

Traction has been used for conditions ranging from muscle strain to radiculopathy. White and Panjabi summarized theoretical and observed changes in the spine with traction as including decreased discal pressure and protrusion, enlargement of the intervertebral foramen, separation of the intervertebral joints (including facet gliding), stretching of joint capsule, freeing adherent nerve roots, and relaxation of muscle spasm.[51]

The "textbook" diagnosis indicating the need for traction is the herniated nucleus pulposus with radiculopathy.[1,5,9,23,33,35,43,44,49,58] Gupta and Ramarao demonstrated decreased disk protrusion in 11 of 14 patients treated with 60–80 pounds of traction using epidurography.[23] Definite clinical improvements were noted in the patients with reduced defects. Another study using epidurography demonstrated that a disk protrusion would flatten with contrast medium drawn back into the disk space under 120 pounds of sustained traction over 20 minutes.[44]

Ramos and Martin obtained negative discal pressures from 100 to 160 mm Hg in five patients with disk herniations at L4–L5 using a VAX-D traction table with 50–100 pounds of traction.[49] The VAX-D is a split table with a tensiometer in the moving caudal section, which creates distraction in the lumbar spine of a prone-lying patient. In their discussion, they asserted "the only non-interventional method to hold any promise of relieving pressure on vital structures of the lumbar region is that of distraction of the lumbar vertebrae by mechanical forces applied along the axis of the spinal column."

The intervertebral space including the foramen has been shown to be enlarged allowing less potential impingement of the spinal nerves.[6,13] Traction has been found to objectively increase height by 6.6 mm compared to a control group treated the same length of time with passively lying supine in hooklying position.[4] Traction may be more specifically effective in patients with a so-called soft disk problem (herniated nucleus pulposus) as opposed a to hard disk lesion with bony hypertrophy causing a medial ridge in the vertebra.[20] When Christensen and associates used 35% or less of body weight traction to treat patients with severe low-back pain over 2 weeks, 5 of 12 patients with nonspecific back pain stopped traction treatment owing to increased symptoms.[10] None of the 16 patients with herniated disks on CT scan had adverse reactions to traction therapy.

Spurling's sign is a nerve root compression test first described in 1944. Distal symptoms are reproduced by extension, side-bending, and rotation to the side of pain, effectively decreasing the space for nerve root egress.[20] It is a very specific but poorly sensitive test that, if positive, could indicate the utility of traction, which would open the intervertebral space and decrease nerve root pressure.

Home cervical traction can often be a part of a comprehensive management program for a cervical disk lesion. Saal and colleagues followed 26 patients treated nonsurgically for disk lesions, all of whom received home cervical traction.[52] They found good to excellent outcomes in 20 patients, with 21 returning to their same job. Ten of these patients had disk extrusions. Another retrospective study of 88 patients in a 3-year period found 87% of those with mild to moderately severe cervical spondylosis (Quebec whiplash criteria) had relief after 3–5 minutes of properly applied home cervical traction.[58] Other studies related good relief with traction.[1,14]

Beurskens notes that it is often difficult to distinguish among disk, facet, or muscular etiologies in nonspecific back pain.[6] Traction has been shown to stretch the facets through gliding[35] and separate the apophyseal joints.[13] Appropriately strong traction may rupture adhesions,[35] release adhesions in the dural sleeve,[50] and aid in stretching ligaments via physiologic creep.[26]

The relief of muscle spasm may be another indication for traction. Muscle relaxation, which occurs during traction has been postulated to occur through fatigue.[18] Hood found surface electromyography (EMG) activity increased during traction on the lumbar spine, but then the activity decreased toward resting levels after 7 minutes.[28] Leutchuman and Deusinger analyzed the sacrospinalis muscle at L3–L4 in patients with low back pain and found muscle activity decreased with time over traction.[41] More than 50% of patients in the study reported relief with traction.

Traction has also been used empirically for pain control to allow a greater tolerance for rehabilitative exercises.[52] In a randomly controlled trial of 35 men and 65 women, patients given traction had improved cervical range of motion and improved flexion and rotation and required fewer pain medications taken and fewer cotreatments or interventions.[73] In a review of the primary care work-up of elderly patients with neck pain, Kriss and Kriss noted that traction was helpful for some patients.[37] Traction has been used specifically in chronic headaches,[3] especially after whiplash injury,[45] with suboccipital musculature relaxation or elongation being the effect desired. Stone and Wharton used a combination device that delivered traction, transcutaneous electrical nerve stimulation (TENS), and massage, obtaining subjective relief of tension headaches.[57]

Wells details the condition of "cervical angina," chest pain mimicking angina with the pain-generating organ most commonly the C7 nerve root. If coexisting coronary artery disease is ruled out, the patient may benefit from intermittent cervical traction.[69]

The effect of decreased pain may be related to improved vascularity, which serves to decrease inflammation at the nerve root.[29] Another potential pain-relieving mechanism is the probable stimulation of large afferent nerve fibers of the muscle and joints that presynaptically inhibit pain fiber transmission at the spinal cord level.[71]

Lastly, traction may act to promote general healing.[3] In animal models of the hip and knee joint, distraction was found to decrease inflammation and the level of abnormal proteoglycan metabolism characteristic of osteoarthritis.

CONTRAINDICATIONS AND PRECAUTIONS

Traction is a very safe modality in the absence of contraindications. Frazer reported an incidence of "untoward sequalae" in 6 out of 25,000 patients (0.02%).[22] The pulling weight capable of creating potential ligament disruption in the cervical spine is 120 pounds,[12] which is well below the usual effective dose of 20–40 pounds of cervical traction.

Traction is contraindicated in the presence of any structural disease secondary to tumor or infection.[58,72] Any instability in which movement would be contraindicated, such as significant spondylolisthesis, prohibits traction.[72] Rheumatoid arthritis with suspected atlantoaxial subluxation is an absolute contraindication.[53] Flexion-extension films should be reviewed before commencing traction if any occult instability is suspected.

Myelopathy,[52] a neurogenic bladder from cauda equina syndrome,[53] and a midline disk herniation that may worsen with traction[32] are contraindications. A person with Lermitter's sign (described in 1932 as an electrical shock sensation felt in the lower extremities when the neck is flexed) should not receive traction.[20]

Vascular compromise, particulary in the cervical region at the carotids or vertebral arteries, is a contraindication to traction.[58] Positive Doppler studies, carotid bruits, and any dizziness or adverse symptoms with Spurling's movement advise against traction.

Patients with abdominal problems such as hernias or peptic ulcers may have problems with lumbar traction.[53] Also, tight pelvic and chest straps may decrease venous return and restrict breathing. Although it is a relative contraindication, claustrophobia may be a real limiting factor to an effective traction dosage for some people. Pregnancy and osteoporosis, depending on the extent and individual condition, may be a relative or absolute contraindication in those individuals affected.[1]

Traction in the first few weeks of an injury may do more harm than good according to some writers,[19,58] especially if the patient has an acute torticollis.[32] Patients with temporomandibular joint dysfunction may have jaw aggravation with the chin straps on some traction units,[21] especially if they are using home traction with too much weight or at an ill-advised angle.[55]

Last, a relative contraindication is accompanying low-back pain. Seated cervical traction posture may aggravate an existing back condition.[58] In a 2-year retrospective study, LeBan et al. noted significant low back pain in 12 of 2200 patients treated with cervical traction of 15–30 pounds.[39] The patients with an earlier history of low back pain, relatively quiescent, developed a positive straight-leg raise on the symptomatic side. LeBan referenced cadaver studies demonstrating traction at the neck stretched the dura down to the level of the sacral nerve roots. He postulated that the increase in lumbar pain was due to nerve root tethering distal to the traction force (Table 1).

TYPES OF TRACTION AND METHODOLOGY

This section will review the types of traction available with methodologies discussed using the most common techniques of motorized traction in the physical therapy clinic. Studies are cited both to demonstrate the wide variety of application and to provide a sense of common agreement across studies and practices as they occur.

Manual and Positional Traction

Manual traction is delivered with the therapist stretching the spine using his or her own body weight.[1,6,16,58] It is viewed as a form of spinal manipulation by Tan and Nordin, who classify it as a nonthrust technique, usually referred to as a *mobilization* in that it does not involve high-velocity at low-amplitude motion.[59] They prefer supine manual traction to mechanical traction and state that mechanical traction should be used only if manual traction is ineffective.

TABLE 1. SUMMARY OF INDICATIONS AND CONTRAINDICATIONS FOR TRACTION

Indications
  Decrease diskal pressure and disk protrusion
  Enlarge intervertebral foramen and relieve impingement
  Improve facet hypomobility
  Stretch the joint capsule
  Free adherent nerve roots
  Relax muscle spasm
  Assist in pain control

Contraindications and Precautions
  Structural disease due to tumor or infection
  Instability such as spodylolisthesis
  Myelopathy and neurogenic bladder from cauda equina
  Midline disk herniation
  Cardiovascular disease
  Claustrophobia
  Pregnancy
  Osteoporosis
  Acute injury
  Any patient with adverse reaction to treatment
  Previous spinal surgery
  Spinal tumors

Cyriax used manual traction extensively as an adjunct or precursor to manipulation.[16] "Taking up the slack" in a joint allows the practitioner to assess the degree of hypmobility and more specifically stretch the desired spinal segment. Harris states that traction may be the most important part of a manipulative maneuver.[24]

Manual traction is also used to test tolerance of a patient for mechanical traction. The practitioner can also apply distraction at varied angles to find the most comfortable or effective postion for mechanical traction.[55]

Abdulwahab advocates manual cervical traction specifically for cervical radiculopathy.[1] Paris uses manual lumbar traction to treat a herniated disk.[46] A simple application of this technique for unilateral radiculopathy is known as a leg pull. Bradnam et al. noted decreased excitability in alpha motor neurons with manual traction.[3] They studied the H-reflex curve and used nontraction manual contact in their control group.

Positional distraction is a technique taught to patients which may be used at home. The patient lies on a bolster or other object in the sidelying position, with the affected side up, creating side-bending away from the impinged site.[55] A 6- to 8-inch bolster is sufficient, and rotation away from the affected side may be added to open further the facets and stretch the musculature. Paris recommends beginning the posture at 5 minutes' duration and progressing up to a maximum of 40.[46]

Continuous Traction

Continuous traction was used in the past in patients hospitalized with acute low-back pain and used very light weights of 20 pounds or so and was completely ineffective in separating vertebrae.[34] The unspoken rationale behind the treatment was often to encourage bed rest in the patient. Prolonged weightlessness is believed to be a cause of back pain in astronauts.[41] The move toward early mobilization and weight bearing for optimal return, coupled with decreased reimbursement for acute hospital stays for low-back pain, have eliminated continuous traction from the current clinical scene.

Gravity and Inversion Traction

Gravity lumbar traction in a tilted bed or table uses 40% of the patient's body weight (the lower trunk and legs) as the tractive force.[7] Inability to vary the force and discomfort of the restraints over a prolonged session are limiting factors. Inversion traction is sometimes difficult to get positioned into and may put undue stress on the cardiovascular system.[40] Again, the force is not easily increased or decreased outside the effects of gravity on the patient's upper body, and the prolonged upside down posture can be uncomfortable.

Motorized Traction

Static or Intermittent?

After selecting motorized traction as a treatment, the clinician is faced with the decision as to whether static or intermittent traction will be more efficacious (Table 2). In general intermittent traction has been favored in the United States, and static traction is the preference in Europe.[55]

Colachis and Strohm found no significant difference in tolerance and effect between static and intermittent traction in normal subjects.[13] In a controlled study of 100 patients, Zylbergold and Piper noted with blind observers that range of motion improvements in the cervical spine were better after intermittent than static traction.[73] Leutchuman and Deusinger noted greater treatment tolerance in an intermittent pelvic traction group.[41] In their study, 30% of patients undergoing static traction had increased post-traction pain (two with a severe increase) compared with 15% in the intermittent traction group. Those with adverse reactions to intermittent traction recovered faster, with diminution of increased symptoms to baseline 2 hours or less after traction.

TABLE 2. IMPORTANT VARIABLES IN STANDARD TRACTION APPLICATION

1. **Static or intermittent?**
   Dynamic pumping to affect disk or steady stretch for ligaments and facets
   Comfort of patient

2. **Position?**
   Supine, prone or seated
   　Supine best for cervical traction
   　Prone may be used for disc patients with better effect

3. **Angle of pull?**
   Greater flexion produces greater distraction and opening of intervertebral foramen, but may increase muscle tension in cervical spine. Greater extension creates more distraction in the upper cervical spine at the OA joint.

4. **Weight?**
   Heavier weight needed to distract disk and hypomobile facets
   Lighter weights may be more appropriate for more irritable/acute states, for pain and edema control
   More comfortably tolerated

On the other hand, Cyriax favored static traction, noting muscular fatigue after only 3 minutes of static traction.[16] He theorized that intermittent traction for relaxing musculature was ineffective because it might excite only the stretch reflex of the sacrospinalis muscle.

If intermittent traction is chosen, the traction cycle can vary from a 7- to 10-second hold with a 5-second rest to a 30- to 60-second hold with a 10- to 15-second rest over a 15–30 minute treatment.[13] Leutchman and Deusinger used pelvic traction with equal periods of 10-second hold and 10-seconds rest.[41] Colachis and Strohm found that varying the duration of hold from 7 to 30 to 60 seconds made no significant difference in the amount of distraction measured for cervical traction at a constant angle of 24° flexion.[12]

The anatomic structure involved may play a part in the decision of hold time. Stretching ligaments and muscles may be done more easily with a longer hold of 20–30 seconds, as in a traditional stretch, whereas changing the fluid dynamics in a disk may call for a more rapid rhythmic pattern.

Frequency of Treatment

Frequency of treatment depends on patient response. If the disk does indeed quickly revert to herniation shortly after the traction session (noted on epidurography),[44] then daily treatments with postural correction and support of active exercises as part of an overtreatment plan may be most effective.[49] Zylbergold and Piper used 10–15 traction sessions over 3–4 weeks.[73] Saunders successfully treated a hypomobile lumbar facet with four sessions involving traction.[54] Jackson claims that relief should be obtained within 15 treatments.[30]

Lumbar Traction on a Table

To be successful, traction must generate sufficient force to overcome properly muscle contraction, spinal curvatures, ligamentous resistance, and friction of the body on the table.[6] At least one half of the body weight on a friction free table is recommended by Judovich.[33] On a flat table, the friction resistance of the body is considerable. A split table decreases the force necessary for traction from 300–400 pounds down to 80–100 pounds.[12]

The amount of force needed to distract the lumbar spine varies from 70 to 150 pounds, according to a review by Pellecchia.[48] Cyriax noted definite movement of lumbar spinal segments at 120 pounds in a 25-minute period.[15] One hundred pounds was the average used in several other traction studies.[27,48,54]

Positioning of the patient is very important for successful lumbar traction. The supine hook-lying position is standard (Fig. 1) with 70° of hip flexion and 18° of angle for the best separation of the vertebral bodies.[13] The patient should be comfortable, because narrowing of the intervertebral spaces has been noted in traction with muscle guarding when the patient cannot relax.[17] A protective scoliosis should be respected, with the gradual resumption of midline posture when tolerated.[66] The straps should be tight to eliminate slipping and placed against the skin with a protecting towel for sanitary reasons. The pelvic belt should overlap the thoracic belt around the lower ribs and should have good purchase on the iliac crests.

A safety release and cutoff switch should be close at hand for the patient to terminate the treatment, if needed. The patient will, of course, be advised of the treat-

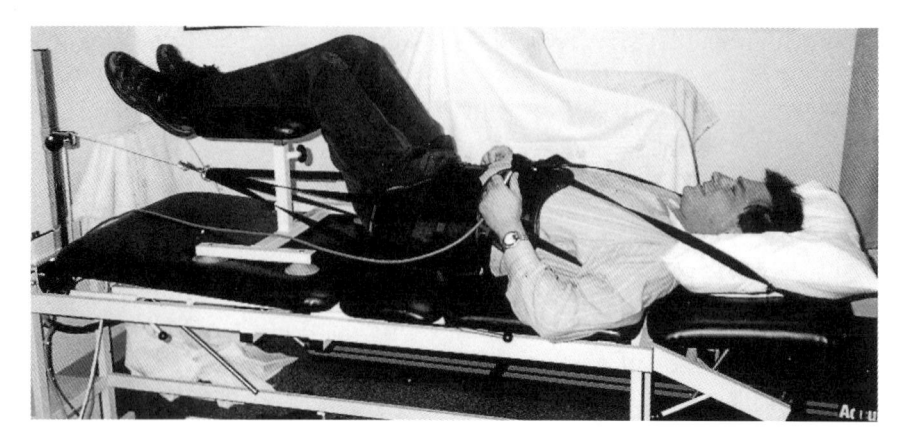

FIGURE 1. Supine traction in semi-fowler position. Note angle of pull, split table, and safety switch in patient's hand.

ment goals and what to expect from the treatment with the understanding that he or she can terminate the session at any time. Traction should be applied smoothly after all slack is taken out of the system and friction is minimized. It is always a good idea to do the first session as a trial treatment at the lower end of the therapeutic range to assess patient response and progress as indicated and tolerated (see Fig. 1).

Prone Pelvic Traction

Prone pelvic traction is a variation on supine traction with the same goals and general guidelines. It is favored by Saunders[55] and is the position for the VAX-D traction machine.[49] The neutral spine is favored in prone traction with a straight pull generally and may be tolerated better in patients who get posterior disk movement in the hook-lying position.

When Humphreys looked at the foraminal space at C5–C6 in traction, he found that traction did not significantly increase the foraminal opening to any additional amount after simply flexing the neck. A correlation was found, however, in neutral, where traction caused a vertebral separation.[29] A neutral spine posture in traction places less load on the posterior components of the back and is favored in the principles of McKenzie.[42]

For proper prone traction, no spreader bar is placed and the patient puts his or her legs through the pelvic straps. The table is raised or the pully is adjusted to effect neutral extension (Fig. 2).

Cervical Traction

More studies have been conducted on cervical traction, and it is generally more widely in use, than pelvic traction. This may be due to the observation that it is easier to set up, with only 7% of friction free body weight required for a physiologic response.[17] It takes 10 pounds of force to overcome the weight of the head,[30] and 25 pounds has been mentioned as the minimum needed for vertebral separation.[30,32] Thirty pounds has been used by several practitioners.[11,18] Judovich found improvement in more than half of 60 patients studied using forces between 25 and 50

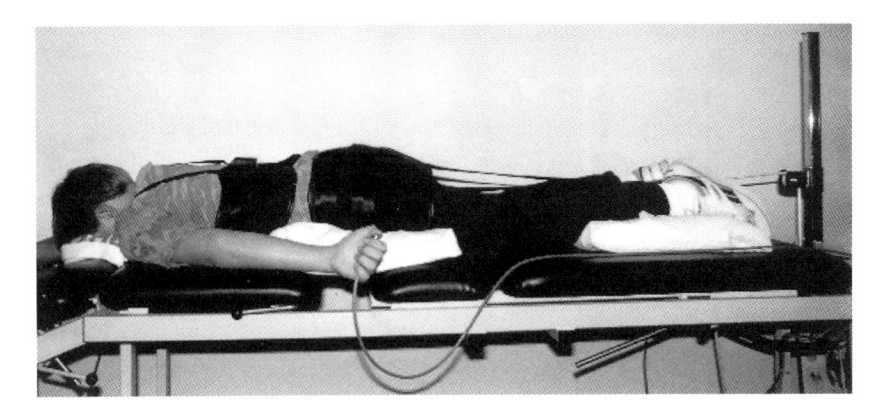

FIGURE 2. Prone pelvic traction. Note no spreader bar and neutral spine position assisted by pillows, straps between patient legs.

pounds.[32] In some patients, pain was increased at 25 pounds but decreased at 35 pounds. Harris used only 15 pounds and achieved relief in patients with whiplash.[24] He treated the patients with three 5-minute cycles of sustained traction, along with moist heat, and allowed the patients to rotate their neck gently during treatment.

Twenty-five degrees to 30° of flexion straightens the normal cervical lordosis, and Colachis and Strohm noted greatest separation at the largest angle (6°, 20°, and 24° degrees were assessed).[11] To stretch the upper spine and subocccipitals, a more neutral posture is used. Excessive extension and compression are to be avoided.

The supine position is generally preferred over sitting[11,17,25] because the patient is more comfortable and the weight of the head is neutralized. It is important for comfort to avoid pressure over the chin if a chin component is part of the head halter (Fig. 3).

New Types of Traction

Several new traction tables and devices are being used currently.[18,26,49,57] In the VAX-D traction device, significant drops in intradiscal pressure have been noted, along with symptomatic relief.[49]

Autotraction is an active technique that seeks to restore normal posture. It was developed by Lind in 1974 and improved by Natchev in 1984. A specialized table and patient training are required.[59] Recently, traction was coupled with an EMG mechanism and a feedback loop. This allowed more rapid progression of a traction protocol by dynamic adjustment of tension in response to muscle EMG in a treatment session.[71]

Home Traction

Traction can used as a home treatment in conjunction with exercises for better resolution of neuromusculoskeletal complaints. Pelvic traction is available but is not as common and is more expensive than a simple home cervical traction kit. These kits use a water weight bag up to 20 pounds in an overdoor position.[1,52,58] A simple buckle and web device with a pulley can convert the traction to supine, and a pull bar can be incorporated so the patient can simulate intermittent traction at

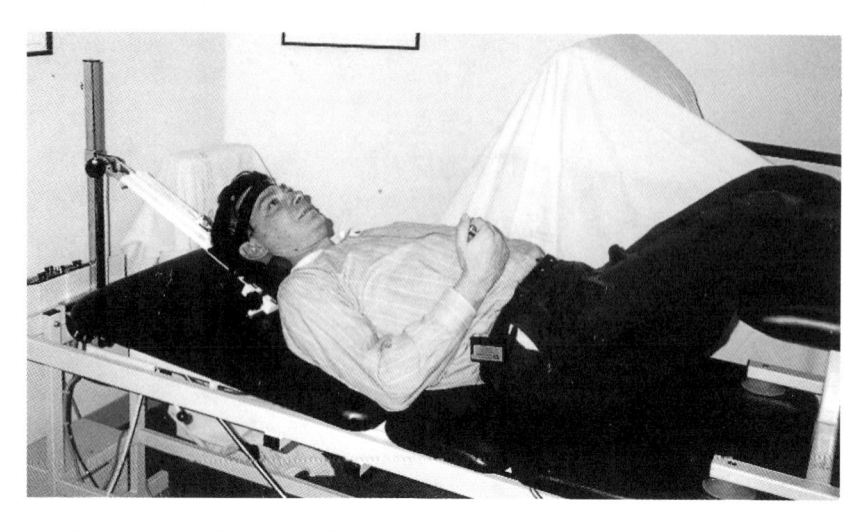

FIGURE 3. Supine cervical traction. Note comfortable lumbar position, angle of pull, and no stress on jaw with head harness apparatus.

home. The Saunders home traction unit relies on a pneumatic pump in the supine position with no strap over the chin.

CONTROVERSIES IN TRACTION USE

Despite, or perhaps because of, the wealth of literature and clinical practice with traction, traction remains a somewhat controversial treatment choice for spinal conditions. Opinions vary as to its utility, ranging from a integral part of rehabilitation[52] to a strong negative reaction. After a review of 31 articles, the U.S. Department of Health and Human Services stated in a report that "spinal traction is not recommended in the treatment of low back pain."[63] Traction is considered an additional trauma to a healing system by Weinberger.[68]

Tan and Nordin state "empirically mechanical traction should only be started if active modalities and manual traction have not achieved the desired end."[59] One difficulty with this position is that if traction is the treatment of choice after all other conservative measures have failed, subjects for traction are those most recalcitrant to treatment and are more likely to fail any additional modality.

In a study published in 1990, 369 orthopaedists and 165 physiatrists were asked if they would use traction in a hypothetical case of a 42-year-old man with acute bilateral low back pain without evidence of radiculopathy.[9] Sixteen percent of those responding stated that they would use traction for nonspecific acute pain and 27% would use traction for a herniated disk. Of those respondents favoring traction, 78% gave nonphysiologic rationales for use (54% to reinforce bed rest and 27% to give psychological support). Seventeen percent did say that they would use traction to decrease nerve root or disk pressure, but the general consensus was reminiscent of the days when continuous traction was in vogue, and the survey writers stated that traction was only delaying recovery by promoting deconditioning and atrophy, and reinforcing passive health-care behavior.

Studies of traction are often fraught with problems. In a review of 21 papers reporting 24 studies, a 100-point scale was assigned to assess the strength and validity of the study (e.g., double-blinded, specific protocol, adequate sample size).[64] Only three studies assessed received over 50 points, and these three showed no improvement with traction in pain, mobility, functional status, or other symptoms.

Beurskens did a pilot study of 28 patients and found a recovery rate in a high traction group of 64% compared with a sham traction group.[6] This study was repeated in a larger trial of 100 patients, and he found no significant differences between the two groups. Both groups did improve over the study.

Humphreys found that traction did not add any additional distraction effects over simply flexing the neck in nine cadaver spines.[29] As all the musculature had been stripped away, this in vitro study may not have taken into account all the structures traction affects in vivo. The effect of traction on muscle activity is still in contention. Hood noted no myoelectric activity in patients without low back pain in supine hook-lying position.[28] After 3–7 minutes of traction, muscle activity increased. It is difficult to speculate on what this could mean for patients with low back pain. The observation that traction has some effect on normal subjects may be the equivalent of saying ibuprofen can cause stomach upset in normal subjects without any inflammation. Using EMG and traction, Wong noted a decrease in muscle activity in both normals and in patients with cervical radiculopathy.[71] A greater decrease was noted in those subjects with high initial resting muscle activity. This indicated a good response to the traction modality.

Some studies that show no change with treatment may be flawed in the use of the modality studied. Klaber-Moffett and colleagues noted greater muscle relaxation in patients treated with 2 pounds of placebo traction versus 6–12 pounds treatment weight.[36] One study using traction as part of a total program for cervical radiculopathy used only 5 pounds of weight.[5] Clearly, if traction is to be accepted or discarded, the decision should be based on both clinical observation and studies that use the modality in its most optimum parameters.

Traction is often used for pain control so that the patient may more rapidly progress in functional exercises,[20,52] but the mechanism of pain relief is still in question. Although some patients get relief for 24 hours or more after traction, disk bulges recur rapidly on epidurography, often within an hour.[44] Although many people obtain relief with auto-traction, the level of disk prolapse remains the same.[61]

In critiquing a study of autotraction, Trudel alluded to the problem of defining the pain generating organ in treating low back pain.[62] Objective findings are often present in overlapping conditions, and many abnormal findings are present in normal subjects without radicular pain.

It may be that the wrong subset of patients is being evaluated for traction. If traction benefits soft tissue structures other than the disk, perhaps more study should be directed to patient populations without radiculopathy.[16] In the case of degenerative joint disease, some structures must be reduced or realigned to provide relief obtained with traction.

Jensen postulates that improvement may be due to change in tissue damage around the herniated material and not the movement of the herniated material itself.[31] This brings up the question of whether pain is mechanical or chemical in nature. If the traction improves blood flow to decrease edema around the disk, then whether the disk is truly reduced may be less an important question than assumed. Also, traction may work at least partly by the mechanical stimulation of large sensory nerve fibers in accordance with the gate theory of pain relief.[41]

The difficulty of relating improving symptoms to changing physiologic effects may be seen in the "release phenomenon." Also known as a "rebound phenomenon," it occurs when a patient notes a significant increase in pain, often at the end of a traction session, when he or she is rising from the table. This is seen as a contraindication to continuing further traction sessions and has been thought of as a sort of "rebound" of disk material back onto the nerve root after distraction. Paris, however, states that it may be a positive sign when pressure is released from a neurovascular structure and is a result of revascularization.[46] Cyriax described this in thoracic outlet syndrome. Although Paris states that the physician should proceed judiciously, the symptom of increased pain (e.g., sensation) may be a very positive indication of traction's beneficial effect.

The problem of ascertaining the efficacy of traction is complicated by the many cointerventions often performed along with traction (other modalities, exercises, corsets or supports, and injections besides any medication or activity changes a patient may make) over the course of treatment.[62] Although these may mitigate or reinforce the effects of traction, any study that focuses only on traction as a sole intervention will not show any lasting relief. Certainly, any patient treated with diabetes would not expect to get improvement on medication alone but would want to incorporate diet control, weight loss, and other measures such as good skin care for total management. Likewise, a patient obtaining improved spinal elongation and disk reduction with traction should receive immediate instruction in maintaining neutral posture and stabilization exercises, along with passive support as needed. Saunders emphasizes this point that man "cannot get well on traction alone. [He] must have total management."[55]

RECENT LITERATURE REVIEW

A number of studies have been published over the past 5 years involving traction. These have ranged from literature reviews and case studies to studies of new methods of traction or assessing traction with EMG results.

In 1996 Beurskens and colleagues published a study of the efficacy of traction in nonspecific back pain in 12 weeks and 6-month follow-up.[6] They did this study because a previous pilot study of 24 individuals had shown better improvement in traction than those in a control group. In their larger study of 151 patients, no significant improvement in the high-dose traction group was found compared with the sham traction group. Cointerventions were not allowed except for pain medication taken before the study. No significant difference was found between the two groups, and the researchers concluded that traction was not efficacious for nonspecific low back pain.

In 1997, two studies came out using new technologies to improve traction outcomes. Stone and Wharton combined traction with TENS, massage, vibration, and acupressure to treat tension headaches and neck pain.[57] Although they noted no improvement in fibromyalgia trigger points, they did achieve relief based on subjective patient response. Combining EMG biofeedback with traction resulted in greater decrease of muscular hypertonus and a more rapid rise to a theraputic dosage of traction, according to the work of Wong and associates.[71]

The same year, an excellent case study on relief of chronic whiplash headache was conducted by Olson.[45] She detailed the history and failure of previous conservative measures, along with a good rationale for including traction in the rehabilitative program as well as corrective exercises. Home traction was an important component of the overall rehabilitation program.

In 1998, Humphreys and colleagues found that flexion angle was the main determinant of enlargening the foraminal space at C5–C6, and traction added little additional effect.[29] In a review of nonoperative treatment on neck and arm pain, Dreyer and Boden cited traction as not scientifically proved but nonetheless commonly used and thought to be beneficial modality in radicular pain.[19]

There were several favorable studies on traction in 1999. On a retrospective study of 58 patients, Swezey, Swezey and Warner found that 87% of patients improved using a simple over-the-door apparatus 5 minutes daily with an average weight of 11 pounds.[58] They made a strong case for safe, cost-effective treatment for patients with conditions such as mild to moderate degenerative changes on x-ray study and neurologic signs.

A study in Germany compared interferential electrical treatment with low-weight traction (10–20 kg), coupled with massage on a special table.[70] Both treatments resulted in equivalent pain relief in 152 patients studied.

Corso and Brosky treated a 42-year-old patient with traction and other modalities, noting improvement at 6 weeks in impairments, functional limitations, and disabilities.[14] Abdulwahab used electrodiagnostic testing of the H-reflex to show the diminishment of nerve root compression in traction.[1]

PERSONAL REFLECTIONS AND EXPERIENCE

These writers have found traction to be a highly beneficial modality in many spinal conditions. The physical therapist can recall only two cases in over 10 years of application of significantly increased pain for several days that mandated the abandonment of traction. In retrospect, although these patients appeared to be good candidates, their disk pathology may have been worse than clinical assessment or imaging studies indicated. Likewise, the traction application may have been less than ideal.

Traction is viewed by some as a passive modality that benefits the patient only, at best, while on the table. These writers see traction as an active part of a total rehabilitation program. We agree with Saal that traction can play a major role in relieving pain and allowing patient to begin active exercises more quickly, comfortably, and safely.[52] The repetitive pull–relax of intermittent traction mimics joint mechanics in patients who lack the present ability to mobilize the spinal segments by themselves.

Patient selection is, of course, critical. All contraindications are ruled out first, and our philosophy is to observe for general hypermobility as a relative contraindication. Also, we are reluctant to place a patient on traction if he or she seems to have a dependent, passive attitude to rehabilitation. The rationale for traction is explained in a active manner. "This treatment will help you move your back in a pain-free manner. You may experience some soreness because you have not been able to move normally for a while."

When soft tissue has been positively affected or disk pressure removed, it is imperative to have the patient maintain good posture and progress with active exercises. If the patient sees traction as one part of the whole treatment program, he or she is less likely to become dependent on the physician or therapist and ignore the home program. Also, the referring physician and treating therapist need to work closely together in defining and monitoring the utility of the traction in progressing toward rehabilitation goals.

Manual traction is often a good indicator of a patient's response to traction, and, if traction is useful in the clinic, an inexpensive over-the-door water weight bag device has, in our experience, helped well over 50% of those taking it home. Weight used is often between 10 and 15 pounds, with the patient gradually increasing weight and duration until an effective dose is reached. The key to success, again, is proper patient selection and education on positioning at home. The patient should be able to verbalize and demonstrate good set-up of the home equipment before leaving the clinic with it. For those with low back pain with unilateral leg pain, we have found positional distraction to be of some benefit. This can be taught as part of the home exercise program. Although not usually dispensed in our clinic, we have found some patients over the years who have benefitted from home pelvic traction.

If the goal of traction is soft tissue stretching, our clinic prefers a 20–30-second stretch with a 10–15-second rest in intermittent traction. We tell patients that this is comparable to their hamstring stretches. Sometimes, we will do 10 minutes of intermittent traction and 5 minutes of static traction, if tolerated, at a slightly lower poundage. A table that allows the physician or therapist to leave a slight pull in the rest phase of intermittent traction (e.g., 90 over 50 pounds) is potentially less irritating than a 90-pound swing in pressure every 20 seconds. Varying the traction angle in three dimensions for the desired effect is also important.

In summary, traction is a modality with a long history of use in physical medicine. There are many conditions in which traction can be used profitably and many variables in employing the modality. Provided the patient is selected appropriately, traction is safe and effective. In view of the widespread prevalence and severity of low back problems encountered in neuromusculoskeletal practice and the literature and clinical evidence for traction as a part of a comprehensive program in back rehabilitation, there is every reason to consider traction as a part of a well thought out physical therapy program. To rule out traction based solely on personal preference or lack of equipment denies a patient his or her full potential for improving more rapidly. Likewise, continued research and clinical practice are needed to validate when and how traction should continue to be used.

REFERENCES

1. Abdulwahab SS: The effect of reading and traction on patients with cervical radiculopathy based on electrodiagnostic testing. J Neuromusculoskel Sys 7:91–96, 1999.
2. Braat MM, Roser S: The treatment of headaches. N Y State J Med 53:687–693, 1953.
3. Bradnam L, Rochester L, Vujnovich A: Manual cervical traction reduces alpha motor neuron excitability in normal subjects. Electromyogr Clin Neurophysiol 40:259–266, 2000.
4. Bridger RS, Ossey S, Fourie G: Effect of lumbar traction on stature. Spine 6:522–524, 1990.
5. Brouillette DL, Gurske DT: Chiropractic treatment of cervical radiculopathy caused by herniated cervical disc. J Manipul Physiol Ther 17:119–123, 1994.
6. Buerskens AJ, de Vet HC, Koke AJ, et al: efficacy of traction for nonspecific low back pain. Spine 22:2756–2762, 1997.

7. Burton C: Low Back Pain, 2nd ed. Philadelphia, J.B. Lippincott, 1980.
8. Caillet R: Neck and Arm Pain, 2nd ed. Philadelphia, F.A. Davis, 1981.
9. Cheatle MD, Esterhai JL: Pelvic traction as treatment for acute back pain. Spine 16:1379–1381, 1991.
10. Christensen T, Bliddal H, Hansen SE, et al: Severe low-back pain. 1: Clinical assessment of two weeks conservative therapy. Scand J Rheumatol 22:25–29, 1993.
11. Colachis SC, Strohm BR: Cervical traction. Arch Phys Med Rehabil 46:815, 1965.
12. Colachis SC, Strohm BR: Cervical traction: Relationship of traction time to varied traction force with constant angle. Arch Phys Med Rehabil 46:815–819, 1965.
13. Colachis SC, Strohm BR: Effects of intermittent traction on separation of lumbar vertebrae. Arch Phys Med Rehab 50:251–255, 1967.
14. Corso DR, Brosky JA Jr: Non-operative management of cervical radiculopathy. Phys Ther case rev 2:139–144, 1999.
15. Cyriax JH: Treatment of lumbar disc lesions. Br Med J 2:1434, 1950.
16. Cyriax JH: Textbook of Orthopedic Medicine: Treatment of Soft Tissue Lesions, 8th ed. London, Bailliere Tyndale, 1982.
17. Deets D, Hinds K, Kopp S: Cervical traction: A comparisim of sitting and supine positions. Phys Ther 51:255, 1977.
18. Delaceda F: Effect of angle of tractionpull on upper trapezius muscle activity. JOSPT 1:205, 1980.
19. Dreyer SJ, Boden SD: Nonoperative treatment of neck and arm pain. Spine 23: 2746–2754, 1998.
20. Ellenberg MR, Honet JC, Treanor WJ: Cervical radiculopathy. Arch Phys Med Rehabil 75:342–352, 1994.
21. Franks A: Temporomandibular joint dysfunction associated with cervical traction. Arch Phys Med Rehabil 8:38–40, 1967.
22. Frazer EH: The use of traction in backache. Med J Aust 41: 694–697, 1954.
23. Gupta R, Ramarao SV: Epidurography in reduction of lumbar disc prolapse by traction. Arch Phys Med Rehabil 59:322, 1978.
24. Harris R: Traction. In Licht S (ed): Massage Manipulation and Traction. Baltimore, Waverley Press, 1963.
25. Harris P: Cervical traction: Review of the literature and treatment guidelines. Phys Ther 57:910, 1977.
26. Harrison DD, Jackson BL, Troyanovich S, et al: The efficacy of cervical extension-compression Traction combined with a diversified manipulation and drop table adjustments in the rehabilitation of cervical lordosis: A pilot study. J Manip Physiolog Ther 17:454–464, 1994.
27. Hickling J: Spinal traction technique. Physiother 58:58, 1972.
28. Hood C, Hart D, et al: Comparison of electromyographic activity in normal lumbar sacrospinalis musculature during continuous and intermittent pelvic traction. JOSPT 2: 137, 1981.
29. Humphreys SC, Chase J, Patwardhan A, et al: Flexion and Traction Effect on C5–C6 Foraminal Space. Arch Phys Med Rehabil 79:1105–1109, 1998.
30. Jackson B: The cervical syndrome. Springfield, IL, Charles C Thomas, 1958.
31. Jensen R, Bliddal H, Hansen SE, et al: Severe low-back pain. II: Changes in CT scans in the acute phase and after long-term observation. Scand J Rheumatol 22:30–34, 1993.
32. Judovich BD: Herniated cervical disc: A new form of traction therapy. Am J Surg 84:646–656, 1952.
33. Judovich BD: Lumbar traction therapy and dissipated force factors. Lancet 74:411, 1954.
34. Judovich BD: Lumbar traction therapy. JAMA 159:549–550, 1955.
35. Kekosz VN, Hilbert L, Tepperman PS: Cervical and lumbopelvic traction. Postgrad Med 80:187-194, 1986.
36. Klaber-Moffett JA, Hughes GI, Griffiths P: An investigation of the effects of cervical traction: Part 2: The effects on the neck musculature. Clin Rehabil 4 287, 1980.
37. Kriss TC, Kriss VM: Neck pain: Primary care workup of acute and chronic symptoms. Geriatrics 55:47-57, 2000.
38. Kumar S: Spinal deformity and axial traction. Spine 21:653–655, 1996.
39. LeBan MM, Macy JA, Meerschaert JR: Intermittent cervical traction: A progenitor of lumbar radicular pain. Arch Phys Med Rehabil 73:295–296, 1992.
40. LeMarr J, Goldig L, Crehan K: Cardiorespiratory responses to inversion. Phys Sportsmed 11: 51–57, 1983.

41. Leutchuman R, Deusinger RH: Comparison of sacrospinalis myoelectric activity and pain levels in patients undergoing static and intermittent lumbar traction. Spine 18:1361–1365, 1993.
42. McKenzie R: The Lumbar Spine. Waikanae, New Zealand, Spinal Publications, 1981.
43. Masturzo A: Vertebral traction for the treatment of sciatica. Rheumatism 1:62, 1955.
44. Matthews N: Dynamic discography: A study of lumbar traction. Ann Phys Med 9:275, 1968.
45. Olson V: Whiplash-associated chronic headache treated with home cervical traction. Phys Ther 77:417–424, 1997.
46. Paris S: Introduction to Spinal Evaluation and Manipulation [course notes]. St. Augustine, FL, Institute Press, 1990.
47. Paris S: Foundations of Clinical Orthopedics [course notes]. St. Augustine, FL, Institute Press, 1990.
48. Pellecchia G: Lumbar traction: A review of the literature. JOSPT 20:262–266, 1994.
49. Ramos G, Martin W: Effects of vertebral axial decompression on intradiscal pressure. J Neurosurg 81:350–353, 1994.
50. Rath W: Cervical traction: A clinical perspective. Orthop Rev 13:430–439, 1984.
51. Rechtiea J, Andary M, Holmes T, Weiting JM: Manipulation, massage and traction. In Gans B (ed): Rehabilitative Medicine: Principles and Practice, 3rd ed. Philadelphia, Lippincott-Raven, 1998, pp 541–547.
52. Saal J, Saal JA, Yurth EF: Nonoperative management of herniated cervical intervertebral disc with radiculopathy. Spine 21:1877–1883, 1996.
53. Salcido R, Hart D, Smith AM: Traction In Braddom R (ed): Physical Medicine and Rehabilitation. Philadelphia, WB Saunders, 1996, pp 436–442.
54. Saunders HD: Unilateral lumbar traction. Phys Ther 61:221, 1981.
55. Saunders HD: Spinal traction. In Evaluation, Treatment and Prevention of Musculoskeletal Disorders. Minneapolis, Viking Press, 1988.
56. Shore NA, Shaefer MG, Hoppenfeld S: Iatrogenic TMJ difficulty: Cervical traction may be the etiology. J Prosth Dentistry 41:541–542, 1979.
57. Stone RG, Wharton RB: Simultaneous multiple-modality therapy for tension headaches and neck pain. Biomed Inst Tech 31:259–262, 1997.
58. Swezey RL, Swezey AM, Warner K: Efficacy of home cervical traction therapy. Am J Phys Med Rehabil 78:30–32, 1999.
59. Tan JC, Nordin M: Role of physical therapy in the treatment of cervical disk disease. Orthop Clin North Am 23:435–449, 1992.
60. Tesio L, Merlo A: Autotraction versus passive traction: An open controlled study in lumbar disc herniation. Arch Phys Med Rehabil 74:871–876, 1993.
61. Tesio L: Author's response [letters to the editor]. Arch Phys Med Rehabil 75:234–235, 1994.
62. Trudel G: Autotraction [letters to the editor]. Arch Phys Med Rehabil 75:234, 1994
63. U.S. Department of Health and Human Services: Acute Low Back Problems in Adults. Washington, DC, U.S. Government Printing Office, 1994, AHCPR publication 95-0642.
64. van der Heijden GJ, Beurskens AJ, Koes BW, et al: The efficacy of traction for back and neck pain: A systematic blinded review of randomized clinical trial methods. Phys Ther 75:93–104, 1995.
65. van Valberg AA, et al: Joint distraction in the treatment of osteoarthritis. II. Effects on cartilage in a canine model. Osteoarthritis Cartilage 8:1–8, 2000.
66. Waitz E: The lateral bending sign. Spine 6:388–397, 1981.
67. Webster's New Collegiate Dictionary. Springfield, MA, Merriam, 1977, p 1237.
68. Weinberger LM: Trauma or treatment? The role of intermittent traction in the treatment of cervical soft tissue injuries. J Trauma 16:377–382, 1976.
69. Wells P: Cervical angina. Am Family Phys 55:2262–2264, 1997.
70. Werners R, Pysent PB, Bulstrode CJ: Randomized trial comparing interferential therapy with motorized lumbar traction and massage in the management of low back pain in a primary care setting. Spine 15:1579–1584, 1999.
71. Wong AM, Lee MY, Chang WH, Tang FT: Clinical trial of a cervical traction modality with electromyographic biofeedback. Am J Phys Med Rehabil 76:19–25, 1997.
72. Yates D: Indications and contraindications for spinal traction. Physiotherapy 58:58–65, 1972.
73. Zylbergold R, Piper MC: Cervical spine disorders: A comparison of three types of traction. Spine 10:867–870, 1985.

Chapter 13
Joint Mobilization

Ida Hirst, PT

When the normal mechanics of joint motion are altered, pain and early signs of joint degeneration often occur. This chapter explores the effects of altered mobility, reviews normal joint function, and provides basic information on appropriate treatment techniques that can be applied. The word *manipulation* has been used loosely in medicine to mean passive movement of any kind. In this chapter, *manipulation* will be defined as a sudden movement or thrust, of small amplitude, performed at a speed that renders the patient powerless to prevent it.[9] *Joint mobilization* is defined as passive movements performed in such a way that, at all times, they are within the control of the patient so that he can prevent the movement if he so chooses. Joint mobilization techniques are applied in the presence of restricted joint motion. The practitioner must make certain, however, that a painful joint exhibits restriction of the capsule and requires mobilization. Often, active range of motion is limited or painful, but the cause of the limitation is found in other periarticular structures. The effective examination procedures to make an accurate diagnosis and to provide the most effective treatment are covered.

HISTORY

Much literature is available on various techniques and methods of joint manipulation and mobilization. Important contributors include Cyriax, James and John Mennell, Maitland, Kaltenborn, and Cookson and Kent.[2,3,6,9,11,12]

For a period of time, the use of passive mobilization techniques almost became a forgotten art. This is thought to be a result of the techniques provoking pain when they were used too aggressively. Maitland contributed tremendously to the advancement of standardized educational programs and tutelage available to physical therapists and other members of the medical community, teaching safe and gentle treatment techniques around the world.[9] This in part has helped to make these techniques popular once again.

Controlled studies on the effectiveness of joint mobilization have been few.[14] The primary evidence for the efficacy of this type of treatment comprises clinical experience, case histories, and inference.[5] Further controlled studies are necessary to assess the benefits of joint mobilization.

PHILOSOPHY OF JOINT DYSFUNCTION

Joint injury, including conditions, such as osteoarthritis, instability, and the after effects of sprains and strains, are not diseases but dysfunctions. These dysfunctions are manifested as either an increase, a decrease, or abnormality of motion.

When the dysfunction manifests as limited motion, the treatment of choice is mobilization of joint structures, stretching muscles and fascia, and sometimes strengthening of muscles. When the dysfunction is manifest as increased movement, laxity, or instability, the treatment is not mobilization of the joint in question but stabilization. This may be accomplished through correction of joint limitations in neighboring joints that may be contributing to the joint's need for compensation or through postural training and exercise.

Joint dysfunction responds well to conservative treatment. Even after degeneration has occurred and resulted in a loss of joint space, cartilage can be made to regenerate by removing restrictions, stretching the joint capsule, and promoting normal and frequent use.[1]

The effects of continuous passive motion (CPM) have been studied on the healing of full thickness articular cartilage defects. Salter et al. published the results of experimental continuous passive motion on defects in the distal joint surfaces of the femur in 20 immature rabbits. With continuous passive motion, healing through the formation of new hyaline cartilage (chondroneogenesis) occurred in over half of the induced defects within 4 weeks.[15]

EFFECT OF IMMOBILIZATION ON ARTICULAR AND PERIARTICULAR STRUCTURES

Each structure responds uniquely to immobilization. It is important to understand each structure's response to effectively manage the patient during the rehabilitation process.

Cartilage

Cartilage does not have a direct blood supply. It relies on the compressive and distractive forces of joint motion to obtain nutrients and oxygen. When a joint is immobilized, the cartilage weakens and begins to lose its stiffness and resilience to compression. Areas in which the articular cartilage does not make good contact with the articular cartilage on the opposite joint surface develop fibrous changes, or pannus formation, and loss of cartilage results. This accounts for the loss of vertical height in the joint space with degenerative changes. Radiographs exhibit degenerative changes including spurring after as little as 4 weeks of immobilization.[4]

Synovium

In 2 weeks of immobilization, the blood vessels in the subsynovial region proliferate, and increased synovial fluid is produced. After 4 weeks, there is a marked increase in the number of synovial cells, hyperemia is present, and pannus begins to form over the noncontact articular cartilage. Within 6 weeks, the amount of fibroblasts and collagen within the joint increases, giving a fibrotic appearance.[1]

Joint Capsule

The joint capsule begins to show signs of increased thickness after 5 weeks of immobilization. Folds of capsular tissue adhere to each other and further restrict motion.[1]

Ligaments and Tendons

Disuse atrophy of the surrounding ligaments and tendons occurs. The tensile or breaking strength reduces, and the strength of the structure's insertion at the bone diminishes. Ligaments demonstrate a decrease in fiber bundle thickness. Tissue samples taken from immobilized sites are found to have a reduced amount of aerobic enzymes.[1]

Bone

Bone density is maintained through weight bearing. Weight-bearing bones require at least 2–3 hours of vertical weight bearing each day in order to maintain density. After a period of immobilization when weight bearing is prohibited, the capacity of the bone to withstand stress is diminished.[1]

Muscle

Similar effects take place at the voluntary muscle groups surrounding the involved immobilized joint. Muscles atrophy, vascularization decreases, and fuel stores and mitochondria within the muscle decrease. The aerobic capacity diminishes, there is loss of volitional control of the muscle and the capacity to withstand tensile forces reduces.[1]

Not all of these structures recover at the same rate. During the rehabilitation process the program must be adapted to allow recovery of the lowest metabolic systems first, progressing over time to the higher metabolic systems.

JOINT MOBILIZATION AND CLASSIFICATION OF MOVEMENT

There are five classifications of joint movement as outlined by Dr. Mennell.[11]

1. **Active joint movement**. These are the classical gross motions taught by anatomists, or joint motion that can be actively performed by a voluntary muscle.

2. **Passive joint movement**. The movement in which a joint is passively put through the range of motion normally under voluntary control.

3. **Joint play movement**. This movement is not under voluntary control but is necessary for the performance of painless, free, voluntary movement. Examples of these motions are long axis traction, rotation, anterior and posterior gliding, and medial and lateral gliding.

4. **Articulary movement**. This is also a nonvoluntary motion. A joint with limited joint play is taken through the full range of motion, and then a series of passive, rhythmic repetitions of movement are applied by a practitioner to restore normal synovial joint play movement.

5. **Specific joint manipulation**. This movement describes the action in which a joint with limited synovial joint play is taken through the full range of movement present, at which point a manipulative thrust is applied to restore the full normal range. Full joint play allows pain-free active motion.[12]

Traction

The use of traction is an important component of manual therapy. The force of pull is determined by the purpose for which the traction is being applied. The manual therapist Kaltenborn describes three stages of traction[6]:

- **Stage 1 traction (piccolo)**. The traction is so small that only the compressive effect in the joint is released while the joint pressure is neutralized. The joint surfaces are not actually separated.

- **Stage 2 traction ("taking up the slack")**. The joint is distracted using little force to separate the joint surfaces just as far as the soft tissues allow.
- **Stage 3 traction (mobilization treatment)**. A continuation and extension of the stage 2 distraction of the joint is applied with enough force to stretch the soft tissues.

Traction is used as a treatment for the relief of pain, and for this reason it is best to use either stage 1 or stage 2. The traction is held for approximately 10 seconds, with a rest of 2–3 seconds before repeating.[6]

Compression

When symptoms from a joint surface disorder are present, joint compression is used both to test and to treat certain disorders. When symptoms can be reproduced with joint compression, treatment can include compression to a degree that does not provoke a painful response. The compression is combined with oscillating movements to the joint back and forth for 1 or 2 minutes. As the joint responds favorably to the treatment, the degree of compression can be progressed. This has been especially beneficial in the treatment of patellofemoral joint disorders.[9]

Joint Positions

The term *0-position* is used to describe the anatomically defined basic position or "normal" position as a basis for the measurement of joint movement. This is different from the resting position. *Resting position* is the position where the joint capsule, ligaments, and muscles related to the joint are most relaxed and where the joint capsule gives the most amount of space. The *close-packed position*, on the other hand, is the position in which the capsule and ligaments are in maximal tension. It occurs at one extreme of the most habitual movement of that particular joint. In this position, the concave and convex joint surfaces are in complete congruence and the two bones of the articulation cannot be separated by traction.[11]

Planes and Axes of Movement

When performing and teaching joint mobilization, the axes of motion must be understood, as must the plane in which the motion is performed. The four planes of motion are as follows:

Median plane—Divides the body vertically into two "equal" lateral parts
Sagittal plane—Any plane parallel to the median plane
Frontal (coronal) plane—Divides the body vertically into an anterior and posterior part
Horizontal plane—Divides the body across into an upper and lower part
Each plane has two main axes that run at right angles to each other.

When the mobilization is applied to the joint, it is applied as a movement of traction, translation, or rotation. Traction separates the two joint surfaces perpendicularly. With translatory movement, all of the points on the moving articular surface move in the same direction at the same rate of speed. With rotatory movement, the farther a point on the articular surface is from the axes of motion, the greater the speed of motion and the greater the distance covered. Examples of rotatory movement are passive and active joint motion.

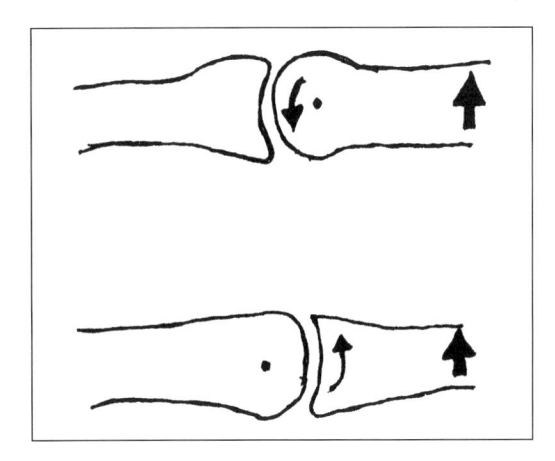

FIGURE 1. The bone on the left is the side being stabilized. The bone (or extremity) on the right is the side receiving mobilization. The large arrows indicate the direction the extremity is moving. The small curved arrows depict the direction that the joint surface needs to go to accomplish this movement. The convex surface is moved in the opposite direction of the bone movement (*top*). The concave surface is moved in the same direction as the bone movement (*bottom*).

Direction of Treatment

The direction of treatment is determined by the shape of the joint surface being mobilized. One surface is always considered concave and one considered convex. The axis of motion is always found on the side that is convex (Fig. 1).

The principles to remember are:

- When mobilizing a concave joint surface on a convex joint surface, mobilize in the same direction the bone or extremity is trying to go.
- When mobilizing a convex joint surface on a concave joint surface, mobilize the joint surface opposite the direction the extremity is trying to go.[8,9]

TREATMENT SEQUENCE AND PRINCIPLES OF TECHNIQUE

1. **Communication**. One of the most important contributions practitioners can make to the successful management of a patient's symptoms is taking time to understand the patient. Verbal and nonverbal communication must be considered to understand the patient's complaints clearly. This information must be correlated with the objective findings of the examination and used to assess the effectiveness of the chosen treatment.[9]

2. **Patient positioning**. The patient must be positioned in a comfortable manner, with the extremity relaxed and properly stabilized. The patient must have complete confidence in the therapist's grasp, and the position should take full mechanical advantage of levers.

3. **Therapist positioning**. The therapist also must be positioned correctly for successful mobilization with good technique. Without correct positioning, the therapist will fatigue rapidly, and the intended result will not be achieved. Wherever possible, the therapist should embrace the parts to be moved or stabilized. In

addition, the therapist should hold around the joint so as to feel the joint movement as the technique is performed. The therapist's position must afford complete control of the movement, and the patient must feel confident that the joint will not be hurt by being moved further than he or she expects.

4. **Stabilization**. It is important to determine which joint surface is to remain stable and which is to be moved. If proper stabilization is not achieved, the treatment may provoke pain.

5. **Direction of treatment**. Ideally, mobilization is initiated from the resting position. Sometimes, however, this must be modified to treat in the position in which there is the least amount of pain. The structure of the joint surface determines the direction of treatment. It is advisable to begin with joint traction, which reduces joint contact, followed by movement parallel to the joint surface. The direction should first be toward the motion least impaired, followed by that which is most impaired.

6. **Taking up the slack**. The joint play movement is taken up with direct and steady pressure in the direction you wish to treat.

7. **Mobilization**. Articulary mobilization consists of repeated, nonvoluntary movements applied by a skilled therapist. The motion applied begins from the joint's resting position and continues to the position where the slack is taken up, and then back again. The degrees or "grades" of mobilization pressure applied are discussed later in this chapter. Any part of a range of movement may be used in treatment, and widely varying amplitudes and speeds may be chosen. A painful joint is best treated with a slow, smooth, even rhythm; whereas a stiff, small joint is treated best with sharp, staccato type movements. Some patients have difficulty relaxing completely, even when pain is minimal. If large-amplitude treatment movements are hindered because of this, a "broken rhythm" can be used with varied amplitude in an attempt to trick the muscles.

When attempting to increase the range of movement in a stiff joint with pain present at the extremes of motion, passive stretching is applied slowly up to the point that pain becomes a limiting factor. This position is held until the pain subsides, after which an additional slow stretch is added until the pain increases again. Small, slow, oscillatory movements are then applied just short of this new limit of movement.

The initial treatment must be performed in the painless part of the range in one of the least painful directions. The number of oscillations given is determined by the degree of irritability present. The average time spent passively moving joints that are not excessively painful is approximately 4–5 minutes. A highly irritable joint should be moved less with the treatment time anywhere between 30 seconds and 2 minutes.

8. **Testing**. Both the voluntary active (or passive) range of motion and the nonvoluntary range of motion, also known as the joint play, should be tested for the effectiveness of the treatment after an articulary mobilization procedure has been completed.[6,9]

New Technique

Brian Mulligan, a physical therapist from New Zealand, has recently popularized a relatively new technique for joint mobilization that can be applied to spinal and peripheral joints.[13a] He has called these techniques natural apophyseal glides (NAGs), sustained natural apophyseal glides (SNAGs), and mobilization with movement (MWM). With these techniques, the therapist manually sustains pressure in a lateral glide, rotatory glide, or otherwise while the patient actively moves the joint into the direction in which increased movement is desired. Although research to prove the effectiveness of these techniques has not been completed, Mulligan believes that they improve the mechanical position of the joint allowing for pain-free motion, thus restoring the mechanical ability of the joint to move throughout its normal range. After moving repetitively (usually 3 sets of 10 movements during one treatment) with the joint supported using the glide necessary to improve mechanical position or alignment, the motion is generally dramatically improved. This allows the patient to function within the new range and avoid loss of the range gained between treatment sessions.

INDICATIONS AND CONTRAINDICATIONS TO JOINT MOBILIZATION

Joint mobilization is used as a treatment modality when limited mobility is expected to be reversible. Such is often the case with osteoarthritis.[9] Radiographs are required to determine whether or not there is structural alteration or damage to the joint resulting in limited mobility. If there are structural alterations but the degree of mobility restriction is suspected to be greater than these alterations, joint mobilization is indicated to improve functional mobility.

Another indication for joint mobilization is joint pain. Pain can be reduced by using a gentle force in the pain-free range. This is thought to stimulate afferent mechanoreceptor pathways to the central nervous system, reducing pain. If the disorder produces pain throughout the range, the mobilization should also be applied through range, also known as a large-amplitude mobilization. However, if pain occurs only at the end of range, then treatment is directed at the end of range with a low-amplitude movement. This low-amplitude movement at the end of range is known as grade IV mobilization and is discussed later in this chapter.[9]

Studies indicate that the use of early mobilization following fracture improves the clinical and functional recovery, resulting in a more rapid and complete return of range of motion and strength.[13]

Contraindications to joint mobilization include joint hypermobility, as in rheumatoid arthritis and other conditions in which the patient does not have active voluntary muscular control for stability, and compromised ligamentous joint stability. Care must be taken when treating patients during pregnancy because of the hormonal effects on ligaments. This is especially the case at the joints of the spine and sacroiliac region. Joint mobilization should also be avoided when a joint is acutely swollen and inflamed.[9]

GRADES OF ARTICULARY MOVEMENT

In order to communicate and document treatment techniques in a concise and simple manner, grades of articulary mobilization have been established. This is especially helpful if more than one therapist is treating the same patient. The grading system used may differ from one school of thought to another, but Maitland's grading system (below) is commonly used[9]:

Grade I. A small-amplitude movement performed at the beginning of range. This is approximately the first 20% of joint play.

Grade II. A large-amplitude movement performed within the range but not reaching the limit of the range. It is performed between 20% and 60% of the available joint play. If the movement is performed at the beginning of this range, it is expressed as II−, and if it is taken deeply into the range, yet still not reaching the limit, it is expressed as II+.

Grade III. A large-amplitude movement performed up to the limit of the range. This movement can also be expressed with plus and minus values. If the mobilization knocks vigorously at the end of range, it is graded a III+, but if it nudges gently at the limit of the range it is expressed as III−.

Grade IV. A small-amplitude movement at the limit of the range, well into resistance. This can also be expressed as IV+ and IV−, depending on the vigor, using the same criteria described for grade III.

Grade V (joint manipulation). This is a high-velocity, short-amplitude thrust from the limit of range to beyond. This grade of movement will not be explored further in this chapter.

If the normal range of joint movement or joint play is restricted by a joint disorder, grades III and IV are restricted to the new limit of the range, and grade II movements are restricted to smaller amplitudes. Similarly, in the case of a hypermobile joint, these movements are altered.

EXAMINATION

A thorough examination is necessary to determine the source of joint pain and the appropriateness of joint mobilization. Limited joint motion can be present for a variety of reasons. The examiner must avoid assumptions and allow time for good communication with the patient. Connective tissue disorders of the skin and neuromuscular disorders should be ruled out before assuming that the limitation is due to an articulary disorder. During the exam, the periarticular structures are examined to determine the source of pain. This is done through active and passive range of motion, isometric resistance, traction, compression, and palpation testing. During passive range of motion, the noncontractile tissues are tested. If the pain that was present during active range of motion disappears with passive range of motion, then a reason other than joint dysfunction should be suspected. If pain present during passive range of motion disappears with distraction, articular causes of the pain should be expected. Compression to the joint should again reproduce the pain. When traction or distraction to the joint increases pain, pain most likely is originating in the ligamentous or muscular structures, placed on stretch. A muscular origin of pain can be confirmed by applying isometric resistance to the muscle in question. Keep in mind, however, that muscle activity increases joint compression and will increase pain in a painful joint. If the pain is of muscular origin, this can be further confirmed through palpation.

The examination must also include a detailed **history** including the mechanism of injury, subsequent symptomatology, nature of symptoms, pain description and pattern, aggravating and relieving factors, functional loss, and past pertinent medical care. **Function** is then assessed including active and passive range of motion. The patient's willingness to move as well as the quality of motion should be determined. Observe any crepitus. Check end-feel and stability. The contractile structures should be tested for pain and weakness. Isometric resisted movements create tension only in the contractile structures, while the "inert" structures remain static. This helps in differential diagnosis. Strength should be graded using the 0 to normal or 0 to 5 method. Traction and compression can be used to assess the anatomic joints, including the intra-articular structures, as can gliding or translatory movement.

The examination continues with **palpation** of the skin, muscle, tendons, bursae, tendon sheaths, joints, nerves, and blood vessels. If necessary, **neurologic tests** can be included to rule out peripheral and central neurologic involvement. Based on the findings, additional radiography and laboratory tests should be included.

The clinician should then determine if there is a correlation between the objective findings and the complaints of the patient. Do the joints have a normal pain-free range of movement and stability? Could there be other causes of the pain: neuromuscular, vasogenic, autonomic, psychogenic, or a combination? What treatment can be done? What structures are responsible for the limited joint motion? How does this affect my decision on mobilization techniques available to me? Before a definite diagnosis has been made, a trial treatment may be given. After a few days, based on the results, a positive diagnosis can be made.

In some situations, the use of classic articulary mobilization techniques are not the best choice of treatment to restore range of motion and function to the compromised joint. When structural changes have taken place in the periarticular structures, such as shortening of the capsule, ligament, or adhesive formation, low-load prolonged stress to the tissues may be more effective. This is administered in the form of CPM, splinting, and active stretching exercise.[10]

CASE STUDY

A 35-year-old man sustained a comminuted fracture to the left distal radius as a result of a motorcycle accident. Surgical open reduction with internal fixation was performed followed by 6 weeks of immobilization. At 8 weeks, physical therapy was initiated. At the onset of care, active and passive range of motion were limed as follows: flexion, 30°; extension, 5°; radial deviation, 5°; ulnar deviation, 15°; supination, 10°; pronation, 60°. The incision sites had healed nicely, but heavy scar tissue was present over the volar aspect of the wrist, contributing to the loss of mobility into flexion and extension. Functionally, the patient complained of difficulty holding objects such as a plate of food due to the limited supination and lack of functional grip strength. He was a meat cutter by trade, and his goal was to return to work without restrictions.

The initial emphasis of physical therapy was placed on restoring range of motion. Because supination was severely restricted, it was decided to augment his home range of motion exercise program with a CPM device to be worn through the night as tolerated and during waking hours when not actively using the hand. The patient also performed active and active-assisted range of motion exercises, as well as passive stretching into all planes of motion at the wrist, forearm, and hand. This was performed three times a day by the patient independently.

186 Joint Mobilization

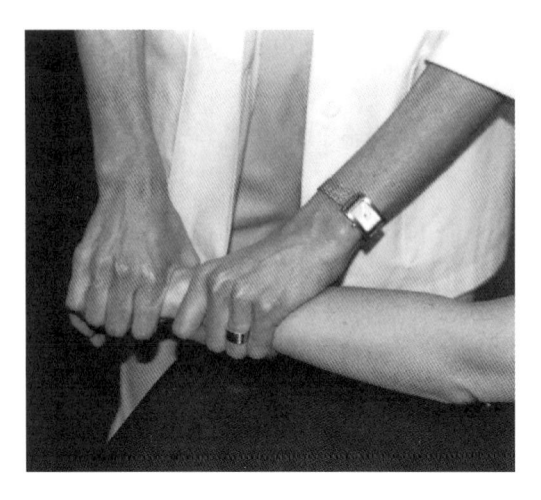

FIGURE 2. Radiocarpal joint: volar glide.

The patient attended physical therapy appointments three times per week over the course of 8 weeks, where the physical therapist performed manual joint mobilization techniques (Figs. 2 and 3). This consisted of stage 3 traction to the radiocarpal joint combined with small-amplitude, staccato mobilization at end-range (grade IV) flexion, extension, ulnar, and radial deviation. Grade IV mobilization was also applied to the radioulnar joint both proximally and distally at end range supination and pronation. Similar mobilization forces were applied to the metacarpophalangeal and interphalangeal joints of each finger as well as to the carpometacarpal joint of the thumb with goals of achieving full finger flexion and thumb opposition. Finger extension had remained intact so did not require treatment. Following the mobilization directed at restoring joint play, passive sustained stretching was performed to each joint. This entailed a steady

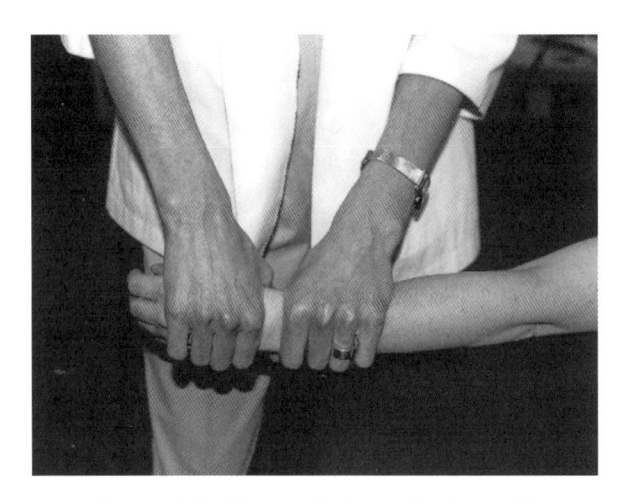

FIGURE 3. Radiocarpal joint: radioulnar glide.

sustained hold of the joint at the end of range up to the patient's pain tolerance. Once pain reduced, additional force was applied gradually to the new end of range and repeated for a total of 3–4 end-range positions, based on the patient's tolerance. This was directed at the periarticular structures that had shorted over the course of immobilization required following the fracture and surgical reduction or stabilization.

At the end of 8 weeks of treatment, forearm–wrist supination had improved to measure 85°. It was decided to increase efforts to restore wrist extension because this would allow the patient a more functional wrist position to perform the heavy gripping required for his occupation. The CPM device used for the purpose of increasing supination was returned to the vendor and replaced with a dynamic splint (Dynasplint) designed to place continuous low-grade pressure on the wrist into extension, thereby increasing total time spent receiving passive sustained stretch at the periarticular structures that were restricting this motion.

Manual therapy continued as described above, diminishing to two sessions per week as additional exercise was implemented directed at restoring strength to the forearm, wrist, and hand.

After 12 weeks of care, range of motion measures were: flexion, 70°; extension, 50°; radial deviation, 20°; ulnar deviation, 35°; supination, 85°; and pronation, 85°. Motion was no longer changing significantly between sessions. The patient was able to return to work as a meat cutter approximately 4 months from the injury. To determine the need for continued care to maintain the gains in mobility and strength, the Dynasplint was discontinued, and the frequency of treatment was reduced from twice per week to once per week, then down to once every 2 weeks, with a final session after 1 month without care for reassessment. Range of motion had been maintained by the patient's active use of the wrist and with his home exercise program. Periodically, the patient would experience bouts of pain accompanied by mild swelling over the tendons at the dorsal and radial aspect of the wrist, especially those tendons responsible for thumb extension and abduction. This was treated with the application of ice and rest because this was always preceded by heavy use of the wrist and hand. Pain and swelling were attributed to inflammation of the tendons not yet accustomed to resistive activity.

The patient was discharged and advised to contact his doctor and physical therapist if a loss of function at the wrist and hand developed. Follow-up at 1 year postinjury found the patient continuing his occupation with near normal use of his wrist and hand.

INDIVIDUAL JOINTS

Each joint must be understood in relation to these criteria for effective and safe treatment. In order to provide effective treatment, the shape of the joint surfaces must be understood, normal joint mobility and the resting and close-pack positions must be known. The shoulder girdle is one of the most complex and most frequently encountered peripheral joints. The specifics of the shoulder girdle complex are outlined here, but the same type of information must be understood for each peripheral joint requiring treatment (Table 1).[8]

TABLE 1. NORMAL PERIPHERAL JOINT POSITIONS

The Fingers: PIP, DIP, and MCP Joints

0-Position: The fingers are straight with the long axis through the metacarpal and phalangeal bones
Resting position: Slight flexion (approximately 15°)
Close-packed position: PIP, DIP, and MCP joints completely flexed

Voluntary ranges:
    DIP flexion: 90°
    PIP flexion: 120°
    MCP flexion: 90°, abduction: 45°, adduction: 15°

Nonvoluntary ranges:
    Traction
    Dorsal and volar gliding
    Radial and ulnar gliding
    MCP also rotation

The Thumb: Carpometacarpal Joint

Voluntary range:
    Flexion and extension: 50°
    Abduction and adduction: 40°
    Circumduction

Nonvoluntary range:
    Traction
    Rotation
    Dorsal and volar gliding
    Radial and ulnar gliding

The Wrist: Carpal Joints of 8 Bones (Pisiform, Triquetrium, Lunate, Scaphoid, Hamate, Capitate, Trapezoid, and Trapezium)

0-Position: The long axis of the radius and the third metacarpal are continuous
Resting position: Same as 0-position, but with the wrist in slight flexion
Close-pack position: Maximal wrist extension

Voluntary ranges:
    Flexion: 90°
    Extension: 85°
    Ulnar deviation: 45°
    Radial deviation: 20°

Nonvoluntary ranges:
    Dorsal and volar gliding
    Radial and ulnar gliding
    Mobilizing of the individual carpal bones

The Elbow: Humeroulnar and Humeroradial Joints

0-Position: Extended elbow
Resting position: 80–90° flexion at the elbow

Close-pack position:
    Humeroulnar: Maximum extension and maximum supination
    Humeroradial: 90° flexion with the forearm 5 supinated

Voluntary range:
    Flexion: 135°
    Extension: 160–180°

Nonvoluntary range:
    Separation of the joint surface (traction)
    Anterior and posterior glide of the radius

Continued on next page

Table 1. Normal Peripheral Joint Positions (continued)

The Forearm: Radioulnar Joints (Distal and Proximal)

0-Position: Elbow flexed 90° to the side of the body and radio-ulnar joint in supination
Resting position: Midway between pronation and supination, elbow flexed
Close-pack position: With the forearm in 5 supination, the interosseus membrane is maximally tightened.
Voluntary range:
    Pronation: 75°
    Supination: 85°
Nonvoluntary range:
    Distal radioulnar joint: dorsal and volar gliding
    Proximal radioulnar joint: anterior and posterior gliding

The Ankle: Talocrural Joint

0-Position: Right angle between the tibia and the lateral edge of the foot
Resting position: Slightly plantar flexed
Close-packed position: Maximum dorsiflexion
Voluntary range:
    Plantar flexion: 25°
    Dorsiflexion: 15°
Nonvoluntary range:
    Anterior and posterior gliding
    Separation of the joint surfaces

The Knee Joint

0-Position: The long axis of the femur shaft and the tibia are continuous
Resting position: Approximately 45° flexion
Close-pack position: Knee maximally extended
Voluntary range:
    Flexion: 135–150°
    Extension: 135–150°
    Medial rotation: 10–15°
    Lateral rotation: 20–25°
Nonvoluntary range:
    Anterior and posterior gliding
    Traction
    Rotation
    Distal and proximal glide at the patella

The Hip Joint

0-Position: The trunk and thigh in the same frontal plane. Right angle between a line connecting the two ASIS of the pelvis, and a line from the ASIS through the mid patella
Resting position: About 45° flexion and 20° abduction
Close-packed position: Maximum extension from 0°, maximum internal rotation, and maximum abduction
Voluntary ranges:
    Flexion: 120°
    Hyperextension: 10–15°
    Medial rotation: 25–35°
    Lateral rotation: 40–45°
    Abduction: 45–50°
    Adduction: 20–30°
Nonvoluntary ranges:
    Separation of joint surfaces
    Rotation

PIP = proximal interphalangeal, DIP = distal interphalangeal, MCP = metacarpophalangeal, ASIS = anterior superior iliac spine.

Shoulder Girdle

The shoulder girdle comprises four separate functional units: the glenohumeral joint, the scapulothoracic joint, the acromioclavicular joint, and the sternoclavicular joint. The glenohumeral joint is a multiaxial ball and socket joint. The articular surfaces are the glenoid fossa on the scapula and the humeral head. The joint surfaces are reciprocally curved with the convexity of the humerus being much larger than the glenoid cavity. The glenoid cavity is deepened somewhat by the fibrocartilaginous glenoid labrum.

Two of the important ligaments of the glenohumeral joint are the glenohumeral (anterior, middle, and superior), which reinforces the anterior capsule, and the coracohumeral, which helps prevent the humeral head from gliding distally.

Certain tendons strengthen the capsule, most notably those belonging to the rotator cuff (supraspinatus, infraspinatus, teres minor, and subscapularis). The capsule is weakest ventrally and caudally, and there tends to be more subluxation in these directions. The capsule is penetrated by the long head of the biceps tendon, and trauma to the tendon in this area often creates a tear in the corresponding part of the capsule.

The joint capsule is responsible for supplying stability to the glenohumeral joint where there is a high degree of mobility. The anterior capsule is relaxed in the neutral position with the arm dependent at the side, but tightens with external rotation, horizontal abduction, and extension. The inferior capsule is redundant, having many folds that can become adhered to each other when the arm is immobilized in the neutral position. The inferior capsule tightens on flexion and abduction. The posterior capsule tightens on internal rotation and horizontal adduction. With inactivity, all parts of the capsule may become involved, leading to the common diagnosis of adhesive capsulitis.

- 0-Position. The humerus is parallel to the body, the elbow is flexed to 90°, and the hand is in a sagittal plane.
- Resting position. The shoulder is in approximately 70° abduction and 30° flexion. The elbow is flexed, and the forearm is in a position to make a 30–40° angle with the horizontal plane.
- Close-pack position. The shoulder is in maximal abduction and external rotation.
- Voluntary range. Abduction, 120°; adduction, 70°; flexion, 120°; extension, 50°; internal rotation, 60°; external rotation, 80°.
- Nonvoluntary range. The head of the humerus can be mobilized in relation to the glenoid fossa superiorly, inferiorly, anteriorly, and posteriorly, and it also can be rotated and separated (traction) from the fossa (Figs. 4 and 5).

Scapulothoracic Joint

In addition to the glenohumeral joint, the shoulder girdle relies on the scapulothoracic joint for smooth coordinated movement between the thorax and the upper extremity. This is known as **scapulohumeral rhythm**. During the abduction movement of the arm, for each 15° of arm abduction, 10° of motion occurs at the glenohumeral joint, and 5° of rotation occurs at the scapula upon the thorax. When the arm has been abducted to 90° in relationship to the erect body, this is accom-

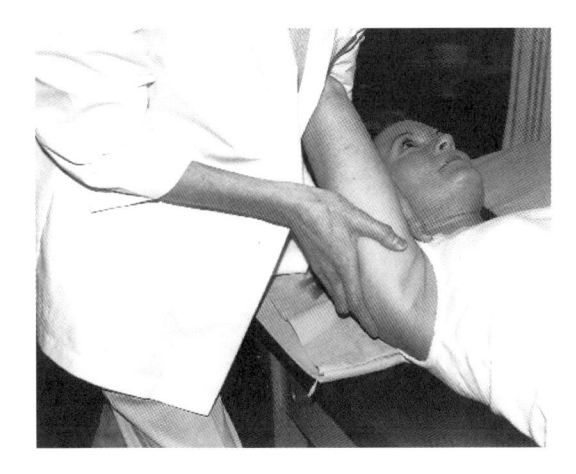

FIGURE 4. Glenohumeral joint: anterior glide.

plished by 30° rotation at the scapula and 60° of the humerus at the glenohumeral joint, a 2:1 ratio (Fig. 6). These relationships are crucial to understanding shoulder dysfunction and the appropriateness of joint mobilization as a treatment modality.

Acromioclavicular and Sternoclavicular Joints

The acromioclavicular joint functions much the same as a triaxial ball and socket joint; however, it does not have convex–concave articular surfaces. Instead, it has a lax capsule and a disc (usually) that changes shape easily and is mechanically defined as a compound plane gliding joint. Its close-pack position is at 90° abduction.

The sternoclavicular joint also functions around three axes in relation to the manubrium. It should be treated as a saddle joint, but because of its lax capsule and a disc that easily changes shape, it can function around these three axes, much the same as a ball and socket joint. The three axes are:

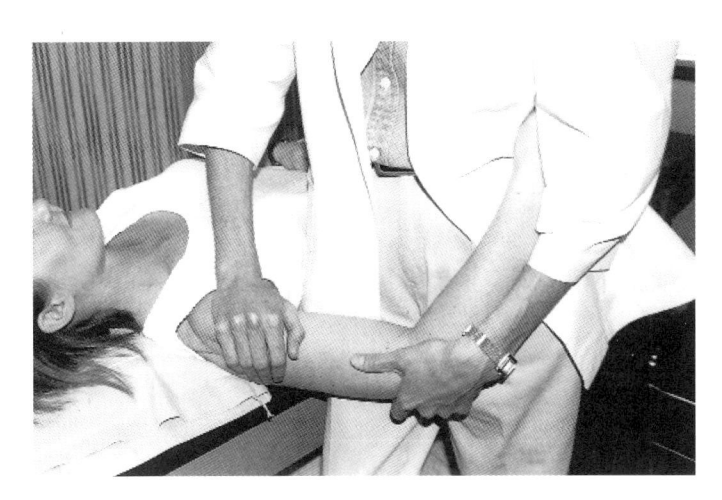

FIGURE 5. Glenohumeral joint: posterior glide.

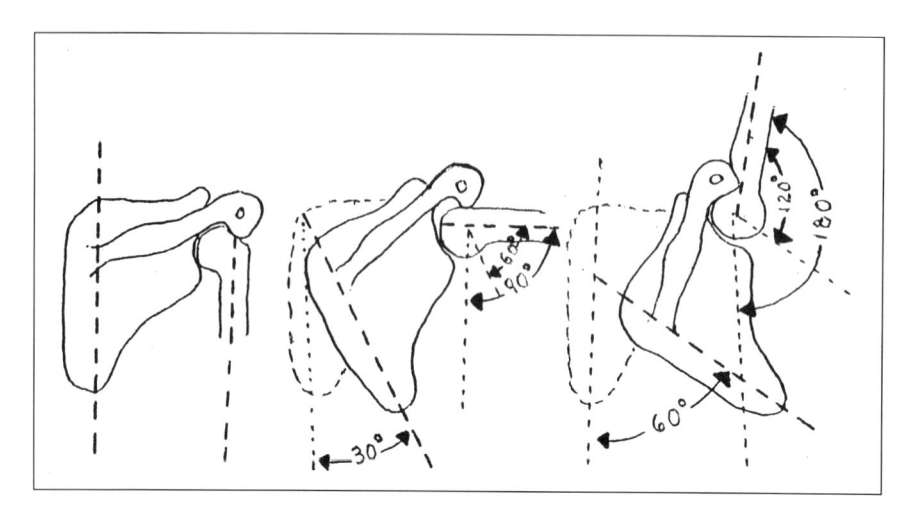

FIGURE 6. Scapulohumeral movement with arm elevation.

1. The **sagittal axis** (through the medial end of the clavicle). The clavicle moves in a cranial and caudal direction with its convex surface around the sagittal axis.
2. The **vertical axis** (longitudinal through the body and the manubrium). The clavicle with its disc moves in an anterior and posterior direction, with its concave surface around the vertical axis.
3. The **longitudinal axis** (through the clavicle). The clavicle rotates around its own longitudinal axis.

REIMBURSEMENT

Joint mobilization is recognized in the Physical Medicine Sections of the Current Procedural Terminology (CPT) manuals as "manual therapy." The CPT code for manual therapy at this time is 97140 and is paid in increments of 15 minutes. The average reimbursement for this procedure is approximately $20.00 per 15 minutes.

CONCLUSION

Peripheral joint mobilization is a manual skill that practitioners have been studying and improving for decades. Many of the materials used as references were published in the 1950s and 1960s, but they remain the most respected texts on manipulation of the extremities used by treating therapists today. This chapter is meant only as an introduction to understanding the mobilization process. For more details on any specific peripheral joint, the reference section will be helpful for further study. The new therapist must receive manual training in the laboratory from an experienced therapist in order to learn the skills required for safe and effective treatment.[7] Physical therapists do not currently have access to the diagnostic testing required to rule out more serious pathology or other contraindication to joint mobilization. The physical therapist relies on the patient's physician to perform these screening procedures before referring the patient for PT care. Most patients receive manual joint mobilization two to three times per week from the treating therapist. This is complemented by an exercise program to be performed several times a day as prescribed by the physical therapist. In particularly resistant cases of capsulitis, joint mobilization is required 4–5 days per week to achieve progress. Treatment frequency is then gradually reduced until the patient is able to maintain range of motion independently.

REFERENCES

1. Akinson WH, Woo SLY, Amiel D, et al: The connective tissue response to immobility: Biomechanical changes in periarticular connective tissue of the immobilized rabbit knee. Clin Orthop 93:356–422, 1973.
2. Cookson JC, Kent BE: Orthopaedic manual therapy: An overview. Part 1: The Extremities. Phys Ther 59:136–146, 1979.
3. Cyriax J: Textbook of Orthopaedic Medicine, Vol. II, 7th ed. London, Bailliere Tindall, 1965.
4. Ekholm R: Nutrition of articular cartilage. Acta Anat 12:77, 1955.
5. Goldstein M: Introduction, summary, and analysis. In Goldstein M (ed): The Research Status of Spinal Manipulative Therapy. Washington, DC, US Government Printing Office, 1975, pp 3–7.
6. Kaltenborn FM: Mobilization of the Extremity Joints. Oslo, Norway, Olaf Noris Bekhandel Universitetsgaten, 1980.
7. Lee M, Moseley A, Refshalage K: Effect of feedback on learning vertebral joint mobilization skill. Phys Ther 70:97–104, 1990.
8. MacConaill MA: The movements of bones and joints: The significance of shape. J Bone Joint Surg 35B:290–297, 1953.
9. Maitland GD: Peripheral Manipulation, 3rd ed. London, Butterworth, 1991.
10. McClure PW, Flowers KR: Treatment of limited shoulder motion: A case study based on biomechanical considerations. Phys Ther 72:929–936, 1992.
11. Mennell J: Science and Art of Joint Manipulation. Vol. II. London, Churchill, 1952.
12. Mennell JM: Joint Pain. Boston, Little, Brown, 1965.
13. Millet PJ, Rushton N: Early mobilization in the treatment of Colle's fracture: A 3-year program study. Injury 26:671–675, 1995.
13a. Mulligan BR: Manual Therapy, NAGs, SNAGs, and MWMS, 4th ed. Wellington, New Zealand, Plane View Services Ltd, 1999.
14. Olson VL: Evaluation of joint mobilization treatment: A method. Phys Ther 67:351–356, 1987.
15. Salter RB, Simmons DF, Malcolm BW, et al: The effects of continuous passive motion on the healing of articular cartilage defects: An experimental investigation in rabbits. J Bone Joint Surg 57A:570–571, 1975.

Chapter 14
Taping Techniques as an Adjunct to Rehabilitation

Wendy S. Burke, DPT, OCS, and Cindy Bailey, DPT, OCS, SCS, ATC

There are three basic taping (strapping) techniques and uses of tape: athletic taping, rigid proprioceptive taping, and taping with Kinesiotex tape ("Kinesio" taping). All three techniques have a different history, require a different type of tape, and are used for a different purpose in patient care and rehabilitation.

ATHLETIC TAPING TECHNIQUES
History

The use of tape and taping techniques has been an effective modality and adjunct to physical training and therapeutic intervention for centuries. Historically, taping for physical support, injury prevention, and injury treatment has been used since the age of the ancient Roman gladiators. Taping for organized sports and athletic injuries began in the 1890s with collegiate athletic competition. Since the 1950s, the use of athletic taping techniques has been studied extensively. Although certified athletic trainers use taping techniques for nearly all body parts, the predominant techniques researched have been those of the ankle, wrist, hand, and knee.

Uses of Athletic Taping

Athletic taping techniques can be categorized according to their use: acute, rehabilitative, functional, or prophylactic. Compressive taping techniques are used in the acute injury phase to limit the joint motion and control edema. Rehabilitative techniques are used following injury or surgery to protect the joint and provide increased proprioception of the injured area while healing occurs. Once the athlete's injury is beyond the initial inflammatory stage and he or she is beginning active motion, functional proprioceptive techniques are used. Taping techniques are applied during early return to activities to protect the injured part from further damage. Often, even after full recovery of the injury, the participant or the coach continues to want the area wrapped prophylactically to prevent injury while the participant is engaged in functional or athletic endeavors.[51,73,77,78]

The use of taping techniques has long been a normal part of athletic injury management.[6,8,11,15,23,26,27,43,51,54,56,60,69,72,77,78] Originally, it was thought that taping techniques could "hold" two bones closer in approximation and, consequently, control whether or not the ligaments became reinjured. However, radiographic studies indicate that the bones do not maintain the same relationship in a weight-bearing dynamic position that they do in the non–weight-bearing static position after taping.[42]

When taping is used to restrict motion, several authors have found that the tape's effectiveness is decreased within 30 minutes of beginning physical activity.[30,48,51–53,59,78] These changes were attributed to body perspiration and the tape stretching or loosening during weight-bearing activities. Taping techniques are currently believed to be effective in injury rehabilitation and prevention because of an increase in proprioception, not limitation in joint range of motion as was once believed.[1,6,8,11,14,15,19,20,23,26,27,35,40,43,51,54,56,60,66,68,69,72,77,78]

Taping techniques used for athletics have several drawbacks.[43] First, a trained professional is required for correct application of the tape. Second, supply costs are high because the tape is used only for that particular practice or game and then is removed. Finally, frequent reapplication of the tape causes skin irritation.

Because of these drawbacks, several braces have been manufactured to provide athletes with an alternative to taping. The effectiveness of bracing versus taping has been compared by several authors, and no significant differences were found between bracing and taping in the *un*injured joint.[10,11,33,35,37,40,55,57,69,72,73,79] In addition, gait analysis and the landing patterns of the foot during side shuffle and single leg jump were used to assess whether the proprioceptive input from the tape changed the joint kinematics.[14,35] Researchers found that the effect of bracing and taping on the selected biomechanical variables associated with landing were specifically limited to a reduction in muscle action. This supports the theory that taping/bracing increases the effectiveness of proprioceptive feedback on the muscular system and reassures the players that their landing patterns would not be altered whether they chose to wear a brace or tape their ankle joints.[35]

Although the ankle is the most common joint taped with athletic tape and the most often studied, athletic taping techniques are used for nearly all body parts, including the shoulder, acromioclavicular joint, elbow, wrist, hand, fingers, knee, and foot. The type of technique used depends on the assessment of the injured tissue for irritability, stage of healing, and treatment goal (Fig. 1).[1,3,5,6,9,22,29,31,34,36,38,48,61,67,70,71,75]

Types of Athletic Tape

The tape itself has undergone a number of design and manufacturing changes based on the desired control of the joint and the skin's ability to tolerate the tape. The most commonly used athletic tape is Zonus, also known as "coach" tape (Fig. 1). Most athletic tapes are made of cotton and are easily torn by hand. The tape does not stretch lengthwise or along its width but has a small amount of flexibility along the bias. The tape is moderately breathable, which allows for the sweat and toxins in the skin to escape. However, application of the tape is generally applied over a thin foam-like material called underwrap. The purpose of the underwrap, or prewrap, is to protect the skin from the adhesive backing of the tape. When the tape is applied over the underwrap, the skin can no longer breathe and becomes highly irritated after a period of time. Therefore, athletic tape is applied for only short periods of time. Some of the many other types of tape that are used in athletics include Elasticon, Elastaplast, Blister Tape, Leukotape, Cover Roll, and Kinesiotex. In addition, adhesive-backed protectants such as moleskin or adhesive felt are also commonly used.

RIGID PROPRIOCEPTIVE AND SUPPORTIVE TAPING TECHNIQUES

History

Throughout the history of injury care, body and posture taping techniques have been used predominantly by certified athletic trainers rather than physical therapists.

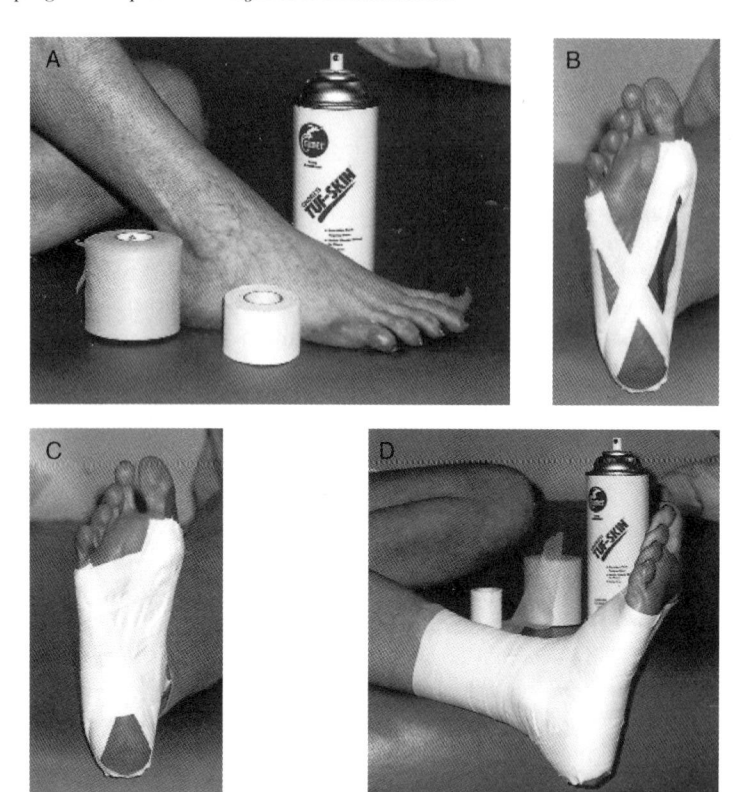

FIGURE 1. Traditional athletic taping technique for the ankle joint. *A*, Supplies for traditional athletic taping: Tuf-Skin, Zonus tape, and foam underwrap. *B*, Athletic taping for arch and the ankle joint. Initial taping strips. *C*, Athletic taping as the arch and foot is filled in with more tape. *D*, Completed athletic taping for the ankle.

However, the use of tape as a modality in general rehabilitation was popularized in the 1980s by Australian physiotherapist Jenny McConnell, MAPA, MMTAA. She developed a taping technique for the treatment of patellofemoral syndrome by using two different kinds of tape, Cover-Roll and Leukotape. Her evaluation methods and the use of tape for anterior knee pain revolutionized treatment for patellofemoral syndrome and opened new thinking processes in knee rehabilitation.[21,24,47,65,76]

Uses of Proprioceptive Taping

Initial studies and theories of the use of taping for patellofemoral syndrome were designed to alter the relationship of the patella in the trochlear groove to improve patellar tracking and decrease anterior knee pain. Clinically, McConnell developed an entire evaluation and treatment method for patellofemoral syndrome. Her assessment of the patella in a static and dynamic position changed the course of symptomatic care for this syndrome throughout the world.[18,58]

More recent studies indicate that changes in the patellar position within the trochlear groove by tape may occur in a static position. However, this patellofemoral relationship is not maintained once the patient bears weight in a functional, closed kinetic chain.[7,50,64] It also has been theorized that the tape allows the quadriceps muscle to function more efficiently by altering the timing of contraction between the vastus medialis (VMO) and vastus lateralis (VL),[21] although alteration in the timing of the VMO and VL remains somewhat controversial during functional activities.[16,32,65]

Other studies show evidence to support an increase in overall quadriceps muscle power and output in taped subjects testing vertical jump with electromyography (EMG).[25,81] Gait in patients with anterior knee pain was tested with both taped and untaped knees. Researchers found a significant reduction of pain (78% by visual analogue scale), increased stride length during ramp ascent, and improved loading response with knee flexion in taped patients. The authors concluded that the subjects, when taped, were more willing to load the knee joint. Thus, the pain reduction allowed increased quadriceps activity, and improved tolerance to patellofemoral joint reaction forces.[63]

McConnell-type taping techniques with Leukotape and Cover Roll have been expanded beyond repositioning the patella to techniques for muscle facilitation and inhibition. When using a rigid proprioceptive tape, the tape can be applied perpendicular to the muscle fibers to inhibit overactive muscles such as the upper trapezius and VL. Taping parallel to the muscle fibers with the joint in a more aligned or neutral position facilitates muscle activation. As part of the complete treatment, surface EMG biofeedback is used in conjunction with taping for retraining the associated musculature.

McConnell created many additional techniques that are effective for the foot, ankle, shoulder, and spinal radiculopathy. Taping techniques for the foot and ankle are used to control excessive pronation and lower extremity alignment. McConnell developed taping techniques for treatment of a variety of shoulder dysfunctions including glenohumeral instability and rotator cuff tears. Clinical techniques have been developed using Leukotape and Cover Roll to "unload" tissues near irritated nerve roots in order to decrease radicular symptoms in the upper and lower extremities. This is accomplished primarily by creating a small "pouch" of soft tissue around the irritated nerve. In other cases, the "drag" effect of gravity is lessened by slightly lifting the tissue along the radicular pathway, thus decreasing the tension on the nerve and its surrounding tissues.

Types of Rigid Proprioceptive and Supportive Tape

Two different types of tape placed one on top of the other are used for rigid proprioceptive taping techniques: athletic tape over prewrap or underwrap or, more commonly, Leukotape over Cover Roll. The bottom tape is called, ironically, Cover Roll. Cover Roll is thin, cotton, and highly breathable. Scissors are required to cut each strip. A lengthwise split in the backing allows the paper backing to be peeled off easily. Cover Roll is not designed to stretch lengthwise, and if pulled will cause the center of the tape to constrict and become thinner. It also stretches along the width and bias and, again, loses its integrity and shape. During application, care must be taken not to stretch Cover Roll, or blisters may form on the skin.

Leukotape, the second layer of tape, is rigid and barely breathable. This tape

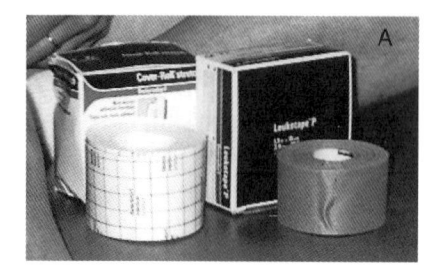

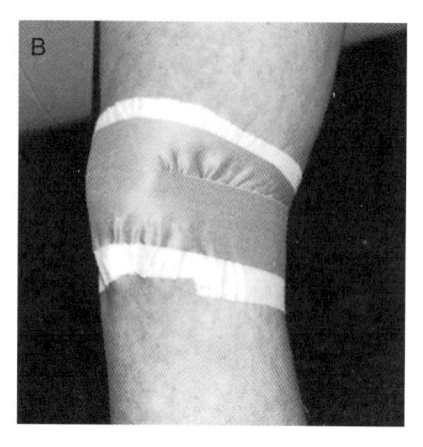

FIGURE 2. Rigid proprioceptive technique (McConnell technique). *A*, Rigid proprioceptive taping (McConnell technique) for patellofemoral pain using Cover Roll and Leukotape. *B*, Completed taping technique for medial glide of the patella using McConnell technique.

does not stretch along its length or width. Its adhesive is extremely sticky and has a propensity to tear layers of skin away if it is not applied and removed properly. In addition, reapplication after tape removal is often not tolerated because of skin sensitivity. Skin irritation occurs around the edges of the tape from friction between the skin movement and the tape (Fig. 2).

KINESIOTEX TAPING METHODS

History

Kenzo Kase, D.C., created Kinesio taping methods for treatment of standard orthopedic patients. Kase was trained in the United States as a chiropractor, but he practiced in Japan, where he found that the traditional tapes available to him did not provide the results he desired. He developed and manufactured a more elastic tape (Kinesiotex) in an effort to decrease pain, decrease edema, assist in muscle function, and ultimately improve joint function. During its first 10 years, Kinesiotex was used primarily for medical practitioners in standard clinical settings in Japan. In the 1980s, Kinesiotex taping techniques were introduced to the athletic population on Japanese Olympic volleyball players. The accounts of its effectiveness spread to other athletes and care practitioners.

Today, Kinesiotex tape is used in every professional sport in Japan, including sumo wrestling, yet 75% of its use remains in the nonathletic population. The tape was introduced to the United States in 1995 through intercollegiate athletics. Kinesiotex tape is now used by medical practitioners in Japan, throughout the U.S., Europe, and South America.

Theory for Use

Kinesio-taping techniques approach treatment of muscles, nerves, joints, and orthopaedic conditions in a new way. The tape is flexible and has other physical

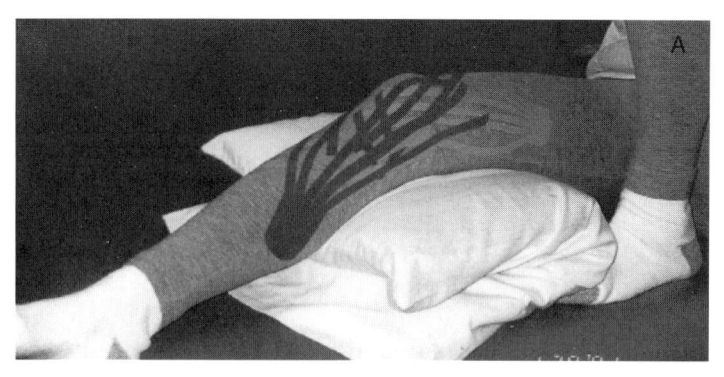

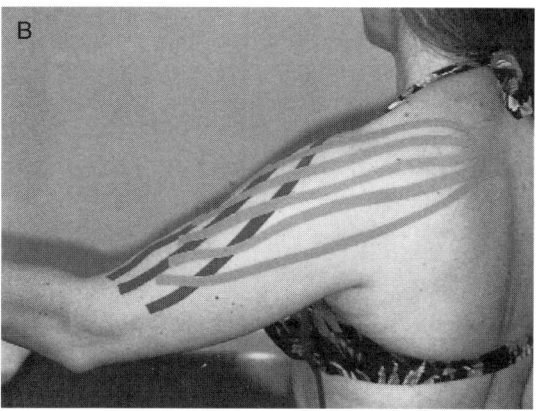

FIGURE 3. Kinesio-taping technique for edema. *A*, Kinesio-taping technique for edema in the knee. This is particularly effective for postoperative edema. *B*, Kinesio-taping technique for upper extremity (shoulder) lymphedema. This is effective for postoperative edema and lymphedema after mastectomy.

properties that affect the neurologic, proprioceptive, musculoskeletal, and lymphatic systems. The theory behind Kinesiotex taping is based on aiding the body's own natural healing processes. Kinesiotex taping techniques vary based on the structure involved, its stage of healing, and treatment goals.

One of the greatest differences in application of Kinesiotex taping compared with other methods is in the treatment of edema (Fig. 3). When treating edema, traditional taping methods employ tape for compression. In contrast Kinesiotex is applied lightly to the surface of the skin to facilitate the lymphatic system. The tape itself has a bit of elasticity and once applied to the skin, gently lifts the skin directly under the tape to facilitate extracellular fluid drainage. This lifting of the skin has two effects. First, it creates an area of lower pressure under the tape and allows the flow of interstitial fluid from an area of higher pressure to an area of lower pressure. Second, there are tiny filaments under the skin that are attached to the lymphatic valves within the lymphatic vessels. Lifting the skin assists in opening the thin subcutaneous lymphatic valves and channels. Kase and Hashimoto conducted a study using Doppler ultrasound to measure the fluid flow in patients with and without circulatory insufficiency. They found that there was an increase in flow after application of Kinesiotex taping methods and no adverse side effects.[44–46]

More recently, studies have been conducted involving patients with lymphedema to determine the tape's role in association with manual lymphatic drainage. The Vodder Institute, which developed an established accepted methods for manual lymphatic drainage has endorsed the Kinesio-taping methods as an effective adjunct in the treatment of lymphedema. Currently, several research studies are underway to test the effectiveness of manual lymphatic drainage with and without the Kinesiotex taping techniques.

Kinesiotex taping differs from traditional taping methods used in the treatment of muscle weakness and muscle spasm. Traditional athletic taping places the joint in a neutral position, and the tape works through proprioception and skin irritation to limit end ranges of motion. By doing this, the associated muscles are not subjected to as much stretching and healing is promoted although full motion patterns are sacrificed. Kinesiotex tape is applied directly to the dysfunctional muscle. Therefore, knowledge of muscle anatomy is essential for application.

The Kinesiotex taping methods for treatment of muscle spasm weakness also differ from traditional athletic taping techniques. The tape has an elastic component, and like a rubber band, will attempt to achieve zero tension by recoiling toward the anchor, or starting spot. Therefore, application of the tape from muscle origin to its distal insertion helps facilitate the muscle. In the opposite situation, application of the tape from the distal to the proximal attachment has a tendency to inhibit or decrease the muscle activity. This distinction is important clinically during rehabilitation of an injury. For example, in lateral epicondylitis, the application of Kinesiotex taping differs depending on the acuity and treatment goals. If the muscle is in spasm and treatment is directed at resting the wrist and elbow, taping for muscle inhibition would be indicated. However, once the muscle has healed and a controlled exercise program is initiated, taping to facilitate the muscle would then be appropriate. A limited number of studies have been conducted measuring EMG muscle activity with the tape applied in each direction. The studies show that there is more EMG activity when the taping technique is applied for facilitation and less EMG activity when it is applied for muscle inhibition (Fig. 4).[44,46]

Properties and Uses of Kinesiotex Tape

Kinesiotex is manufactured and designed with a number of unique qualities. The thickness and weight of the tape was designed to be similar to the thickness and weight of skin. Like skin, Kinesiotex has an elastic component to it that allows it to stretch 30–40% beyond its original length.

The type and pattern of the adhesive is another unique feature. The heat-activated adhesive allows the tape to be worn for several days. The tape may also be worn in the shower and pool without coming off. Not only is Kinesiotex designed to breathe, but the pattern in which the adhesive is applied helps to wick away sweat, salts, and toxins from the skin, thereby causing fewer skin reactions. In an effort to decrease skin irritation, the tape contains no latex and is hypoallergenic. This makes Kinesiotex tape more acceptable for patients with sensitive or more fragile skin (e.g., patients with diabetes, fibromyalgia, and rheumatoid arthritis).

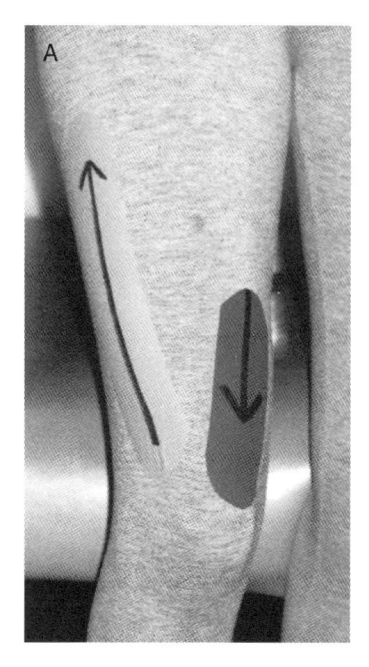

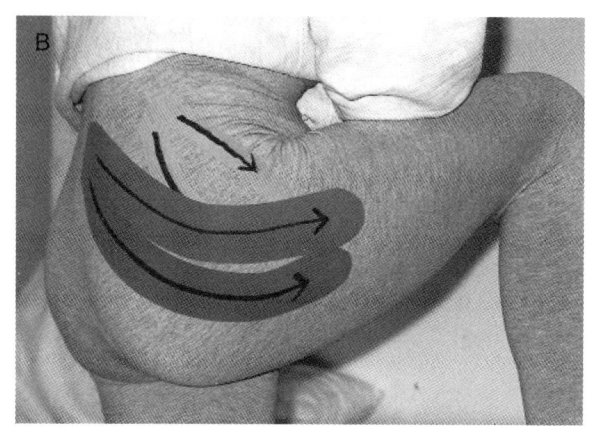

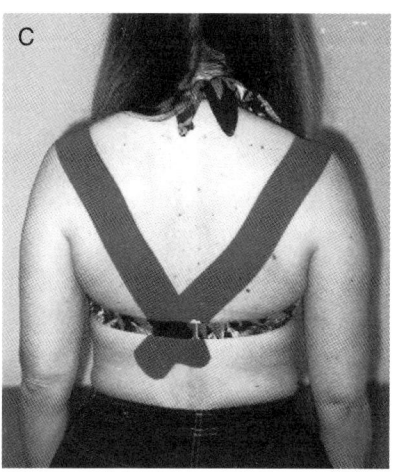

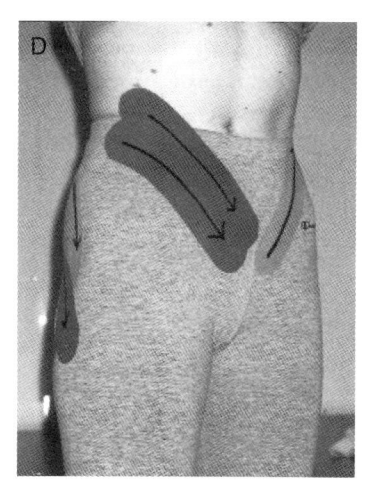

FIGURE 4. Kinesio-taping technique for muscle facilitation and inhibition. *A*, Vastus medialis facilitation (*right*) and vastus lateralis inhibition (*left*). *B*, Facilitation of gluteus medius (*top*) and gluteus maximus (*bottom*). *C*, Scapular positioning and postural facilitation. *D*, Abdominal oblique muscle facilitation.

The tape is available in different colors: neutral, blue, and pink. The colors are intended to follow the Eastern medicine theories of light, color, and healing. Theoretically, pink absorbs more light and generates a warming effect. Blue reflects light and produces a cooling effect. In limited clinical studies, athletes blinded to the color applied have a tendency to choose blue, and patients with rheumatologic diseases generally preferred the pink tape.

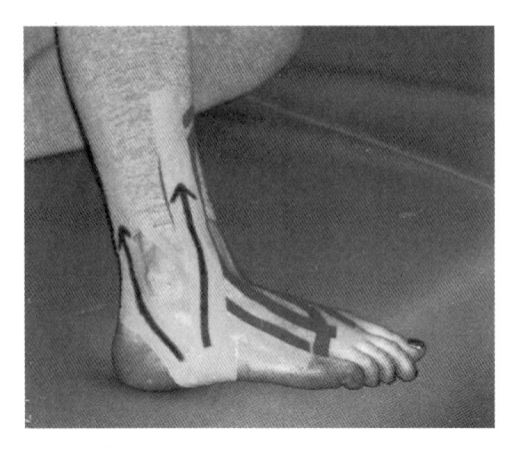

FIGURE 5. Kinesio-taping technique. Combination of edema taping and muscle inhibition for lateral ankle sprain.

One final difference in the Kinesiotex tape from other types of tape is its ability to be cut lengthwise without losing integrity or any of its unique qualities. Therefore, many of the different taping techniques use the tape cut into different shapes (I, X, Y, and V). A 2-inch strip of Kinesiotex can be cut lengthwise into two 1-inch strips or several narrower strips if needed for application on children or petite patients whose muscles are smaller. Cutting the tape lengthwise in multiple strips is part of the taping technique for lymphedema and allows for application around sutures, wounds, or bony prominences (Fig. 5).

APPLICATION DIFFICULTIES AND TIPS

Difficulties with application and adherence occur with all three types of taping techniques (Table 1). Increased body hair prevents the tape from adhering and makes removal of the tape painful. If the body part is particularly hairy, the hair needs to be shaved or clipped before application. Shaving with a razor, electric or manual, may cause skin tenderness and cuts. One solution is to have the patient shave the area the night before and use lotion to help resolve the skin irritation. Another suggestion is to use a Panasonic hair clipper, which clips the hair close to the skin without disrupting the skin. This is advocated particularly for those patients with lymphedema where any break in the skin from shaving could cause an infection.

Tape adherence can also be problematic. For athletic taping techniques, a tape adherent is used under the prewrap. For Kinesio-taping on persons who may be perspiring, the use of a spray or wipe-on adherent (e.g., tincture of benzoin, Tuf-Skin, QDA) is helpful. Otherwise, application of the tape 30 minutes before activity is advised in order for the body's heat to activate the tape's adhesive. In general, it is recommended that the skin be dry and free of oils. If the patient has been sweating or has naturally oily skin or if oils have been used for other manual techniques, soap and water or an alcohol wipe is effective in removing the excess oil.

TABLE 1. TAPING APPLICATION DIFFICULTIES

Problem	Solution
Body hair	Shaving (use razor or Panasonic clipper)
Dry skin	Light lotion several hours before taping application
Oily skin	Alcohol wipe or soap and water
Removal	Peel off parallel to the tape, not perpendicular Peel the skin off the tape Use baby oil, alcohol, or adhesive remover at the edge as you roll it off
Blister	Proper application technique Avoid wrinkles and creases in the tape, particularly with Cover Roll and athletic tapes
Skin irritation	Use tapes that allow motion and breathe for skin toxins to escape

Dry skin, such as with diabetes, is a problem for Kinesiotex tape because its main effect is accomplished by its ability to attach to the top layer of skin. If the skin is too dry, a layer of dead skin cells will stick to the tape, and the tape will be less effective. If a client has this problem, have them apply a moisturizer several hours prior to the expected taping application.

Removal of any tape can be difficult. It is recommended, regardless of the taping technique used, that the tape be peeled off parallel along the skin and not perpendicular to the skin. When the tape is removed quickly and by pulling away from the body it can tear off layers of skin. This not only is destructive to the skin, but also prevents reapplication until the skin is healed. If an area of tape is particularly adherent, it is helpful to peel the skin from the tape rather than the tape from the skin. Peeling tape off after a shower while wet may also help. Applying alcohol, lotion, baby oil, or other adhesive solvents (e.g., Goo Gone) to the edges of the tape–skin barrier should also ease in its removal.

Occasionally, a blister may form on taped skin from wrinkles or creases in the tape, moisture under the tape, or friction between the tape and skin. Blisters tend to be more of a problem with Leukotape, Cover Roll, and athletic tape than with Kinesiotex tape. Careful and proper application techniques generally prevent blisters from forming. Patient education regarding when and how to apply the tape will prevent the patient from getting friction blisters. With Kinesiotex, blisters can occur if the tape has been stretched, particularly when there is edema or if tension is applied to the ends of the tape. Again, proper application technique with the correct amount of tension will eliminate this problem.

Skin irritation or hypersensitivity occurs most commonly with the rigid taping techniques. The tape does not allow the skin to breathe, and the salts and toxins in sweat cannot escape. This causes an irritation to the skin. Patients with fair skin or with systemic diseases, particularly autoimmune disorders, are at risk for developing hypersensitivity. For people with sensitivity, hypoallergenic athletic and Cover Roll tapes are available. Kinesiotex tape is latex free and hypoallergenic. Application of lotion and several days of rest from taping may be necessary before retaping. Another option would be to use a prewrap for athletic taping, Cover Roll for Leukotape, or skin protectant for any taping before application. If the risks of sensitivity to tape outweigh the benefit of taping, alternative treatments should be administered.

SUMMARY

Taping techniques have been an integral and effective part of injury rehabilitation for decades. Traditional athletic taping techniques are applied with the joint in neutral position and are designed to limit the end ranges of motion while the injured area heals. These techniques are used in the acute, early rehabilitative, and functional stages of recovery, as well as for injury prevention. Although the taping techniques were initially thought to reposition bony alignment, it has been shown that the effect of the tape is predominantly proprioceptive. Athletic taping techniques are generally used during the functional activity and then removed.

McConnell pioneered the use of rigid proprioceptive techniques for rehabilitation of the patellofemoral syndrome. Her taping techniques initially were designed to reposition the patella on the trochlear groove for improved muscular activity. However, like the athletic taping techniques, once the limb is in a weight-bearing functional position, the tape cannot control the bony alignment. The clinical results were attributed to proprioceptive input to the muscular skeletal system. Typically, two different tapes are used, Leukotape and Cover Roll.

Kinesiotex taping methods were developed by Kenzo Kase in Japan as an alternative to the current taping techniques. The tape itself is designed to be similar to skin in the thickness, weight, and flexibility in an effort to enhance the body's own systems. Kinesiotex taping methods are used to assist the musculoskeletal, lymphatic, neurologic, and proprioceptive systems in recovery from injury. The taping techniques may change within the same client for the same diagnosis, depending on the acuity of the injury and goal of treatment. The treatment for edema is the most significant difference between Kinesiotex and athletic or rigid proprioceptive techniques. Rather than taping the joint in neutral position and with compression, the tape is applied with the joint moving through its available range to facilitate the lymphatic channels. Just like the other taping techniques, Kinesiotex has a significant effect on muscle activity through the proprioceptive system (Table 2).

TABLE 2. TAPES AND THEIR USES

Type of Therapeutic Tape	Uses	Tapes Used	Manufacturer
Athletic	Support Limit motion Edema compression	Zonus tape Elastic adhesive Elastic nonadhesive Prewrap Wraps	Johnson & Johnson Mueller Cramer
Rigid	Support Limit motion Rigid proprioceptive input	Cover Roll Leukotape	Buers Dorf Smith & Nephew Endura fix
Kinesiotex	Edema (lymph assist) Pain control (point specific) Flexible proprioceptive input Muscle facilitation Muscle inhibition	Kinesiotex	Kinesiotex

Application and removal of the tape are of concern in all three of the taping techniques. Body hair, oily skin, and dry skin can make tape application difficult. Shaving causes skin irritation which can be aggravated by taping. Overly dry or oily skin decreases the tape's ability to adhere. Removing the tape can be difficult if the adhesive is strong or the skin is frail. Clients must be instructed in proper removal of the tape in order to decrease the irritation and prevent the skin from tearing. Blisters are possible with any kind of taping technique and are more common if there are wrinkles in the tape during application.

Taping is a clinically effective modality and is widely used in a variety of musculoskeletal conditions and diagnoses. A complete evaluation of the patient's condition and stage of healing is integral in determining not only the taping technique to be used, but whether or not it is the most appropriate modality for the care of the patient at that moment. A proper evaluation and musculoskeletal diagnosis will lead the practitioner to the proper taping technique and the most appropriate type of tape.

REFERENCES

1. Agnew PS: Taping of foot and ankle for Korean karate. J Am Podiatr Med Assoc 83:534–536, 1993.
2. Alt W, Lohrer H, Gollhofer A: Functional properties of adhesive ankle taping: Neuromuscular and mechanical effects before and after exercise. Foot Ankle Int 20:238–245, 1999.
3. Anderson K, Wojtys EM, Loubert PV, Miller RE: A biomechanical evaluation of taping and bracing in reducing knee joint translation and rotation. Am J Sports Med 20:416–421, 1992.
4. Baker MM, Juhn MS: Patellofemoral pain syndrome in the female athlete. Clin Sports Med 19:315–329, 2000.
5. Benaglia PG, Sartorio F, Ingenito R: Evaluation of a thermoplastic splint to protect the proximal interphalangeal joints of volleyball players. J Hand Ther 9:52–56, 1996.
6. Beynnon BD, Renstrom PA: The effect of bracing and taping in sports. Ann Chir Gynaecol 80:230–238, 1991.
7. Bockrath K, Wooden C, Worrell T, et al: Effects of patella taping on patella position and perceived pain. Med Sci Sports Exerc 25:989–992, 1993.
8. Bonci CM: Adhesive strapping techniques. Clin Sports Med 1:99–116, 1982.
9. Braakman M, Odrwald EE, Haentjens MH: Functional taping of fractures of the 5th metacarpal results in a quicker recovery. Injury 29:5–9, 1998.
10. Burks RT, Bean BG, Marcus R, Barker HB: Analysis of athletic performance with prophylactic ankle devices. Am J Sorts Med 19:104–106, 1991.
11. Callaghan MJ: Role of ankle taping and bracing in the athlete. Br J Sports Med 31:102–108, 1997.
12. Cameron MH: Patellar taping in the treatment of patellofemoral pain: A prospective randomized study. Am J Sports Med 25:417, 1997.
13. Capasso G, Maffulli N, Testa V: Ankle taping: Support given by different materials. Br J Sports Med 23:239–240, 1989.
14. Carmines DV, Nunley JA, McElhaney JH: Effects of ankle taping on the motion and loading pattern of the foot for walking subjects. J Orthop Res 6:223–229, 1988.
15. Cass JR, Morrey BF: Ankle instability: Current concepts, diagnosis, and treatment. Mayo Clin Proc 59:165–170, 1984.
16. Cerny K: Vastus medialis oblique/vastus lateralis muscle activity ratios for selected exercises in persons with and without patellofemoral pain syndrome. Phys Ther 75:672–683, 1995.
17. Chomiak J, Junge A, Perterson L, Dvorak J: Severe injuries in football players. Influencing factors. Am J Sports Med 28:S58–S68, 2000.
18. Clark DI, Downing N, Mitchell J, et al: Physiotherapy for anterior knee pain: A randomised controlled trial. Ann Rheum Dis 59:700–704, 2000.
19. Cordova ML, Ingersoll CD, LeBlanc MJ: Influence of ankle support on joint range of motion before and after exercise: A meta-analysis. J Orthop Sports Phys Ther 30:170–182, 2000.

20. Cox JS: Surgical and nonsurgical treatment of acute ankle sprains. Clin Orthop 198:118–126, 1985.
21. Crossley K, Cowan SM, Bennell KL, McConnell J: Patellar taping: Is clinical success supported by scientific evidence? Man Ther 5:142–150, 2000.
22. Cushnaghan J, McCarthy C, Dieppe P: Taping the patella medially: A new treatment for osteoarthritis of the knee joint? BMJ 308(6931):753–755, 1994.
23. Distefano V, Nixon JE: An improved method of taping. An interposition material allows extended use of adhesive tape in a sports medicine setting. J Sports Med 2:209–211, 1974.
24. Engstrom BK, Renstrom PA: How can injuries be prevented in the World Cup soccer athlete? Clin Sports Med 17:755–768, 1998.
25. Ernst GP, Kawaguchi J, Saliba E: Effect of patellar taping on knee kinetics of patients with patellofemoral pain syndrome. J Orthop Sports Phys Ther 29:661–667, 1999.
26. Ferguson AB Jr: The case against ankle taping. J Sports Med 1:46–47, 1973.
27. Firer P: Effectiveness of taping for the prevention of ankle ligament sprains. Br J Sports Med 24:47–50, 1990.
28. Fitzgerald GK, McClure PW: Reliability of measurements obtained with four tests for patellofemoral alignment. Phys Ther 75:84–92, 1995.
29. Forster KK, Schmid K, Reichelt A: Sports-induced acute epicondylitis of the elbow and conservative therapy. Sportverleta Sportschaden 11:16–20, 1997.
30. Fumich RM, Ellison AE, Guerin GJ, Grace PD: The measured effect of taping on combined foot and ankle motion before and after exercise. Am J Sports Med 9:165–170, 1981.
31. Gerrard DF: External knee support in rugby union: Effectiveness of bracing and taping. Sports Med 25:313–317, 1998.
32. Gilleard W, McConnell J, Parsons D: The effect of patellar taping on the onset of vastus medialis obliquus and vastus lateralis muscle activity in persons with patellofemoral pain. Phys Ther 78:25–32, 1998.
33. Gross MT, Batten AM, Lamm AL, et al: Comparison of DonJoy ankle ligament protector and subtalar sling ankle taping in restricting foot and ankle motion before and after exercise. J Orthop Sports Phys Ther 19:33–41, 1994.
34. Hadley A, Griffiths S, Griffiths L, Vicenzino B: Antipronation taping and temporary orthoses. Effects on tibial rotation position after exercise. J Am Podiatr Med Assoc 89:118–123, 1999.
35. Hopper DM, McNair P, Elliott BC: Landing in netball: Effects of taping and bracing the ankle. Br J Sports Med 33:409–413, 1999.
36. Host HH: Scapular taping in the treatment of anterior shoulder impingement. Phys Ther 75:803–812, 1995.
37. Hume PA, Gerrard DF: Effectiveness of external ankle support. Bracing and taping in rugby union. Sports Med 25:285–312, 1998.
38. Hunter LY: Braces and taping. Clin Sports Med 4:439–454, 1985.
39. Jerosch J, Bork H, Hoffstetter I, Bischof M: The influence of orthoses on the proprioception of the ankle joint. Knee Surg Sports Traumatol Arthrosc 3:39–46, 1995.
40. Jerosch J, Hoffstetter I, Bork H, Bischof M: The influence of orthoses on the proprioception of the ankle joint. Knee Surg Sports Traumatol Arthrosc 3:39–46, 1995.
41. Jerosch J, Thorwesten L, Bork H, Bischof M: Is prophylactic bracing of the ankle cost effective? Orthopedics 19:405–414, 1996.
42. Karlsson J, Andreasson GO: The effect of external ankle support in chronic lateral ankle joint instability. An electromyographic study. Am J Sports Med 20:257–261, 1992.
43. Kase K: Illustrated Kinesio-taping, 3rd ed. Albuquerque, Universal Printing & Publishing, 1994.
44. Kinesio-taping Association: Kinesio-taping Perfect Manual. Albuquerque, Universal Printing & Publishing, 1998.
45. Kinesio-taping Association: Instructors Certification course notes. Kinesio-taping Association.
46. Karlsson J, Sward L, Andreasson GO: The effect of taping on ankle stability. Practical implications. Sports Med 16:210–215, 1993.
47. Klipstein A, Bodnar A: Femoropatellar pain syndrome: Conservative therapeutic possibilities. Ther Umsch 53:745–751, 1996.
48. Konradsen L, Ravn JB: Prolonged peroneal reaction time in ankle instability. Int J Sports Med 12:290–292, 1991.

49. Kowall MG, Kolk G, Nuber GW, et al: Patellar taping in the treatment of patellofemoral pain: A prospective randomized study. Am J Sports Med 24:61–66, 1996.
50. Larsen B, Andreasen E, Urfer A, et al: Patellar taping: A radiographic examination of the medial glide technique. Am J Sports Med 23:465–471, 1995.
51. Larsen E: Taping the ankle for chronic instability. Acta Orthop Scand 55:551–553, 1984.
52. Laughman RK, Carr TA, Chao EY, et al: Three-dimensional kinematics of the taped ankle before and after exercise. Am J Sports Med 8:425–431, 1980.
53. Leanderson J, Ekstam S, Salomonsson C: Taping of the ankle: The effect on postural sway during perturbation, before and after a training session. Knee Surg Sports Traumatol Arthrosc 4:53–56, 1996.
54. MacCartee CC Jr: Taping treatment of severe inversion sprains of the ankle. Early return to functional activities. Am J Sports Med 5:246–247, 1977.
55. MacKean LC, Bell G, Burnham RS: Prophylactic ankle bracing versus taping: Effects on functional performance in female basketball players. J Orthop Sports Phys Ther 22:77–81, 1995.
56. Mascaro TB, Swanson LE: Rehabilitation of the foot and ankle. Orthop Clin North Am 25:147–160, 1994.
57. McCaw ST, Cerullo JF: Prophylactic ankle stabilizers affect ankle joint kinematics during drop landings. Med Sci Sports Exerc 31:702–707, 1999.
58. McConnell Patellofemoral Treatment Plan. McConnell Seminars, course notes. 1990.
59. Morris HH, Musnicki W 3d: The effect of taping on ankle mobility following moderate exercise. J Sports Med Phys Fitness 23:422–426, 1983.
60. Myburgh KH, Vaughan CL, Isaacs SK: The effects of ankle guards and taping on joint motion before, during, and after a squash match. Am J Sports Med 12:441–446, 1984.
61. Peters TA, McLean ID: Osteochondritis dissecans of the patellofemoral joint. Am J Sports Med 28:63–67, 2000.
62. Pope MH, Renstrom P, Donnermeyer D, Morgenstern S: A comparison of ankle taping methods. Med Sci Sports Exerc 19:143–147, 1987.
63. Powers CM, Landel R, Sosnick T, et al: The effects of patellar taping on stride characteristics and joint motion in subjects with patellofemoral pain. J Orthop Sports Phys Ther 26:286–291, 1997.
64. Powers CM, Mortenson S, Nishimoto D, Simon D: Criterion-related validity of a clinical measurement to determine the medial/lateral component of patellar orientation. J Orthop Sports Phys Ther 29:372–377, 1999.
65. Powers CM: Rehabilitation of patellofemoral joint disorders: A critical review. J Orthop Sports Phys Ther 28:345–354, 1998.
66. Refshauge KM, Kilbreath SL, Raymond J: The effect of recurrent ankle inversion sprain and taping on proprioception at the ankle. Med Sci Sports Exerc 32:10–15, 2000.
67. Rettig AC, Stube KS, Shelbourne KD: Effects of finger and wrist taping on grip strength. Am J Sports Med 25:96–98, 1997.
68. Robbins S, Waked E, Rappel R: Ankle taping improves proprioception before and after exercise in young men. Br J Sports Med 29:242–247, 1995.
69. Robbins S, Waked E: Factors associated with ankle injuries. Preventive measures. Sports Med 25:63–72, 1998.
70. Rooks MD: Rock climbing injuries. Sports Med 23:261–270, 1997.
71. Roser LA, Miller SJ, Clawson DK: Effects of taping and bracing on the unstable knee. Northwest Med 70:544–546, 1971.
72. Rovere GD, Clarke TJ, Yates CS, Burley K: Retrospective comparison of taping and ankle stabilizers in preventing ankle injuries. Am J Sports Med 16:228–233, 1988.
73. Rovere GD, Curl WW, Browning DG: Bracing and taping in an office sports medicine practice. Clin Sports Med 8:497–515, 1989.
74. Scranton PE Jr, Pedegana LR, Whitesel JP: Gait analysis: Alterations in support phase forces using supportive devices. Am J Sports Med 10:6–11, 1982.
75. Shamus JL, Shamus EC: A taping technique for the treatment of acromioclavicular joint sprains: a case study. J Orthop Sports Phys Ther 25:390–394, 1997.
76. Shelton GL: Conservative management of patellofemoral dysfunction. Prim Care 19:331–350, 1992.
77. Tropp H, Askling C, Gillquist J: Prevention of ankle sprains. Am J Sports Med 13:259–262, 1985.
78. Vaes P, De Boeck H, Handelberg F, Opdecam P: Comparative radiologic study of the influence of ankle joint bandages on ankle stability. Am J Sports Med 13:46–50, 1985.

79. Verbrugge JD: The effects of semirigid Air-Stirrup bracing vs. adhesive ankle taping on motor performance. J Orthop Sports Thys Ther 23:320–325, 1996.
80. Warme WJ, Brooks D: The effect of circumferential taping on flexor tendon pulley failure in rock climbers. Am J Sports Med 28:674–678, 2000.
81. Werner S, Knutsson E, Eriksson E: Effect of taping the patella on concentric and eccentric torque and EMG of knee extensor and flexor muscles in patients with patellofemoral pain syndrome. Knee Surg Sports Traumatol Arthrosc 1(3-4):169–177, 1993.
82. Wilkerson GB: Comparative biomechanical effects of the standard method of ankle taping and a taping method designed to enhance subtalar stability. Am J Sports Med 19:588–595, 1991.
83. Wright IC, Neptune RR, van den Bogert AJ, Nigg BM: The influence of foot positioning on ankle sprains. J Biomech 33:513–519, 2000.
84. Yamamoto T, Kigawa A, Xu T: Effectiveness of functional ankle taping for judo athletes: A comparison between judo bandaging and taping. Br J Sports Med 27:110–112, 1993.

Chapter 15

A Practical Guide to Biofeedback

Daren Drysdale, BCIA, BSC, and Kazuko Shem, MD

Although biofeedback has not been used or recognized as much as physical or occupational therapies, it has been available as a noninvasive therapeutic option since the 1960s for management of conditions that are frequently seen in the field of physical medicine and rehabilitation. This chapter is neither a comprehensive review of the clinical practice of biofeedback nor of the research currently available in the biofeedback field. It is instead an overview or "how to" for potential referring sources (i.e., physiatrists) when one is considering whether to send a patient for biofeedback therapy.

Contained throughout the chapter is text that may come in useful when explaining biofeedback to a potential client. The text is taken from examples used in both authors' practices. It should be helpful when referring a client and will prepare him or her for the approach he or she needs to adopt to make the therapy successful.

DEFINITIONS

Biofeedback

Biofeedback has been defined in many ways with what seems like an ever-increasing level of complexity. Olson describes it as follows:

> As a process, applied biofeedback is a group of therapeutic procedures that utilizes electronic or electromechanical instruments to accurately measure, process and feed back to persons information with reinforcing properties about their neuromuscular and autonomic activity, both normal and abnormal in the form of analogue or binary, auditory and/or visual feedback signals. Best achieved with a competent professional, the objectives are to help persons develop greater awareness and voluntary control over their physiological processes that are otherwise outside awareness and/or under less voluntary control, by first controlling the external signal, and then by use of internal physiological cues.[6]

This definition, although comprehensive, is hardly suitable in the clinical setting where a referring physician must explain biofeedback to the patient/client. A more suitable definition for the average client may come in the form of the musical mirror metaphor. The explanation might go something like this:

> In order for you to learn, you must get feedback about the event that has just taken place. For example, if you want to learn to play a piano, you must be able to tell if you have hit the right key. If the wrong key is hit by accident, the bum note lets you know that the wrong key has been hit. The feedback is essential. Without the feedback, you cannot tell if the notes are being played

correctly or in the right order. The piano effectively functions as a mirror allowing you to see if you are playing the music correctly.

Biofeedback is similar in that it is an instrument or group of instruments that act as a mirror and allow you to see if you are using your physiology correctly. The various instruments allow you to see or hear events in your body that you normally can't sense and by becoming aware of them you can learn to control them.

The analogy continues when it is explained to a client that the time line expected for the therapy would be similar to the time line expected when learning a new musical instrument.

If you want to play Carnegie Hall, you had better expect to put in a few years of practice. This does not mean that you will be in therapy for that length of time, but you will have to put what you learn into practice for the rest of your life to make the therapy work. If you learn to hold muscles correctly, you will have to continue to hold yourself that way. If you learn to relax more effectively, you will have to change your lifestyle to allow you to do it. If you learn to breathe more efficiently, the point is to continue to do so.

It is important to stress here that biofeedback is not a passive modality. It requires active participation on the part of the patient. Nothing is "done" to the patient. Examples of passive modalities include massage, acupuncture, and ultrasound. Biofeedback is an active modality that is designed solely to increase awareness and help bring about behavioral change at both a psychological and physiologic level.

Psychophysiology

The term *psychophysiology* is an interesting blend of what, until recently, has been considered two different approaches to medicine: psychological and physiological. It is, however, inevitable and appropriate, given the blurring that occurs between the edges of mind and body, that we try to shape physiologic behavior through psychological intervention. Think of the cardiac surgeon who looks at a patient who has just undergone a triple bypass; the surgeon knows that, because of body composition, the patient must change his or her behavior, lifestyle, and outlook on life or the patient's chances of living for the next 5 years are severely diminished. Is this person's condition psychological or physiologic? To view it another way, if a person has poor posture that causes pain in the lower back and the solution is to habituate the correct posture, is the problem best addressed through physiologic or psychological intervention? At a more esoteric level, is the electroencephalography (EEG) technician who is examining the beta activity from the left hemisphere looking at electrical activity generating thought or at thought generating electrical activity?

For a psychophysiologist, these arguments become redundant. In a psychophysiologist's universe, the Cartesian split does not exist. The patient with back pain needs psychological support to overcome the poor posture. The patient needs training to recognize what correct posture feels like. The overweight patient with a heart condition needs to learn how to change the habits of a lifetime, and the

EEG technician is observing the fact that there can be no psychology without physiology and vice versa. The simple premise at the root of the psychophysiologic gestalt is that psychology and physiology are not separate processes. This premise is the basis of all psychophysiologic intervention.

HISTORY

Biofeedback was introduced as a clinical tool in the 1960s. By 1969, the Biofeedback Research Society, chaired by Barbara Brown, met in San Diego. The meeting was the culmination of research from a number of people who had been in contact since just after the World War II. Numerous researchers had been at work in their own fields and they began to realize that they were reading each other's material. They observed an association between behavior therapy, stress research, biomedical engineering, diagnostic electromyography (EMG), consciousness training, cybernetics, and other seemingly unrelated disciplines. This cross-pollination of disciplines was necessary for the research and development of psychophysiology. In 1976, the organization changed its name to the Biofeedback Society of America, and more recently, the association has become known as the Association for Applied Psychophysiology and Biofeedback (AAPB).

The concept that connected these distinct disciplines was the realization that organisms learned by using feedback and that it is possible to control physiology by using the feedback loop.

Basmajian noted:

> In the more mature 1950s and early 1960s, my team was using feedback signals to train exquisite controls in normal muscles of handicapped persons to substitute for lost limbs and to augment the strength of weakened parts of the body.... I found that when our subjects were provided with instant visual and acoustic feedback from the EMG, they could learn to perform elaborate tricks with the tiniest units of the muscle: the motor units.[1]

Throughout the 1960s, 1970s, and 1980s, many researchers replicated Basmajian's experiments, and the outcome has been a solid foundation for EMG biofeedback. As a result, surface EMG is referred to as the "workhorse" of the biofeedback field. The other modalities commonly used in the biofeedback field include EEG, skin conductance, heart rate, peripheral skin temperature, blood volume pulse, and respiration rate. In fact, any physiologic system that can be fed back to the client can be used. However, it is useful to remember that the mechanism used for the feedback should be noninvasive if at all possible.

MODALITIES

Electromyography

In rehabilitation, the most commonly used biofeedback modality is surface EMG (measured in microvolts), and physical therapists who use surface EMG refer to it as the gold standard. It effectively eliminates any guesswork on the part of therapist and can function as a limited diagnostic tool. The most important function, however, is that the information can be fed back to the clients so that they can learn to control specific musculature. This makes surface EMG extremely effective in continence training, stroke and spinal cord injury rehabilitation, and relaxation training.

Historically, one of the problems with surface EMG has been the artifact picked up by the sensors from nontargeted muscles. The most common artifacts experienced by clinicians include electrocardiogram signals picked up during a broad bilateral hook-up of the upper trapezius or signals detected from musculature that sits below the targeted surface muscle. Kasman et al. have created a surface EMG atlas that, by method of illustration and text, allows the clinician to identify what muscles are causing artifact at any given site.[5]

Explanations to the client regarding EMG are reasonably simple. It is, however, important to point out to any client who has previously undergone needle EMG or nerve conduction studies that surface EMG does not involve invasive techniques. This is particularly important if the patient is being referred for relaxation training. The explanation of the surface EMG to a client might resemble the following:

> All of the muscles in our body rely on electricity as a signaling system. Surface EMG instruments can pick up and detect those electrical impulses. Using the biofeedback devices, you will be able to see when the muscles tense up and when they relax.

Electroencephalography

EEG is one of the fastest growing areas in the biofeedback arena. It is also one of the most complicated. Claims have been made as to the efficacy of EEG feedback for attention deficit hyperactivity disorder (ADHD), stroke rehabilitation, and epilepsy. Early in the history of biofeedback, some of these claims were considered outlandish. However, in the last decade, this arena has come into its own with numerous researchers investigating the use of spectral EEG, bipolar hook-ups, and monopolar hook-ups. Although EEG feedback shows significant promise, it is usually beyond the reach of the rehabilitation-based clinic, and because of insurance concerns, it falls largely in the domain of the private-pay patient. As the modality gains acceptance in the medical community, these restrictions should change.

Skin Conductance

The normal measurements for eccrine activity are skin conductance (measured in mhos) and skin resistance (measured in ohms). These two measurements are the inverse of each other. Skin conductance is also called electrodermal activity (EDA), basal skin response (BSR), skin conductance level (SCL), or galvanic skin response (GSR). All of these techniques are indirect measurements of eccrine activity, which increases or decreases depending on autonomic arousal. An explanation to the patient of eccrine activity can be summarized in the phrase "breaking out in a cold sweat." The clinician may wish to explain as follows:

> As we become more excited, we sweat more. This indicates increased nervous activity in the body, and this can be controlled. We break out in a cold sweat because our skin gets colder when we get anxious.

Although we may not be concerned about the amount of sweat generated by a particular patient (unless he or she has hyperhidrosis), the eccrine system is a good indicator of sympathetic arousal and is very helpful to clients as they learn to relax.

Heart Rate

One of the more interesting areas in biofeedback training is respiratory sinus arrhythmia (RSA) training. This area of biofeedback most resembles some of the ancient Eastern techniques such as yoga, tai chi, and the martial arts. Indeed, using breathing to control autonomic function has been around since the first person said, "Now, take a deep breath" to help someone to calm down. Most people are aware that you calm down when you breathe regularly, and this process can be evidenced with RSA feedback.

As the client inhales, the heart is sympathetically enervated and the heart rate increases. As the client exhales, the heart is parasympathetically enervated and the heart rate slows down. This is the expected pattern, but often there is dissociation between the patient's breathing pattern and the autonomic functions in the body. An explanation to a patient might go like this:

> Biofeedback will help you learn how to control your heart rate by the way you breathe. You may ask why you would want to control your heart. It's not so much about your heart but what you have to do to control it. The part of the nervous system that speeds the heart up is also responsible for speeding everything up. The opposite is also true; the part of the system used to slow your heart down is the same part that helps you to slow down and heal more efficiently. So, if you learn to breathe and control the heart rate, we know that you will be able to optimize your own ability to heal.

Temperature

Peripheral skin temperature has become one of the most commonly used modalities for psychologists and practitioners interested in myofascial pain. Because vasoconstriction is a function of sympathetic activity, skin temperature readings are indicative of increased or decreased sympathetic activity in the human body. Temperature feedback has been found to be highly effective for treating conditions such as Raynaud's syndrome, migraine-based headaches, anxiety disorders, and essential hypertension.[3] An explanation for this modality to the client might be:

> As you relax the smooth muscles, blood vessels in your skin also relax. Because those muscles relax, the blood vessels become larger, the blood flow increases, and your skin becomes warmer. This is why we lose so much heat from our bodies when we are asleep at night and why we use blankets to trap this heat.

Respiration

Control of respiration has become a popular form of feedback. It is strongly linked to RSA training and takes the form of strain gauges used across the thoracic and abdominal regions of the body. These strain gauges relay information about the ratio of thoracic movement to abdominal movement in addition to the rate of respiration, thus training the patient to breathe diaphragmatically.

What should be emphasized to clients before they begin biofeedback is that respiration involves many muscle groups in the body. Pain in any part of the body affects respiration almost immediately. Another aspect to be emphasized is that breathing is the linking factor between somatic and autonomic activity. The explanation might resemble the following:

Some of the functions in your body are controlled automatically; some of the functions in your body are controlled voluntarily. Breathing is one of the systems in your body that is both voluntary and automatic. If you want to control the autonomic functions in your body, you must use a system that you have voluntary control over.

Miscellaneous

Any other modality that can be used to feed back information to the client about his or her physiology falls into the miscellaneous category. Almost every physiologic activity from eye blinking to gastric activity has been or is currently being investigated. As stated, it is generally recommended that any feedback device be noninvasive.

METHODS AND SPECIFIC PROTOCOLS

Establishing Protocols

Protocols have been developed for specific disorders by various researchers. The common feature, however, is the focus on training for homeostasis. A strong argument could be made that this is the basis of all therapy. However, homeostasis is particularly relevant to biofeedback because we are dealing so immediately with physiologic parameters.

The strongest point of contention has been defining homeostasis for different physiologic systems. The most important thing to realize is that homeostasis is measured in ranges and not set points. For example, one of the most commonly known physiological measures is blood pressure. We know that blood pressure must be around 120/80, but there is flexibility. Everybody's physiology is slightly different. The homeostatic level for heart rate in one person is not homeostasis for another.

Another problem common in biofeedback is the variance between biofeedback devices. Using the blood pressure example, imagine that every make of sphygmomanometer gave a different reading. Over a period of time every clinician would come to know his or her own device, but to compare one device to another, the make and model of the device and the difference between the two would have to be known. Thus, when reading research about modalities such as surface EMG, it is vital for the researcher to note the make and model of the device used and to be specific about the hook-up.

This lack of consistency among EMG devices has been a criticism of biofeedback research and needs some scrutiny. Cram et al. have been attempting to standardize surface EMG hook-ups to allow researchers to cross-reference research.[2] This does not, however, account for the fact that one make or model of biofeedback equipment processes a signal differently from another. This could leave the clinician wondering, for example, if a totally relaxed muscle will read 1, 1.5, or 2 μV. There is no choice then but to become familiar with the instruments, or if you are not the treating clinician, to rely on the report of the psychophysiologist. It is also recommended to ascertain that the equipment being used is at least certified by the Food and Drug Administration (FDA) or its equivalent.

Therefore, when a protocol is established it is imperative that clinicians are able to adapt the information to their own systems. This is not too difficult because no matter what system the protocol is developed on, the measurement ratios will remain the same. If you become familiar with the instrument you use regularly, it is simple to read published research and make the appropriate accommodation for your own system.

Protocols for stroke, spinal cord injury, incontinence, chronic pain, ADHD, complex regional pain syndromes I and II, repetitive motion injuries, computer-related disorders, Raynaud's syndrome, and chronic myofascial pain syndrome among others have been developed. Some of these protocols are specific and some more general. A thorough description of each condition is beyond the scope of this chapter (refer to Basmajian: *Biofeedback Principles and Practices for Clinicians*[1]), but a general overview of some of the protocols is included here.

A General Approach

Today, the largest application of biofeedback is in the field of clinical psychophysiology and psychotherapy, and most of the work is based on a simple premise: train for homeostasis. The most efficient way to train for homeostasis is to involve as many of the nervous system subsections as possible. A standard full hook-up used in psychotherapy or applied psychophysiology might include:

- Two channels of EEG (central nervous system)
- Two channels of surface EMG (somatic nervous system)
- Two channels of temperature (sympathetic nervous system)
- One channel for sweat response (sympathetic nervous system)
- One channel for heart rate (sympathetic/parasympathetic nervous system)

Any variation of the above can be used, or the clinician can add respiration rates, blood pressure feedback, or any modality from the miscellaneous section presented earlier (Figs. 1–4). This type of generalized hook up ensures that every major system in the body is trained in the same way. One of the mistakes frequently made when training a client using biofeedback protocols is the assumption that just because one part of the nervous system is reacting in certain way, the rest of the nervous system is reacting in the same way. For example, the clinician who uses only surface EMG may mistakenly assume that, because muscles relax, the sympathetic system is also quieting down.

The generalized hook-up has many benefits. One of them is the ability for the clinician to see potential problems in other systems that may not be immediately apparent. Biofeedback instruments are by their nature limited and, therefore, not particularly good as diagnostic tools. It is possible, however, for the clinician to become aware of problems in other systems that may not be immediately apparent when the diagnosis is made.

A Typical Training Course for Relaxation-Based Training

A typical training course will begin with a psychophysiologic stress profile (PSP) and run for at least 12–16 sessions. The PSP consists of a series of stress-inducing exercises coupled with stress-reducing exercises. A typical evaluation may occur over a 30-minute period (Fig. 5). This initial baseline will help to establish:

- How effective the client is at relaxing without guidance
- How strong the stress reaction is to a controlled stressor
- The length of the recovery period post stressor

216 A Practical Guide to Biofeedback

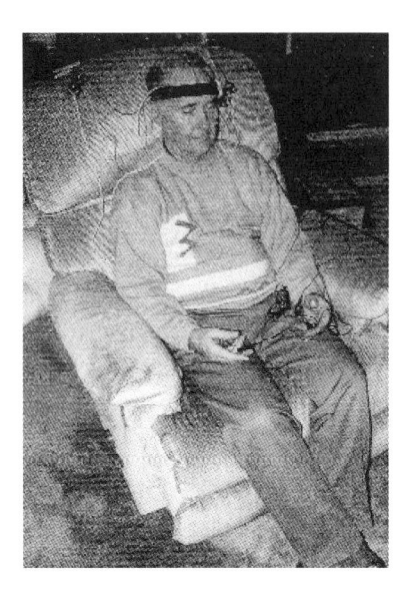

FIGURE 1. General set-up with 2 channels of EEG electrodes, 2 channels of surface temperature probes on both index fingers, galvanic skin response probe (GSR) on the right hand, photoplethysmograph (PPG) probe on the left hand, and two channels of surface EMG electrodes at bilateral temporalis and upper trapezius muscles.

This information is fairly basic, and a PSP is recommended even if the presenting symptom necessitates predominantly body measures such as surface EMG. The information collected in the profile is helpful to the therapist and client as they work together to establish a comprehensive training and treatment plan.

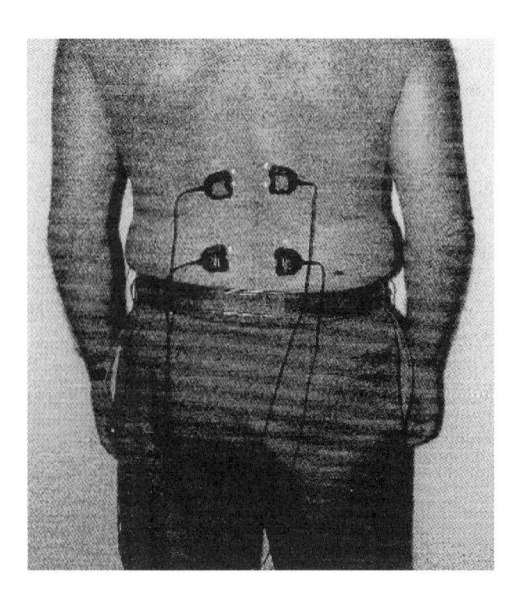

FIGURE 2. Surface EMG electrodes on paraspinal muscles bilaterally at T10 and at L3.

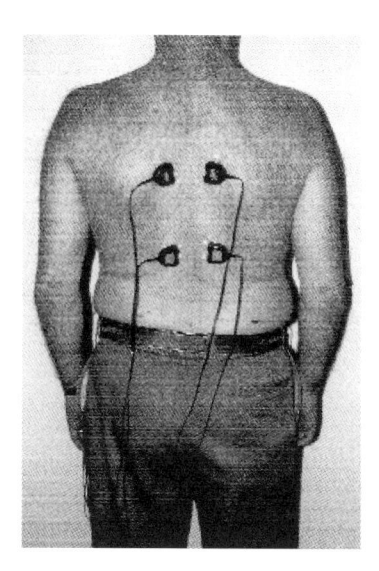

FIGURE 3. Surface EMG electrodes on T6 paraspinals, mid-lower trapezius muscles, and T10 paraspinal muscles bilaterally.

Relaxation training has long been the staple of the psychophysiologist's domain. In order to hear your own body accurately to relearn movements after a stroke, for example, or any of the other rehabilitation goals generally used in rehabilitation clinics, you must first be quiet enough physically and mentally to focus. If you are disturbed by past events or future possibilities, it is difficult to be attentive to the immediate moment when the learning has to take place. Another conversation with a patient might resemble the following:

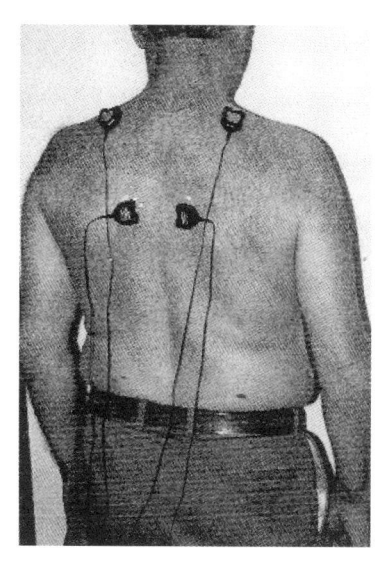

FIGURE 4. Surface EMG channels on upper and lower trapezius bilaterally.

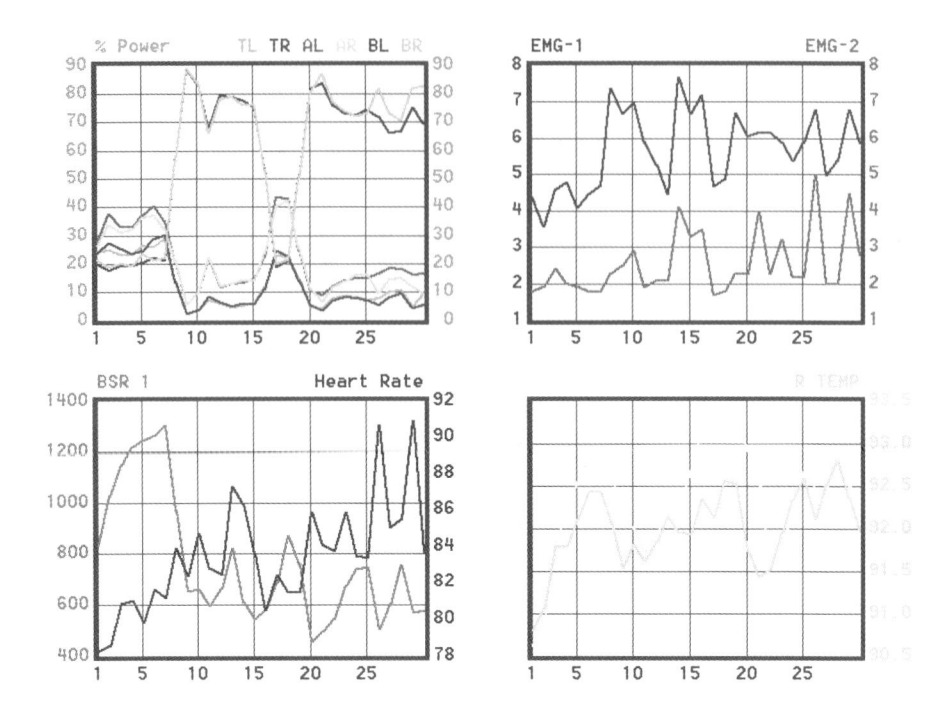

FIGURE 5. Typical initial evaluation.

I know you are having dreams about the accident and are worried about what will happen when you get out of hospital, but you need to learn how to let go of those concerns for awhile so you can concentrate on learning how to use that wheelchair and getting those muscles in your forearm moving so you can feed yourself again.

Another potential problem is convincing the client to learn techniques that may not appear to the client to be related to the presenting symptoms. For example, a client with low back pain might not understand why he should be concerned with the tension in his jaw. The explanation might be something like this:

If you relax your jaw, your whole body will probably relax. There's a trick that professional golf instructors use to teach students to relax when hitting the ball. The instructor puts a potato chip in the student's mouth and then asks the learner to hit the ball without breaking the chip. The question is: are you relaxed enough to walk, talk, and live your life without breaking the chip?

Learning enough control to relax a system is as important as learning enough control to enervate a system. The rule does not change whether we are dealing with musculature, brain-wave activity, or eccrine response. For this reason, relaxation training has become a cornerstone of all biofeedback training.

Most computer-based biofeedback systems average the readings for each modality and track those averages over the course of training. Using these averages, the

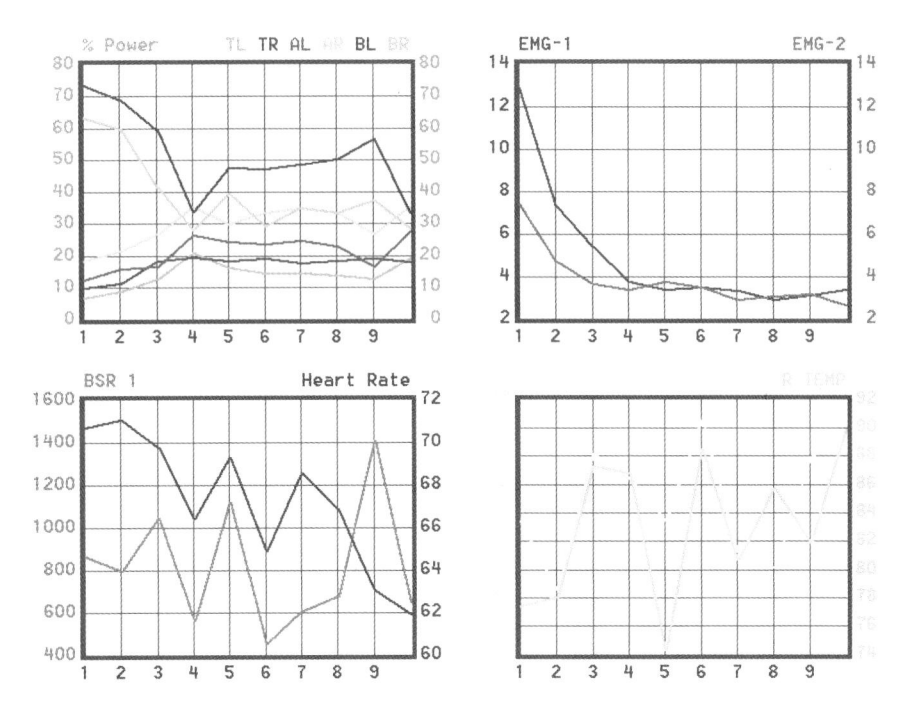

FIGURE 6. Summary of a therapy course over 10 sessions. Session number is displayed along the x-axis, and the session average is displayed along the y-axis.

clinician becomes aware if the therapy is effective or not. Figure 6 shows a summary of a therapy course over 10 sessions.

The most obvious difference is in the readings for surface EMG activity. Over the 10-week period, it is apparent that the client learned basic somatic relaxation. Averages for the shoulder region drop from almost 8 µV to almost 2 µV. This is a 400% reduction in motor unit activity in the area. The temporalis activity drops from 12 or 13 µV to 3 µV, which also represents a 400% drop in activity.

Although the example in Figure 6 shows 10 sessions, this number is sufficient only to teach the techniques. At least 12–16 sessions are needed before a person begins to habituate the newly learned behaviors. Although the readings from the sample show apparent improvement, they are useless if the lessons learned by the patient are not incorporated into his or her lifestyle. The effectiveness of the therapy is based on whether the client habituates the newly learned behaviors. This requires strong concentration on home-based exercises on the part of the client. It cannot be stressed enough that biofeedback is an active therapy and requires active participation by the client.

The final session should be a copy of the baseline session, which will allow the clinician to compare the client's physiology before and after the therapy course. The sessions between the initial evaluation and the discharge evaluation can vary according to therapist, presenting complaint, client's learning ability, and numerous other factors that present themselves in normal clinical settings. A trained psychophysiologist should be flexible enough to adjust the therapy appropriately.

A Typical Training Course for Surface EMG Biofeedback

Surface EMG is the most common form of biofeedback and is frequently encountered in the rehabilitation setting. For many years, physical therapists have been using biofeedback as a modality within general physical therapy, primarily because of the difficulty in billing for biofeedback. It is easier for the therapist to get authorization for physical therapy and include biofeedback as part of the standard physical therapy treatment.

The typical EMG course starts with the initial evaluation. The specifics of the evaluation may vary from therapist to therapist or condition to condition. It is not unusual for some therapists to run 16 channels of surface EMG at once. This level of evaluation allows the therapist to better see the kinesiology involved in the injury. The objective of surface EMG assessment is:

- To clarify aberrant patterns of muscle activity
- To define related physiologic and psychological impairments
- To recognize how objectives 1 and 2 are linked together in preparation for treatment[5]

For example, for a patient with chronic low back pain, the therapist might hook up left and right paraspinal musculature at eight sites along the back. The examination would be used to evaluate symmetric recruitment on both sides of the spine. The patient is asked to perform the same task five times over a 5-minute period. This task should be symmetric in nature such as shrugging shoulders, bending forward, picking up a box, or anterior to posterior pelvic tilt. If the difference between the left and right musculature is greater than 20%, the therapist can conclude that a dysfunction in recruitment exists. Once this has been established, the training is based on eliminating that disparity.

Figure 7 shows surface EMG activity in the left and right upper trapezius muscles. A symmetry test was conducted in which the patient was asked to shrug shoulders five times over a 5-minute period. EMG 1 is the left shoulder, and EMG 2 is the right shoulder. As shown in the figure, there is a discrepancy between the left and right shoulder on the first shrug. The second shrug also shows a discrepancy of approximately 18%. The next three shrugs, however, display symmetry between the left and right sides. This test shows normal discrepancy between the left and right side of the body.

Unlike the patient in Figure 7, the patient in Figure 8 clearly has a problem. Again, EMG 1 is the left shoulder, and EMG 2 is the right. The subject is unable to fully relax the left upper trapezius. The right shoulder muscles relax to a far lower baseline than the left. The musculature on the left is also not recruiting during the shrug. This can be due to fear of pain. It also means, however, that the right side is doing all the work. The baseline levels of the left shoulder increase dramatically for the last two shrugs. The patient reported an increase in pain level, and we can see the corresponding increase in tension in the musculature. Although the baseline level increases, there is still no noticeable correlation between the shrugs and the motor units firing in the left side.

The most difficult task for the clinician in this case is convincing the patient that it is possible to be relaxed despite the fact that he or she may be in pain. The "show and tell" aspect of biofeedback helps this task dramatically. Consistent tension

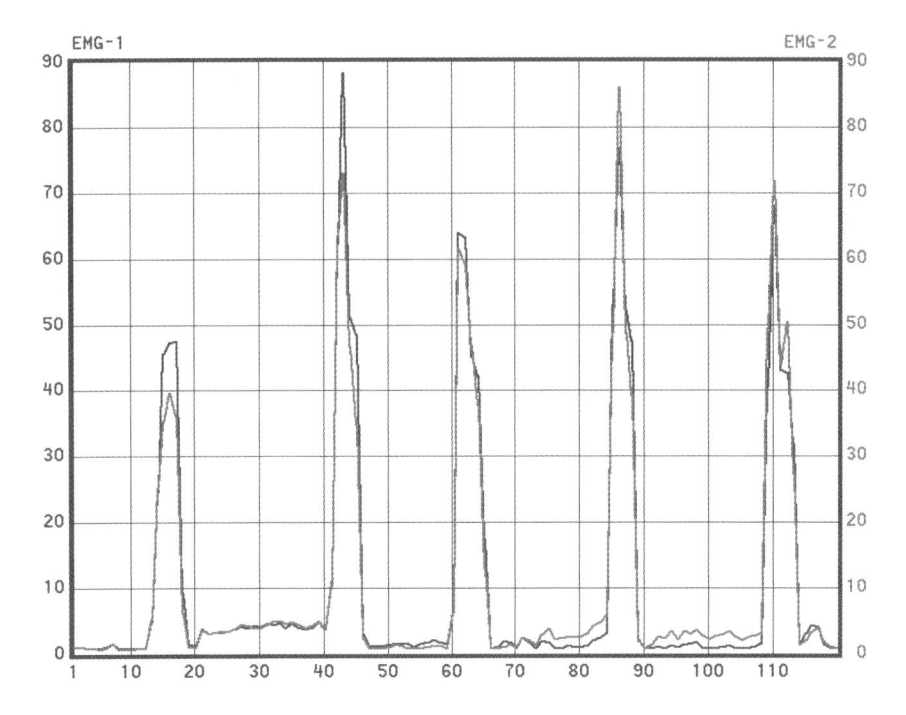

FIGURE 7. Normal EMG activity in both shoulders with only slight discrepancy between right and left sides.

levels, such as those evidenced in Figure 8, will increase the pain dramatically. It is impossible to keep a muscle at these levels of tension without pain being present. The patient begins to discover that the behaviors put in place to help have, in turn, become part of the problem. The treatment goals would obviously involve training to relax the left upper trapezius when appropriate and to coordinate recruitment across both sides of the shoulders.

Specific Disorders

Myofascial Pain

In the area of myofascial pain, Gevirtz and Hubbard seem to believe that trigger points (TrPs) are mediated by excessive sympathetic activity.[4] If this research is borne out, it will be the first conclusive proof that emotional factors have a direct effect on TrP activity. The discovery of spontaneous needle EMG activity and the hypothesis that TrPs are caused by "sympathetically activated intrafusal contractions" may fundamentally change the treatment of chronic myofascial pain.[4] McNulty et al. found that TrPs reacted directly to psychological stressors.[7]

Given this research, the appropriate protocol will address the excessive sympathetic activity by training the client to lower the arousal levels of the sympathetic nervous systems in general and help decrease the amount of muscle activity directly. The modalities indicated include surface EMG, peripheral skin temperature, and general relaxation training.

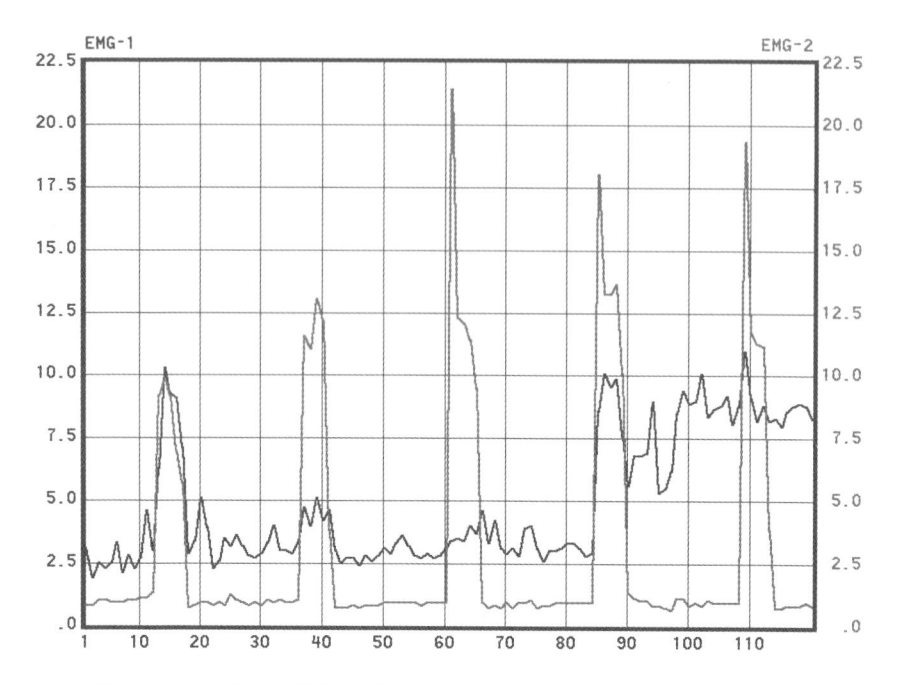

FIGURE 8. Abnormal surface EMC activity in the left upper trapezius muscles with shoulder shrugs (EMG 1, left; EMG 2, right).

General Rehabilitation

Biofeedback as a technique is very adaptive, and the protocol used can vary depending on the stated goal of the therapy. For example, if the anxiety level of the patient is high, the training protocol could be focused on reducing anxiety and improving concentration. If the stated goal were to help recruit muscle fibers, then the protocols are different.

Recently, there has been interest in combining surface EMG feedback with neuromuscular electrical stimulation (NMES).[8] The patient reaching a threshold of surface EMG activity triggers the stimulation. The primary flaw in using only NMES is that the device and muscle are activated by an extrinsic stimulus. In other words, the patient's central nervous system (CNS) does not have to be involved in the contraction. When surface EMG and NMES are combined, the patient is always involved. That way we ensure that the patient's CNS will be actively engaged in the action. This combination of approaches is applicable in a wide range of cases including spinal cord injury, reflex sympathetic dystrophy, patellofemoral dysfunction, and stroke.

Urinary Incontinence

Biofeedback for urinary incontinence has been closely scrutinized recently. Nonetheless, the Health Care Financing Administration (HCFA) has recently announced that biofeedback therapy is covered for the treatment of stress or urge incontinence in patients who failed a documented trial of pelvic muscle exercise training or who are unable to perform pelvic muscle exercises. Insurance carriers may decide whether or not to cover biofeedback as an initial treatment modality.

The protocols for continence training are similar to those of pelvic muscle exercises. In fact, the same pelvic floor musculature is used, and the same exercises are used to target the musculature. The difference is in the addition of biofeedback. An EMG device is used to feed back information to the client about pelvic floor musculature. This allows the patient to see immediately if the exercises are being conducted correctly. Recently, protocols have been developed for combining NMES with the biofeedback.

INDICATIONS

Biofeedback is indicated in a wide range of situations. It is particularly helpful if the client is open to learning and change. Because of the nature of psychophysiology, a good therapist is able to integrate biofeedback into any treatment protocol. From spinal cord injury in which the goal of the therapy is to recruit musculature, to Raynaud's syndrome, in which the goal of the therapy is to decrease sympathetic activity, biofeedback has proved useful. It is best that the referral source is well-versed in the different approaches and is familiar with the protocols. It is also important that the therapist use protocols that have been well established and researched.

CONTRAINDICATIONS

There are very few contraindications to biofeedback. If the patient is particularly resistant, however, or has displayed a history of noncompliance, biofeedback therapy will probably not be effective.

Biofeedback is relatively contraindicated in clients who have moderate to severe depression. The thinking is that biofeedback used as a relaxation protocol will cause a patient to become more depressed as a result of the decreased activity levels. However, symmetry training, as outlined above, may be applicable, and because no relaxation protocol is involved, there is no fear of the patient descending further into depression.

Another potential risk is decompensation. Again, this applies more to the relaxation protocols. A patient who is very stressed and barely coping may begin to decompensate as biofeedback takes effect. This situation needs to be monitored by both the referring source and the clinician. Knowing drug interactions, especially with patients who take psychotropic medication, is essential when managing and treating clients who may be psychotic. The usual contraindications for all therapy including secondary gain, learned helplessness, dependent personality, and recalcitrance are all potential problems. However, none of these potential problems should automatically exclude anyone from participating in the therapy.

One contraindication bears special scrutiny. Secondary gain can be a particular problem when dealing with patients in the workers' compensation system. Conscious self-defeating behavior is almost immediately obvious; however, unconscious self-defeating behavior is more difficult to diagnose. The workers' compensation system inherently rewards people who remain ill and is driven by fear on both sides of the financial fence. The insurance companies are afraid of fraudulent claims, and patients are afraid to improve in case financial support is withdrawn. Careful care and consideration must be applied in this situation.

CONTROVERSIES

Is biofeedback alternative or traditional care? No single question is likely to cause as much emotional outpouring among the biofeedback community as this one. It is very difficult for a biofeedback therapist who is working on a spinal cord injury ward in a large county hospital to consider him- or herself part of the alternative medicine. The opposite is also true. Therapists who have been working inside the complementary community do not see themselves as part of the traditional medical model. Nonetheless, both communities work well together. Indeed, the word *alternative* is becoming obsolete bowing to the newer, more politically correct term, *complementary*.

PRESCRIPTION AND PRACTICE ISSUES

Insurance Coverage

Insurance companies largely drive the U.S. medical system. To a great extent, this prevents a therapy from being considered valid until an insurance company is prepared to pay for it, regardless of whether the medical community deems it well grounded. This is the challenge that faces any new therapy process, and the Association for Applied Psychophysiology and Biofeedback (AAPB), together with the various regional biofeedback organizations, has been fighting to gain acceptance in North America.

In an attempt to make sure that the quality of biofeedback therapy is uniform across the country, the Biofeedback Certificate Institute of America (BCIA) was established. When prescribing biofeedback, make sure that the biofeedback practitioner is BCIA certified. Although this is not a guarantee of good biofeedback therapy, it is a guarantee that the practitioner has gained at least enough elementary knowledge to pass the examination. Because biofeedback is not currently an individual discipline, practitioners' abilities vary widely, and it is important that the person who is referring the client be familiar with the therapeutic modalities that the practitioner uses.

The workers' compensation system gives rise to its own problems. In addition to the clinical challenges posed by secondary gain and other issues, getting authorization for therapy can be difficult. Because of this fact, many therapies are administered under an umbrella code. For example, a physical therapist who wishes to use a reasonably new modality and cannot find the procedure listed in the insurance company's covered procedures can bill under a generic PT code. Licensed professionals have used biofeedback for many years, but because of the difficulty in billing, it has been billed under a generic procedure code for their profession.

Biofeedback Prescription

When prescribing biofeedback, it is important to realize that the success of the therapy is governed by learning theory. Because the therapy is active in nature, the length of the course is influenced by many factors. The first is the motivation of the client, because the patient really has to want to change. There are no instant cures in biofeedback. Instead, it is a powerful learning tool for change. That change can be mostly physiologic or mostly psychological, but in both cases, the effort needed is great. Clients who show a history of passivity may be contraindicated for the therapy.

Other factors that come into play vary depending on the type of biofeedback being prescribed. For example, for a patient with severe depression, using biofeedback to relax is contraindicated; however, if that person also has chronic low back pain, biofeedback for symmetry training is indicated. It is important for the referring source to evaluate each patient carefully and make sure that the type of biofeedback being prescribed is appropriate. Also, the practitioner must have access to psychological and physiologic histories for the patient.

Although it is difficult to say how many sessions should be prescribed, it is safe to say that twelve 1-hour sessions are the minimum number necessary to be effective. It has been more or less established that EEG biofeedback requires a minimum of 30 sessions for behavior to become habituated. With body measures such as EMG and respiration, the number of sessions that is required declines. Most biofeedback clinicians prefer to see patients for at least 16 sessions.

Resources

The AAPB issues a journal called *Applied Psychophysiology and Biofeedback* published by Kluwer Academic–Plenum Publishers. The journal is a good source for the latest research into psychophysiology, although articles about this topic frequently appear in other journals. Biofeedback practitioners regularly submit research to the journals that are dominant in their licensed areas of interest, so relevant articles have been published in better known journals.

The AAPB also publishes a register each year of biofeedback practitioners, and lists sorted by zip code, country, and specialty can all be found within the register. It can also be found at their web site: www.aapb.org. The web site is also a comprehensive research tool that summarizes the latest research and contains a host of links to relevant sites.

The BCIA at www.bcia.org serves as an essential source for those interested in certification. It also acts as a comprehensive source of information for the clinician that may be interested in referring. The site lists the blueprint of knowledge the biofeedback therapist is required to know, as well as the ethical standards the therapist is required to abide by. The European counterpart of the AAPB is the Biofeedback of Europe (BFE). Their web site, www.bfe.org, is also a comprehensive source of information.

CONCLUSION

Biofeedback requires an active participation and habituation of new behavior on the part of the patients. The continuing challenge for the field of biofeedback is getting wider acceptance of biofeedback as a valid option in the treatment of conditions such as chronic pain and neurologic disorders.

Therapists who practice inside traditional medical facilities are well aware of how the system needs to change in order for biofeedback therapy to evolve. Therapists who work outside of traditional medical facilities are also well aware that the system needs to change. A good clinician is convinced of the necessity for good, solid research to prove the biofeedback approach is viable.

REFERENCES

1. Basmajian JV: Biofeedback in physical medicine and rehabilitation. In DeLisa JA, Gans BM (eds): Rehabilitation Medicine: Principles and Practices, 3rd ed. Philadelphia, Lippincott-Raven, 1998, pp 505–520.
2. Cram J, Kasman G, Holtz J: Introduction to Surface Electromyography. Gaithersburg, MD, Aspen Publications, 1997.
3. Green E, Green A: General and specific applications of thermal biofeedback. In Basmajian JV (ed): Biofeedback Principles and Practices for Clinicians, 3rd ed. Baltimore, Williams & Wilkins, 1989, pp 209-211.
4. Hubbard D, Berkoff G: Myofascial trigger points show spontaneous needle EMG activity. Spine 119:1803–1807, 1993.
5. Kasman G, Cram F, Wolf S: Chronic musculoskeletal pain.. In Clinical Applications in Surface Electromyography: Gaithersburg, MD, Aspen Publications, 1997.
6. Schwartz MS, et al: Biofeedback: A Practitioner's Guide. New York, Guilford Press, 1987.
7. McNulty J, Hubbard D, Gevirtz R, Berkoff G: Needle electromyographic evaluation of trigger point response to a psychological stressor. Psychophysiology 31:313–316, 1994.
8. Kasman G, Cram F, Wolf S: SEMG-triggered electrical stimulation. In Clinical Applications in Surface Electromyography: Gaithersburg, MD, Aspen Publications, 1998.

Chapter 16
Acupuncture in the Management of Neuromusculoskeletal Disorders

Alice M. K. Wong, MD, Simon F. T. Tang, MD, and Henry L. Lew, MD, PhD

Acupuncture has been used in traditional Chinese medicine to relieve pain and cure a variety of diseases for more than 2500 years. The ancient Chinese were aware of an increased sensitivity of certain skin areas (called *acupoints*) when an organ or function was impaired. Through experience, 361 acupoints were gradually identified to form a network of 14 channels, called *meridians*. The whole system of meridians brings about the integrity of the body by connecting the internal organs with the superficial parts of the body.[1]

Acupuncture was introduced to the West by Jesuit missionaries to Peking in the 17th century. In the 1930s, de Morant reintroduced acupuncture to France, and the rest of Europe soon became interested, developing research programs to study its clinical applications. Since then, research has confirmed that acupuncture therapy produces an analgesic effect through noxious stimuli that induce endogenous pain relief substances. Animal experiments verified the positive effects on the circulatory, digestive, and urinary systems and for epilepsy control.[2–8]

The interest in acupuncture is growing in the United States, Europe (especially France, Italy, the United Kingdom, Germany, Russia, and some Eastern European nations), and Argentina, but it also has been the object of scientific study in East Asia (China, Japan, and Korea). Acupuncture was brought to the attention of American medical professionals in 1971 when James Reston reported that acupuncture analgesia relieved postappendectomy complications he suffered in China.[1,2] Dr. Howard A. Rusk also expressed interest in acupuncture research in the preface of his textbook *Rehabilitation Medicine*.[9]

A World Health Organization (WHO) interregional seminar drew up a provisional list of 47 diseases that are amenable to acupuncture treatment.[10] Of these 47 disease, 16 are neuromusculoskeletal disorders. Learning acupuncture may be simplified by limiting its use to therapy for neuromusculoskeletal disorders rather than for all fields.

THE SCIENTIFIC BASIS OF ACUPUNCTURE POINTS

Acupoints can be easily determined by anatomic landmarks or by the measurement with subject's own hand or finger called "own body scale." In 1950, Nakatani found that the electric impedance at an acupoint is 1/20 to its surrounding skin area, an area that is easily measured with a simple impedance detector.[4]

Acupoints have been reported with different sizes, from small points to large areas (100–400 μm), and are located subcutaneously, intramuscularly, or in the viscera. Nearly all of them are closely related to nerves, and 84.36% of them are near blood vessels. Local infiltration with an anesthetic agent blocks the effect of acupuncture analgesia only when the anesthetic is injected to a certain depth,

TABLE 1. ACUPOINT CHARACTERISTICS

1. Occupies the position of an acupuncture site
2. Are different sizes, from small points to large area (100–400 µm)
3. Nearly all are related to the nerves
4. Located near vessels (84.36%)
5. Local infiltration with anesthetic agent blocks the effect of acupuncture
    - Classical points: belong to the 14 meridians
    - Trigger points (TPs): Ah's points have the same characteristics as TPs in myofascial pain syndrome

depending on the point treated (Table 1). The depth varies from several millimeters at digits or toes, to several centimeters at proximal parts of the limbs.[2,4]

Other than the 361 classical acupoints, other groups of acupoints exist that are effective in treating particular symptoms. They were named in Chinese in accordance with their position or function. The Chinese names are easier to remember than their English translations, but the difficulties in proper translation may be overcome by readily available commercialized computer programs. Another group of acupoints, called Ah's points (remembered by the phrase "Ah yes, this is the trigger point"), have the same characteristics and locations that are similar to the trigger points of myofascial pain syndrome, but were discovered independently and labeled differently.[11–15]

NEUROMODULATION OF ACUPUNCTURE

The word *acupuncture* is derived from two Latin words, *acus* ("needle") and *punctura* ("puncture"). However, the structure of an acupuncture needle differs from the ordinary injection needle in its fineness (gauge 30–36) and in its blunt tip, which separates the tissue rather than sharp cutting during twirling.[8,10]

The characteristic sensation of acupuncture needling, which is called *de qi*, is a prerequisite for effectiveness (Table 2). It can be evoked only with puncturing and twirling at the acupoint. In general, the manual needling evokes activity in type II and type III fibers (Table 3). Electrical acupuncture stimulation mainly excites type II fibers. Type III and IV fibers might be excited when heavy needing techniques are applied, which may cause resultant occurrence of pain.[2]

The sensations evoked by acupuncture applied to points on a limb to be amputated were recorded by Lu and colleagues and Lin and associates.[15a,15b] In general, sensations described as "numbness" are evoked by direct stimulation of nerves, and "soreness" by needling tendons or periosteum. "Heavy" or "numb" sensations are

TABLE 2. CHARACTERISTIC SENSATIONS ON ACUPUNCTURE NEEDLING

1. **De qi response**—for acupuncture to be effective
    Numbness—evoked by direct stimulation of nerves
    Soreness—evoked by needling tendon or periosteum
    Heavy or numb—evoked by stimulation of muscles
    Pain—when perivascular nerve filaments are stimulated[15a,15b]

2. **Propagated sensation**—a quasinervous structure that entwines blood vessels and is related with the neurliemma or the sheet of Henle possible:
    - Related to sympathetic innervating
    - Spread of excitation in the CNS

TABLE 3. NEUROMODULATION OF ACUPUNCTURE

Technique	Fibers Stimulated
Manual needling, insertion and twirling	Type II and III
Electrical acupuncture	Mainly type II
Heavy needling	Type III and IV

evoked by acupuncture stimulation of muscles, whereas pain is altered when perivascular nerve filaments are stimulated by acupuncture. The propagated sensation according to Cajal is a quasi-nervous structure that entwines blood vessels and is related to the neurilemma or the sheet of Henle.[15c] It is believed to be related to the sympathetic innervation of skeletal muscles. Another possibility is that propagated sensation is the result of processes similar to the spread of excitation in the central nervous system.[2]

The development of electroacupuncture provides good effect on pain control and muscle stimulation (Tables 4 and 5). The use of skin electrodes at the acupoint has increased public acceptance in recent years.[5,6] With surface electrodes, the side effects of acupuncture including local pain, hemorrhage, infection, pneumothorax, broken needle, and syncope (0.2% incidence) can also be avoided.

ACUPUNCTURE FOR MUSCULOSKELETAL INJURY OR DISORDERS

The **Hegu (LI4)** is a point located at the junction of the proximal end of the first and second metacarpal bones, with good general analgesic effect for fascial pain,

TABLE 4. PAIN CONTROL BY ACUPUNCTURE

Theory	Example
Gate control theory (Melzack, Wall, 1965)	Large fiber inputs tend to close the gate
Hyperstimulation analgesia (Melzack)	Ice packs, hot cups, or blistering the skin
Secretion of pain relief substances	
Spinal cord	Enkephalin, dynorphin
Midbrain	Enkephalin
Raphe magnus and reticular paragigantocellularis	Serotonin, norepinephrine
Pituitary-hypothalamus	β-Endorphin

TABLE 5. ELECTROACUPUNCTURE

Stimulation Type	Effects Produced
Low-frequency, high-intensity	Involves the endorphinergic mechanism
	Generates a slow-onset analgesia
	Has long-lasting results
	Has a cumulative effect
	Requires usually only small doses of naloxone to inhibit its analgesic
High-frequency, low-intensity	Involves nonopioid monoaminergic systems
	Generates a rapid-onset analgesia
	Has short-lasting results
	Has no cumulative effect
	Requires unusually large doses of naloxone to inhibit its analgesic effect

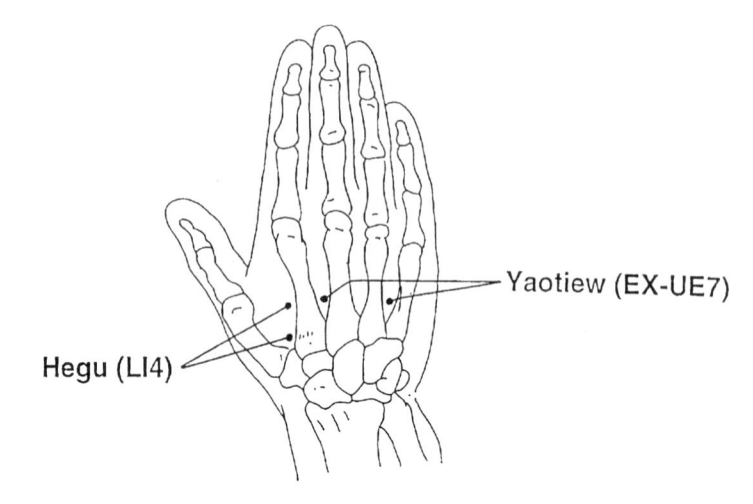

FIGURE 1. Location of the acupoints Hegu (LI4) and Yaotiew (Ex-UE7).

such as headache, toothache, and other painful conditions.[12–20] It is prohibited in pregnant women due to the risk of the abortion (Fig. 1).

Taichong (Liv3) is located between the proximal end of the first and second metatarsal bones (Fig. 2); it also has good analgesic effect, especially in combination with the Hegu.

The **Zusani (ST36)** is located on the lateral side of the anterior tibial muscle below the tibial tubercle (*see* Fig. 2). This point provides good general analgesic effect as well as analgesia for visceral pain.

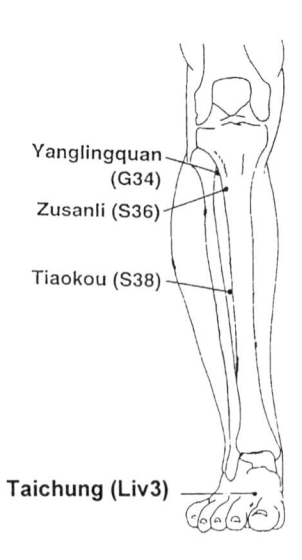

FIGURE 2. Location of the acupoints Taichung (Liv3), Tiaokou (S38), Zusanli (S36), and Yanglingquan (G34).

Acupuncture in the Management of Neuromusculoskeletal Disorders   231

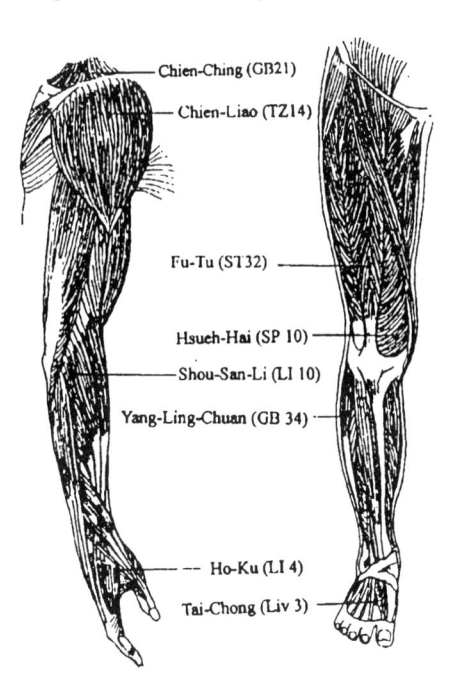

FIGURE 3. The commonly used acupoints of the upper and lower extremities. (From Wong AMK: Clinical trial of electrical acupuncture on hemiplegic stroke patient. Am J Phys Med Rehabil 78:117–122, 1999, with permission.)

Yanglingquan (GB34) is located on the depressed area lateral to the tuberosity of the tibia with the knee flexed 90° (Figs. 2 and 3). It is a very good acupoint for muscle relaxation, which is indicated for traumatic injuries.

Sanyanglo (T8), which is located at the lower third of the forearm on the extensor side between the radius and ulna, is good for treating chest pain, intercostal neuralgia, and pain in the upper extremities.

Huantiao (GB30) is located at the lateral one third of the gluteus maximus, between the greater trochanter of the femur and coccyx (Fig. 4). At 3 or more inches, this is the deepest acupoint. This point is effective for treating back pain and sciatica.

Weichung (B54) is located right in the middle of the popliteal fossa (see Fig. 4). Needling this point treats lumbago, sciatica, leg muscle cramp, and knee stiffness.

Tiaoshan, located at the midpoint of the tibia one of the lateral aspect, is penetrated from **Tiaokou (ST38)** to the back of leg at **Chengshan (B57)** for 2–3 inches (see Figs. 2 and 4). Shoulder pain and acute frozen shoulder can be treated using this acupoint.

The pair of acupoints known as **Yaotiew (Ex-UE7)** is located at the proximal end in between the second and third metacarpal bones and the fourth and fifth metacarpal bones (see Fig. 1). These points are effective for lumbar strain, lumbago, and sciatica.

Acupuncture had been reported to be very effective in acute soft tissue injuries, with excellent results in 71.5% of the patients, 18.9% with good results, and 9.6%

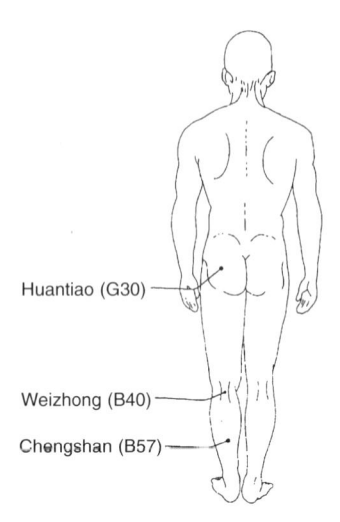

FIGURE 4. Location of the acupoints Huantiao (G30), Weizhong (B40), and Chengshan (B57).

with fair results.[19] However, in chronic soft tissue injuries treated with acupuncture, only 34% of the patients achieved excellent results, 29.3% achieved good results, 27.8% reported fair results, and 9% indicated a poor grade.[19] The author stressed that this phenomenon may be considered important for the attenuation of pain. It has the benefits of noninvasive and better patient tolerance. It is suitable in treating athletic injuries on both body acupuncture and ear acupuncture, especially in combination with an acupoint detector. Some chronic painful conditions including myofascial pain syndrome can be treated by acupuncture in Ah's point (trigger point), commonly seen in the management of sport injuries.

ACUPUNCTURE FOR OSTEOARTHRITIS

Acupuncture is a common alternative to medication in the treatment of osteoarthritis (OA). The long-term effect of acupuncture treatment was studied in patients with OA of the knee. Significant reductions of pain and analgesic consumption in the treatment were noted by comparison with the control group.[21–23] However, a randomized, placebo-controlled study involving 40 patients with OA of the knee showed that both real and sham acupuncture significantly reduced pain, stiffness, and physical disability, but no difference was found between the two groups.[24]

The common acupoints for OA are selected from the points near the joints. For instance, GB34, GB33, SP9, and SP10 for knee OA and SI6 for wrist OA and the multiple OA joints are suggested.

ACUPUNCTURE FOR PAIN CONTROL

Acupuncture and electroacupuncture effects are mediated through a variety of neural and neurochemical mechanisms. Research done in the early 1970s first elucidated the mechanisms for the effect of acupuncture anesthesia.[3–6,25,26] Experiments in rabbits showed that this effect can be transferred from one rabbit to another by cerebrospinal fluid (CSF) transfusion. More recent investigation explored the role of classic central neurotransmitters in the mediation of acupuncture analgesia, including catecholamines and serotonin. The availability of rat models for electroacupuncture, using the tail flick latency as a bioassay, allowed further experiments done to explain the basis for the effect. Differential release of central nervous system (CNS) opioid peptides by electroacupuncture has been noted, with 2-Hz of electroacupuncture triggering the release of enkephalins and beta-endorphins, and a 100-Hz stimulation selectively increased the release of dynorphin in the spinal cord. A combination of both frequencies allows synergistic interaction among the three endogenous opioid peptides and provides a powerful analgesic effect. In addition, multiple acupuncture treatments with the optimal time spacing may result in an accumulation of electroacupuncture effect. A bimodal distribution of analgesic effect can be noted if a large group of rats is given electroacupuncture (low responders and high responders). Low response is caused by at least two mechanisms: a low rate of release of opioid peptides in the CNS and a high rate of release of cholecystokinin octapeptide (CCK-8), which exerts potent antiopioid effects. A newly discovered antiopioid peptide, orphanin FQ, has also been linked to negative feedback control of electroacupuncture stimulation.[27-28]

ACUPUNCTURE FOR PHANTOM LIMB PAIN

Acupuncture therapy for phantom limb pain of amputees may stimulate large sensory afferent fibers and suppress pain perception as explained by the gate control theory of pain. The needle insertion may act as a noxious stimulus and induce endogenous production of opiate-like substances to effect pain control.[29]

In the patient with single-limb amputation, acupoints in the intact, contralateral limb that correspond to or near the painful areas may be used in the perceived phantom limb every day or every other day. In patients with bilateral amputation of lower limbs, the acupoints of the intact upper limbs can be used as reference points to treat patients (e.g., elbow for knee; wrist for ankle). Remarkable reduction of pain scores and shortening of the most severe phantom pain were reported, although these results do not appear to alter the final outcome in the pain score or the duration of phantom limb pain.[30]

With single photon emission computed tomography (SPECT) study, phantom limb pain was possibly associated with cortical activation involving the frontal, temporal, or parietal cortex.[31] Hypoperfusion of bilateral thalami and brain stem was observed after acupuncture therapy.[32]

ACUPUNCTURE FOR STROKE THERAPY

Acupuncture may be enhanced by the functional plasticity of the brain.[33] A study with real versus sham acupuncture in the treatment of paralysis in stroke patients indicated that a significantly greater number of patients had a good response to real acupuncture than sham acupuncture at various lesion sites based on CT scans.[34] Studies on functional reorganization after stroke using positron emission tomography (PET) suggest that considerable reorganization within the brain occurs after stroke, including metabolic activation of contralateral and frontal areas.[35]

Many studies report that acupuncture treatment for stroke patients can produce beneficial effects on motor function recovery, reduction of spasticity, and improvement of poststroke depression.[33,36,37] Decreased ankle spasticity and improved gait cycle parameters have been reported after acupuncture therapy in older patients.[38] The H-reflex recovery time of the paretic side of chronic stroke patients is significantly prolonged after acupuncture therapy.[39,40]

The use of electrical acupuncture through adhesive surface electrodes on GB21, TZ14, LI10, and LI4 in the upper extremity and ST32, SP10, GB34, and Liv3 in the lower extremity help achieve a better functional outcome in stroke patients and shorten the hospital stay for rehabilitation. It can be applied during the acute stage of stroke without the side effects of needle acupuncture, even in patients who underwent anticoagulation therapy.[11]

ACUPUNCTURE FOR SPINAL CORD–INJURED PATIENTS

The animal experiment of first aid acupuncture treatment in spinal cord–injured (SCI) rats at Bl60, Bl54, and GV3 within 15 minutes after surgery was accompanied by minimization of post-traumatic cord shrinkage and a marked sparing of ventral horn neurons.[41] Human clinical studies also show remarkable improvement of spinal paraplegia with acupuncture therapy in 120 patients.[42]

Therapeutic trials of acupuncture therapy for neurogenic bladder of SCI patients at CV3, CV4, and bilateral UB32 (Fig. 5), in addition to conventional intermittent catheterization program (1CP), showed significantly shortened duration for bladder training. There was no difference in duration in treating the neurogenic bladder of upper or lower motor neuron lesion.[43]

NEURAL BASES OF ACUPUNCTURE STUDIED BY FUNCTIONAL MAGNETIC RESONANCE IMAGING OF THE BRAIN

Modern advanced brain imaging such as functional magnetic resonance imaging (fMRI) and PET of the brain has been successfully applied to the study of

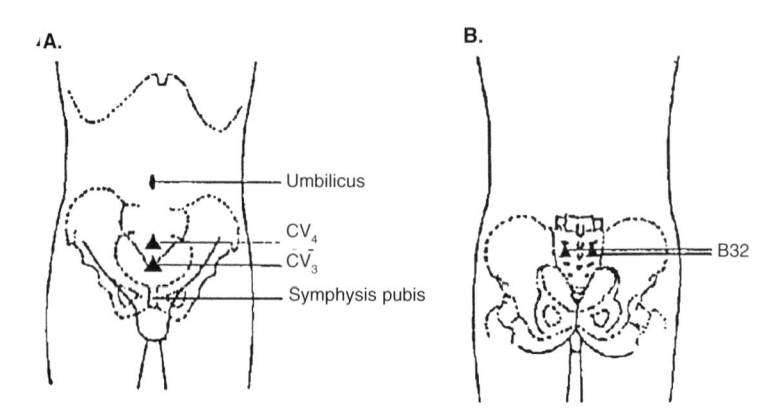

FIGURE 5. Location of the acupoints CV3, CV4, and UB32. A, Anterior view. CV4 is located on the midpoint from the umbilicus to the symphysis pubis. CV3 is located on the upper one-third from CV4 to the symphysis pubis. B, Posterior view. B32 is located at the intervertebral foramen between S2 and S3.

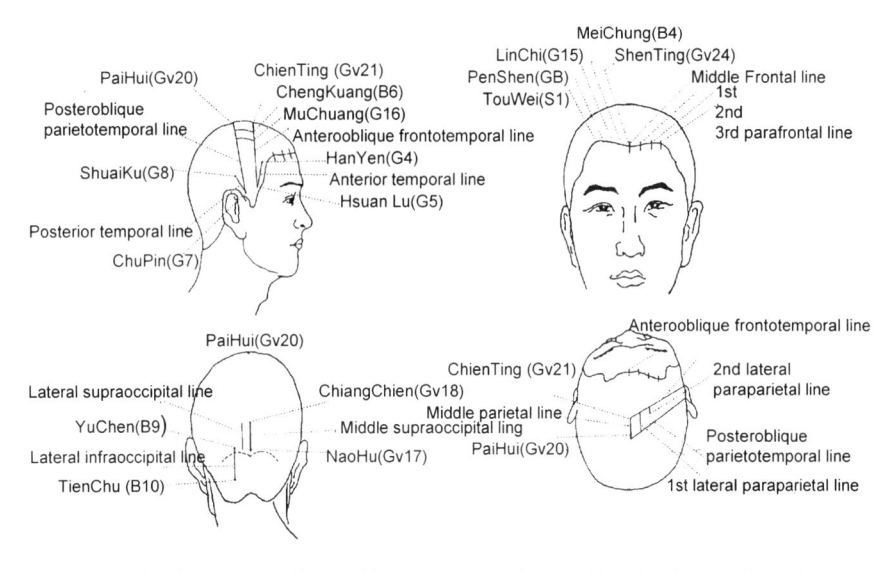

FIGURE 6. The commonly used landmarks and acupoints in the head region.

acupuncture. Many scientists believe that the main thrust of acupuncture may be in the brain. The activation result of acupuncture stimulation of acupoint GB37 (vision-related disease treatment) showed nearly the same result of the direct visual stimulation by an increased signal in MRI. Similarly, for ear or hearing-related acupoint SI5, a similar result of cortical activation pattern of acupuncture stimulation followed closely that of direct auditory stimulation with music.

It might support the hypothesis that acupuncture stimulation of a specific acupoint could deliver information to the corresponding cortical area or areas, thereby activating higher centers of the brain to make necessary alterations to balance hormonal, autonomic nervous systemic, and neurochemical activity.[44]

OTHER TYPES OF ACUPUNCTURE

Scalp Acupuncture

Acupuncture applied to the scalp was developed by the Chinese neurologist S.F. Chiao in 1970.[45] He treated brain injury patients with motor paresis or paralysis by inserting needles into the scalp according to the referral area of Brodmann (Fig. 6).

Vasodilatation in cerebral vessels and an increase of cerebral blood flow were proved by transcranial Doppler sonography in some stroke patients but not in a normal control group.[46] It is used in the treatment of cerebrovascular accident (CVA), head injury, cerebral palsy, and hyperactivity and psychic disorders.[47]

Auricular Acupuncture

In the traditional Chinese literature, scattered statements about ear acupoints can be found, but no meridian specifically is noticed among them. Around 1956, reports appeared both in China and in France that the diagnosis and treatment of some diseases could be attained through needling or stimulating specific points on

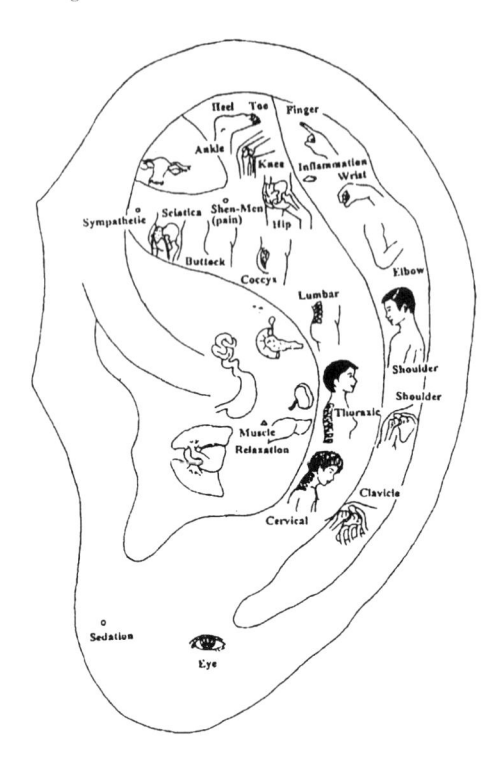

236 Acupuncture in the Management of Neuromusculoskeletal Disorders

FIGURE 7. The acupoints of the ear.

the auricles (Fig. 7). In 1956–1957, Nogier of France first reported his techniques of auricular acupuncture, later refining them in 1972.[48]

Auricular acupuncture can be performed by a small needle (1 mm long) with a ring tail, held in place by tape for 1 or 2 weeks at the ear acupoint. It has better clinical convenience for chronic soft tissue pain and may be applied as an adjunct in the treatment of myofascial pain syndrome. It is also used for treating cerebral palsy.[49]

REFERENCES

1. Lee MHM, Liao SJ: Acupuncture in physiatry. In Kottke FJ, Lehmann JF (eds): Krusen's Handbook of Physical Medicine and Rehabilitation, 4th ed. Philadelphia, W.B. Saunders, 1990, pp 402–432.
2. Wu DZ: Acupuncture and neurophysiology. Clin Neurol Neurosurg 92:13–25, 1990.
3. MacDonald AFR: Acupuncture analgesia and therapy. In Wall PD, Melzack R (ed): Textbook of Pain, 2nd ed. UK, Longman Group, 1989, pp 906–919.
4. Richardson PH, Vincent CA: Acupuncture for the treatment of pain: A review of evaluative research. Pain 24:15–40, 1986.
5. Lewith GT, Kenyon JN: Physiological and psychological explanations for the mechanism of acupuncture as a treatment for chronic pain. Soc Sci Med 19:1367–1378, 1984.
6. Han JS, Sun SL: Differential release of enkephalin and dynorphin by low and high frequency electroacupuncture in the central nervous system. Acupunct SCI Intern J 1:19–24, 1990.
7. Levin MF, Hui-Chan CWY: Conventional and acupuncture-like transcutaneous electrical nerve stimulation excite similar afferent fibers. Arch Phys Med Rehabil 74:54–60, 1993.
8. Shanghai College of Traditional Medicine: Acupuncture: A Comprehensive Textbook [English]. Chicago, Eastland Press, Inc., 1981.

9. Rusk HA: Rehabilitation Medicine, 4th ed. St. Louis, Mosby, 1977, p viii.
10. Chung FS: Fundamentals of Acupuncture and Moxibustion [Chinese]. Taipei, China, Acupuncture Research Institute, 1984, pp 10–11.
11. Wong AMK, Su TY, Tang FT, et al: Clinical trial of electrical acupuncture on hemiplegic stroke patients. Am J Phys Med Rehabil 78:117–122, 1999.
12. Melzack R, Stillwell DM, Fox EJ: Trigger points and acupuncture points for pain: Correlations and implications. Pain 3:2–23, 1977.
13. Lewit K: The needle effect in the relief of myofascial pain. Pain 6:83–90, 1979.
14. Li T: Acupuncture treatment of fibrositis. World J Acupunct Mox 2:23–25, 1992.
15. Milano PGF, Hare BD: The effects of myofascial trigger point injections are naloxone reversible. Pain 32:15–20, 1988.
16. Garvey TA, Marks MR, Wiesel SW: A prospective, randomized, double-blind evaluation of trigger point injection therapy of low back pain. Spine 14:962–964, 1989.
17. Chen A: Effective acupuncture therapy for sciatica and low back pain: Review of recent studies and prescriptions with recommendations for improved results. Am J Acup 18:305–323, 1990.
18. Chung C: The Golden Points: An Illustration of High Effective Therapeutic Points in Medical Acupuncture. Taipei, VA General Hospital, 1990, pp 2–43.
19. Sun FS: Result of electrostimulation in acupoint for soft tissue injury: Report of 932 cases. Chin Acupunct 1:4–6, 1990.
20. Waylonis CW, Wilke S, et al: Chronic myofascial pain: Management by low-output helium-neon laser therapy. Arch Phys Med Rehabil 69:1017–1020, 1998.
21. Fargas-Babjak AM, Pomeranz B: Acupuncture-like stimulation with codetron for rehabilitation of patients with chronic pain syndrome and osteoarthritis. Acupunct Electro-Ther Res Int J 17:95–105, 1992.
22. Creamaer P, Singh BB, Hochberg MC, Berman BM: Are psychosocial factors related to us? Knee osteoarthritis. Altern Therap Health Med 5:72–76, 1999.
23. Archis, Arichi H, Toda S: Acupuncture and rehabilitation (III) effects of acupuncture applied to the normal side on osteoarthritis deformans and rheumatoid arthritis of the knee and on disorders in motility of the knee joint after cerebral hemorrhage and thrombosis. Am J Chin Med 11(1–4):146–149, 1983.
24. Gaw AC, Chang LW, Shaw LC: Efficiency of acupuncture on osteoarthritic pain. A controlled, double-blind study. N Engl J Med 293:375–378, 1975.
25. Goldstein A, Hilgard ER: Failure of the opiate. Proc Natl Acad Sci 72:2041–2043, 1975.
26. Guillemin R: Beta-lipoprotein and endorphins: Implications of current knowledge. Hosp Pract 13:53–60, 1978.
27. Han JS, Terenius L: Neurochemical basis of acupuncture analgesia. Ann Rev Pharmacol Toxicol 22:193–220, 1982.
28. Han JS: Physiology of acupuncture: Review of thirty years of research. In The Neurochemical Basis of Pain Relief by Acupuncture, Vol 2. Hubei Science & Technology Press, 1998, p 771.
29. Melzack R: Folk medicine and the sensory modulation of pain. In Wall PD, Melzack R (eds): Textbook of Pain, 3rd ed. New York, Churchill-Livingstone, 1994, pp 1209–1218.
30. Liaw MY, Wong AMK, Cheng PT: Therapeutic trial of acupuncture in phantom limb pain of amputees. Am J Acupunct 22:205–213, 1994.
31. Liaw MY, You DL, Cheng PC, et al: Central representation of phantom limb phenomenon in amputees studied with single photon emission computed tomography. Am J Phys Med Rehabil 77:368–375, 1998.
32. Liaw MY, You DL, Cheng PT, et al: Observations on brain perfusion before and after acupuncture treatment of phantom limb pain: A case report. Am J Acupunct 24:247–254, 1996.
33. Management M, Johansson K, Johansson BB: Sensory stimulation promote normalization of posture control after stroke. Stroke 25:1175–1181, 1994.
34. Naser MA, Alexander MP, Staiassny-Eder D, et al: Real versus sham acupuncture in the treatment of paralysis in acute stroke patients: A CT scan lesion site study. J Neurol Rehabil 6:163–173, 1992.
35. Chollet F, Dipiero V, Wise RJS, et al: The functional anatomy of motor recovery after stroke in humans: A study with position emission tomography. Ann Neural 29:63–71, 1991.
36. Hu HW, Chung C, Liu TJ, et al: A randomized controlled trial on the treatment for acute partial ischemic stroke with acupuncture. Neuroepidemiology 12:106–113, 1993.

37. Kjendahl A, Sallstrom S: A one-year follow-up study on the effects of acupuncture in the treatment of stroke patients in subacute stage: A randomized, controlled study. Clin Rehabil 11:192–200, 1997.
38. Chen YM, Fang YA: 108 cases of hemiplegia caused by stroke: The relationship between CT results, clinical finding, and the effect of acupuncture treatment. Acupunct Electrother Res 15:9–17, 1990.
39. Yu YH, Wang HC, Wang ZJ: The effect of acupuncture on spinal motor neuron excitability stroke patients. Clin Med J 56:258–263, 1995.
40. Wei H, Tang FT, Wong MK: The effect of scalp acupuncture on motor neuron excitability of stroke patients. J Rehabil Med Assoc Taiwan 23:9–13, 1995.
41. Politis MJ, Korchinski MA: Beneficial effects of acupuncture treatment following experimental spinal cord injury: A behavioral, morphological, and biochemical study. Acupunct Electrother Res Int J 15:37–49, 1990.
42. Ran C, Ba S, Liu X, et al: Acupuncture treatment of spinal paraplegia with acupuncture selected, basing on neuroanatomy. World J Acupuct Mox 2:3–9, 1992.
43. Cheng PT, Wong MK, Chang PL: A therapeutic trial of acupuncture in neurogenic bladder of spinal cord injured patients: A preliminary report. Spinal Cord 36:476–480, 1998.
44. Cho ZH: Neural bases of acupuncture studied by functional magnetic resonance imaging (fMRI) of the brain. Sixth North American Symposium on Acupuncture ((:54–60, 2000.
45. Chiao SF: Scalp acupuncture in branch disease. Chin Med J 3:325–328, 1977.
46. Do GC, Chang TB, Pu EC: The comparison of scalp and body acupuncture in cerebral vascular effect of ischemic stroke. Chin Acup 5:265–266, 1999.
47. Stux G, Pomeranz B: Scalp acupuncture. In: Acupuncture: Textbook and Atlas. Berlin, Springer, 1987, pp 249–252.
48. Leung CY, Spoerel WZ: Effects of auriculo-acupuncture on pain. Am J Chin Med 2:247–260, 1974.
49. Spears C: Auricular acupuncture: New approach to treatment of cerebral palsy. Am J Acupunct 7:49–54, 1979.

Chapter 17

Basic Principles of Injection Techniques

Jeffrey L. Woodward, MD, MS, and Ted A. Lennard, MD

Percutaneous injections are commonly used by pain physicians for the treatment or diagnosis of soft tissue, joint, or neurogenic pain disorders. These may include trigger points in muscle, tender points in ligaments or muscle, inflamed joints, bursa or tendons, or nerve blocks. The injections assist the diagnostician in evaluating the source of pain and usually offer some degree of pain relief. This chapter reviews general principles of injections including medications, techniques, indications, and side effects.

GENERAL CONSIDERATIONS

Positioning and Relaxation

Positioning the patient for comfort and physician accessibility is one of the first steps to good technique. Multiple pads and pillows can be used to optimize positioning and help the patient relax. The physician should communicate to the patient all anticipated procedural steps as they progress. Warning the patient about cool cleansing agents, marks on the skin, and needle sticks diminishes the anxiety level. The physician's conversation should be directed mostly toward the patient, thereby affirming their attention to the task at hand.

Skin Preparation

Adequate skin preparation involves the application of an antiseptic to remove transient and pathogenic microorganisms. This will also reduce any resident flora to a low level. Various agents are available, which include iodophors, hexachlorophene, chlorhexidine, and alcohols. Chlorhexidine (Hibiclens, Hibitane) and iodophors (Betadine) are commonly used and believed to be superior to most agents.[1,2] Alcohol is inexpensive and readily available. Application of isopropyl alcohol destroys 90% of the cutaneous bacteria in 2 minutes, but the typical rushed single wipe reduces approximately 75% of the cutaneous bacteria.[3]

Needle Insertion

The physician can minimize the discomfort associated with a needle insertion with a few simple techniques. Initially, selecting the appropriate size of the needle will reduce unnecessary pain on injection. Small-bore needles (23–30 gauge) should be used instead of large-bore needles (18–22 gauge) if and when possible. When available, the application of topical anesthetics will minimize the initial pain from an injection. As the needle enters the skin, the physician should distract the skin with two fingers. Once at the target site, the needle can be manipulated slightly to avoid injecting into a fixed space or directly against bone. When injecting, one should avoid rapid infusion of the medication into the target area but attempt slow, fractionated dosing.

TECHNIQUES

Soft Tissue Injections

Soft tissue injections that include procedures directed at trigger points, inflamed bursae or tendons, and painful joints typically should be performed in conjunction with a carefully planned exercise and stretching program. Therefore, these types of injections are usually delayed until other simpler measures have been tried, such as medications, local heat or ice, and therapy. When the decision to inject is made, one should be knowledgeable about the regional anatomy and proper indications. On advancement of the needle tip, care should be taken not to inject into the tendon, blood vessel, or nerve.

Nerve Block: Paresthesia versus Nonparesthesia

The two common approaches used to block nerves are the paresthesia technique (PT) and the nonparesthesia technique (NPT). The PT technique purposefully provokes paresthesias of the nerve before injection. The presence of paresthesias indicates that the needle tip is in contact with the nerve and serves as a warning of a pending nerve injury if the needle is allowed to advance any further. Use of PT requires that the patient is conscious and fully cooperative. It also requires that the patient's sensory pathways are intact. In comparison, NPT relies solely on anatomic landmarks. This technique avoids deliberate probing for paresthesias. Because the needle tip may not approximate the nerve like the PT, a greater volume of anesthetic is usually required to accomplish the same therapeutic affect. As expected, the PT is associated with a higher incidence of nerve injuries and should be avoided when possible.[4-6]

MEDICATIONS

Anesthetics

Local anesthetics have a wide range of clinical applications and are safe and effective when used judiciously (Table 1). This margin of safety and effectiveness often depends on the practitioner's knowledge of the properties of the anesthetics. A brief discussion of these concepts follows, although in-depth texts are available to the interested reader.

The mechanism of action of local anesthetics is not entirely understood but is believed to reversibly block nerve transmission by inhibiting ion flux through sodium channels of the axon. As a result, the action potential does not reach threshold, and nerve transmission ceases, resulting in anesthesia. The speed of onset, depth, and duration of this anesthesia are based on multiple factors, including characteristics of the nerve, anesthetic dosage, tissue site injected, and structure of the anesthetic molecule.

Characteristics of the Nerve

The effect of local anesthetics on nerve fibers often depends on physical characteristics of the nerve. For example, many believe that fibers within peripheral nerves are often blocked according to a nerve's diameter, degree of myelination, fascicular arrangement, and conduction velocity. Although it is controversial, this

Table 1. Comparison of Commonly Used Anesthetics

	Onset (Min)	Duration* (Min)	Equivalent Concentration	Toxicity**	Lipid Solubility	Protein Binding
Esters						
Procaine (Novacaine)	5	30–60	2	7	1	5
Chloroprocaine	6–12	30–60	2	8	1	2
Tetracaine (Pontocaine)	15	175	0.25	1	80	85
Amides						
Lidocaine (Xylocaine, Lignocaine)	0.5–1	100	1	5	4	65
Bupivacaine (Marcaine, Sensorcaine)	5	120–240	0.25	2	30	95
Mepivacaine (Carbocaine, Isocaine)	3–5	100	1	4	1	75
Etidocaine (Duranest)	5	120–240	0.25	3	140	95
Prilocaine (Citanest)	1–2	100	1	6	1.5	55

*Varies with route of administration.
**Approximate ranks among the anesthetics listed. From Lennard TA: Fundamentals of procedural care. In Lennard (ed): Physiatric Procedures in Clinical Practice, Hanley & Belfus, 1995, p. 5, with permission.

concept proposes that the smaller B and unmyelinated C fibers are blocked initially, followed by blockage of the small type A delta fibers. This would result in blockade of pain and temperature transmission initially and, later, of proprioception, touch, and motor function. Theoretically, this effect can be altered by the dosage, concentration, and type of anesthetic injected.

Tissue Site Injected

Once injected, anesthetics are transported within the body by simple mechanical bulk flow, diffusion, and vascular transport. The location of injection, especially in highly vascular areas, affects the drug's absorption, duration of action, and toxicity. Highly vascular regions of the body (oral mucosa, intercostal region, epidural space) should be injected with caution because small concentrations of anesthetics can result in rapid absorption, leading to elevated plasma concentrations and toxicity.

Anesthetic Structure

Anesthetics consists of two rings, a hydrophilic and lipophilic entity, that are linked by either an ester or amide bond. The hydrophilic entity facilitates transportation of the anesthetic in extracellular fluids. Once delivered to neural tissue, the lipophilic entity aids in transport into the neural structure by imparting lipid solubility to the molecule. If structural alterations are made to enhance lipid solubility, faster diffusion of the anesthetic molecule through the nerve cell membrane occurs that results in increased potency and duration of action. This duration of action can also be affected by changing a molecule's affinity for proteins. Generally, the higher the degree of binding to tissue and plasma proteins, the longer the duration of action. The ester amide linkage between the hydrophilic and lipophilic rings imparts unique characteristics to the anesthetic molecule. This linkage defines the two distinct classes of anesthetic agents, esters and amides.

Ester Anesthetics. Ester anesthetics are hydrolyzed rapidly by the plasma enzyme cholinesterase, resulting in short half-lives of the anesthetics, which subsequently reduce the risk of systemic toxicity. The metabolites, including paraaminobenzoic acid (PABA), are secreted mainly unchanged in the urine and have a small but possible allergic potential.

Amide Anesthetics. Amide anesthetics, by comparison, are hydrolyzed by liver microsomal enzymes to inactive products and excreted by the kidney. Up to 30% of these agents can be excreted unchanged in the urine. Toxicity from the amide group is more common in patients with diminished hepatic blood flow, for example, those with congestive heart failure or hepatic enzyme dysfunction or those taking beta blockers. The incidence of allergies to amides is very low, and, in general, amide anesthetics are believed to be safer than ester anesthetics.

Corticosteroids

Mechanism of Action

The primary mechanism of action of corticosteroids is at the cellular level (Table 2). These drugs appear to bind to intracellular receptors, alter gene expression, and ultimately regulate cellular processes.[7,8] Their anti-inflammatory effect results from several different factors including inhibition of phospholipase, alterations in lymphocytes, inhibition of cytokine expression, and stabilization of the cellular membrane.[9]

The conversion of phospholipids to arachidonic acid is critical to the formation of the inflammatory mediators such as LTB-4, LTC-4, LTD-4, LTE-4, and various prostaglandins. This initial step is facilitated by the enzymatic action of phospholipase A_2. Corticosteroids inhibit the action of phospholipase and thus prevent the formation of arachidonic acid and subsequently the inflammatory mediators.

Corticosteroids also alter the function of lymphocytes. These drugs appear to alter the chemotactic or chemoattractant mechanism found in the inflammatory response after tissue injury.[10] An apparent retention of white blood cells in the lym-

TABLE 2. COMPARISON OF COMMONLY USED GLUCOCORTICOID STEROIDS

Agent	Anti-inflammatory Potency*	Salt Retention Property	Plasma Half Life (Min)	Duration**	Equivalent Oral Dose (mg)
Hydrocortisone (Cortisol)	1	2+	90	S	20
Cortisone	0.8	2+	30	S	25
Prednisone	4–5	1+	60	I	5
Prednisolone	4–5	1+	200	I	5
Methylprednisolone (Medrol, Depo-Medrol)	5	0	180	I	4
Triamcinolone (Aristocort, Kenalog)	5	0	300	I	4
Betamethasone (Celestone)	25–30	0	100–300	L	0.6
Dexamethasone (Decadron)	25–30	0	100–300	L	0.75

*Relative to hydrocortisone.
**S = short, I = intermediate, L = long.
From Lennard TA: Fundamentals of procedural care. In Lennard TA (ed): Physiatric Procedures in Clinical Practice. Philadelphia, Hanley & Belfus, 1995, p. 6, with permission.

phatic system indirectly limits their ability to migrate to the damaged tissue.[10] Lymphocytic function and availability is diminished to the point at which a 70% reduction in circulating lymphocytes can be observed with a typical dose of the drug.[11] The effects of corticosteroids on lymphocytes differ between humans and laboratory animals such as rats and mice. Following a dose of corticosteroids, a transient elevation in the white blood cell count may be observed. In the absence of infection, this elevation may be attributed to the demargination of neutrocytes from the endothelium and an increased rate of cellular release from the bone marrow.[7,12]

Interleukin 1 (IL-1) and tumor necrosis factor (TNF) are integral components to the cell-mediated immune response to injury. The expression of these cytokines can be effectively inhibited by corticosteroids.[13] IL-1 originates from macrophages, monocytes, and various parenchymal cells and induces the production of endothelial based proteins. This results in thrombus formation and ultimately the activation of inflammatory and immune cells. IL-1 also affects procoagulant proteins, adhesive factors, and the metabolism of arachidonic acid within the endothelial cell. TNF stimulates the production of various chemotactic mechanisms from neutrophils and granulocytic proteins.

Corticosteroids also affect the permeability of the vascular wall. This membrane stabilization effect alters fluid shifts and decreases cellular and fluid movement from the vascular space. Lysosomal enzymes are also prevented from being released.[14–16] The end result is alteration of fluid retention at the site of tissue damage.

PERIPHERAL INJECTION TECHNIQUES

Peripheral joint and soft tissue injections are commonly used by physical medicine practitioners for both diagnostic and therapeutic benefit. These injections are often used to aid in the treatment of conditions associated with active localized inflammation. When these peripheral injections are used carefully, the risks to the patient can be less than nonsteroidal anti-inflammatory drug (NSAID) use. Peripheral injections include needle placement that is intra-articular, peritendinous or ligamentous, intrabursal, perineural, or intramuscular. Diagnostic information is usually obtained using short- and long-acting anesthetics, allowing the physician to compare preinjection and postinjection pain and functional status immediately after injection. Corticosteroid pain-relieving effects that may occur within 7–10 days following the injection may also provide diagnostic information. However, the corticosteroid effects are certainly beneficial for the pain relief and potential improvement in injury healing. Some of the conditions encountered in clinical practice that may be treated with peripheral injection include shoulder impingement and adhesive capsulitis syndromes, lateral epicondylitis, de Quervain's tenosynovitis, trigger finger tenosynovitis, greater trochanteric bursitis, myofascial pain syndromes, and articular disorders, including rheumatoid arthritis and osteoarthritis.

Peripheral injections that are performed strictly for diagnostic block information typically contain only local anesthetic solutions followed by immediate postinjection pain relief evaluation. A more dramatic and definitive pain response often occurs when a higher concentration of anesthetic is used, such as 2% lidocaine or 0.50–0.75% bupivacaine solutions. It is often helpful to use these higher concentration anesthetics in mixtures with corticosteroids so that the final anesthetic concentration is adequate to provide postinjection pain relief after dilution with the steroid solution. Following direct intravascular injection, the volumes typically used for intra-articular and peritendinous injection are small enough to make postinjection anesthetic toxic or side effects rare. Before peripheral corticosteroid injection, the patient should be informed of the possibility of skin depigmentation or localized fat atrophy as a cosmetic side effect, particularly from repeated corticosteroid injection at the same location, before proceeding with these procedures.[17]

INTRA-ARTICULAR INJECTIONS

For any peripheral intra-articular injection, strict aseptic technique should be followed to reduce the risk of postinjection intra-articular infection. For any intra-articular injection, fluoroscopic guidance and radiopaque contrast may be used to confirm intra-articular position of the needle tip and are most helpful for less accessible joints such as the shoulder and hip. Before intra-articular infiltration of corticosteroid, aspiration of any excess synovial fluid may be necessary for both pain relief and laboratory evaluation for diagnostic purposes. Any of the common corticosteroid preparation solutions can be used for intra-articular joint injection. The advantages to the use of triamcinolone hexacetonide is its higher potency at lower volumes of solution, which is helpful for smaller joint injections, and because this particular corticosteroid is the least water-soluble preparation, and it may provide the longest duration of effectiveness within the peripheral joint space.[18]

Contraindications of peripheral intra-articular injections must be heeded strictly because of the potentially devastating effect of intra-articular infection following injection. Obvious contraindications include pre-injection joint infection or infection of soft tissues overlying the joint. A patient with generalized infection should also be considered inappropriate for corticosteroid injection until after effective systemic antibiotic treatment. Patients who are actively taking anticoagulants may be susceptible to serious bleeding episodes, and either the anticoagulant should be discontinued for an adequate period of time before joint injection or the prothrombin time test should be completed before joint injection therapy.

Before any peripheral intra-articular injection, the skin should be prepared aseptically. Antiseptic solution should be spread widely around the entry site and allowed to dry. Local skin and subcutaneous tissue anesthesia may be obtained using 1% lidocaine and a 27-gauge skin needle. If joint aspiration is necessary before injection, the joint should be initially entered with a 20- or 18-gauge needle to allow aspiration of viscous joint fluids. If no joint aspiration is required, the joint may be entered using a 25- or 22-gauge needle. No significant resistance to intra-articular steroid infiltration should be felt, otherwise the needle tip should be repositioned until minimal resistance to the injection is appreciated.

Temporomandibular Joint

The temporomandibular joint (TMJ) is a common location of chronic joint discomfort. The $^5/_8$-inch-long 25-gauge needle is the most appropriate for TMJ injection. The needle should be placed just inferior to the zygomatic arch and just anterior to the tragus of the ear. Care must be taken during joint injection so as not to injure the relatively large cartilaginous articular disk within this joint. The superficial temporal artery passes superficial to the TMJ, and an attempt to palpate this vessel should be made before the injection and careful aspiration through the needle should be performed before injection of any anesthetic or corticosteroid solution.[19] TMJ anesthetic or steroid infiltration should be done only when no significant resistance to injection is identified and only small total volumes of injectate are used, with a total of approximately 1 ml recommended.

Glenohumeral Joint

The glenohumeral joint can be accessed from either an anterior, posterior, or superior approach. The anterior approach allows the needle to pass closest to substantial neurovascular structures. Fluroscopic guidance is very helpful to confirm intra-articular placement within the glenohumeral joint at the time of injection. The challenge of the glenohumeral joint injection stems from the relatively oblique, not truly anteroposterior, orientation of the glenohumeral joint. For the anterior approach, the inferolateral border of the coracoid process is palpated, and the needle is inserted approximately 1 cm below the inferior edge and 1–2 cm lateral to the most lateral aspect of the coracoid process. External rotation of the humerus can sometimes provide easier access into the anterior glenohumeral joint. Aspiration through the needle during advancement of the needle toward the glenohumeral joint can allow identification of intravascular needle placement during this injection approach. A posterior approach to the glenohumeral joint has the advantage of allowing the injectionist to perform the procedure without direct visualization by the patient, which can reduce patient apprehension. The posterior approach involves needle insertion 2–3 cm below the posterolateral angle of the acromion process, with the needle directed anteromedially directly toward the palpable coracoid process (Fig. 1). Angling the needle slightly upward if firm resistance

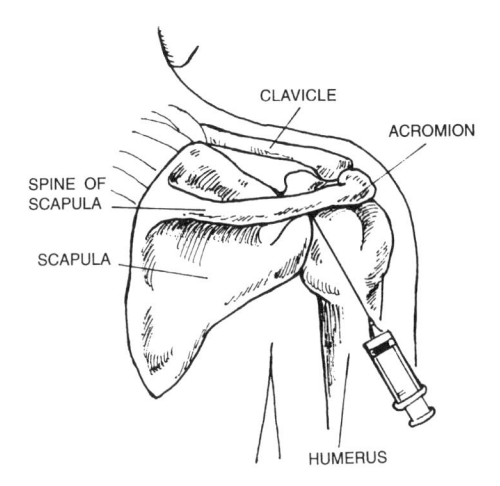

FIGURE 1. Anatomic landmarks and needle orientation for posterior glenohumeral joint injection. (From Obermiller JP, Lox DM: Peripheral joint injections. In Lennard TA (ed): Pain Procedures in Clinical Practice, 2nd ed. Philadelphia, Hanley & Belfus, 2000, pp 124–138, with permission.)

is noted at the shoulder joint may allow greater ease of injection placing the needle in the upper recess of the shoulder joint, away from the head of the humerus.

Acromioclavicular Joint

The acromioclavicular joint is usually injected using a 25-gauge needle with a $5/_8$-inch needle length usually the easiest to manipulate into the joint. This joint is often injected for diagnostic purposes, and for these procedures, only anesthetic solution is used. The joint is palpated, and the tip of the distal clavicle is located. The needle is inserted directly into the joint from either a superior or anterosuperior angle into the joint space, and adequate intra-articular infiltration often can be obtained with entry just within the joint capsule and without deeper needling of this very tight joint space (Fig. 2). Fluroscopy with the use of contrast is often helpful in determining whether actual intra-articular infiltration of either anesthetic or steroid has been accomplished.

Elbow Joints

Humeroulnar elbow joint injection can be safely performed from a posterolateral elbow approach. The posterolateral approach is performed by inserting the needle just lateral to the palpable triceps tendon and directing the needle tip into the joint space, which is palpable between the olecranon of the ulna and the trochlea of the humerus. Flexion of the elbow to about 50° during the injection can allow easier access into the posterior aspect of this joint. The needle tip should not be directed any further laterally than the posterior aspect of the lateral epicondyle. The humeroradial joint is formed by the capitulum and the head of the radius and can be a source of traumatic or osteoarthritic pain. This joint is palpable just distal to the lateral epicondyle. The needle should be directed into the joint with a

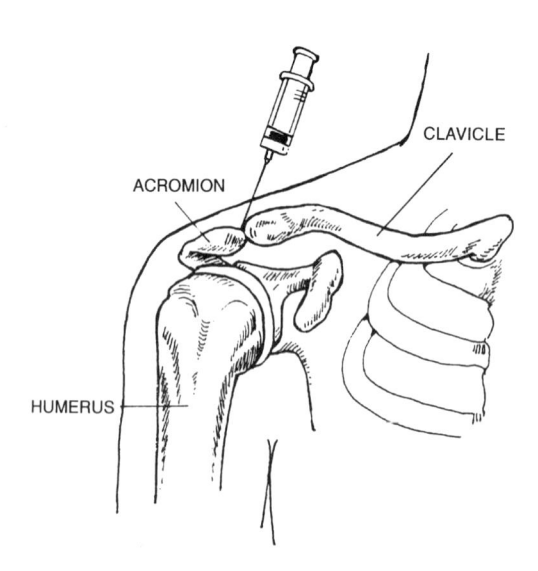

FIGURE 2. Superior approach to the acromioclavicular joint. (From Obermiller JP, Lox DM: Peripheral joint injections. In Lennard TA (ed): Pain Procedures in Clinical Practice, 2nd ed. Philadelphia, Hanley & Belfus, 2000, pp 124–138, with permission.)

straight lateral or slightly posterolateral approach direction, and injection should be performed only when no significant resistance to infiltration is palpable.

Wrist Joints

Several specific articulation sites can be injected at the wrist depending on the location of the patient's pain with the safest approaches at the dorsal aspect of the wrist, which avoids both the radial and ulnar arteries. Entry into the wrist joints from a dorsal approach may be facilitated by having the patient place the wrist in a slightly flexed position, and the wrist should be firmly stabilized during the injection. The radial dorsal wrist can be entered by inserting the needle through the interval between the distal radius and the scaphoid and lunate bones with the point of entry just radial to the palpable extensor digitorum communis tendon to the index finger along the ulnar edge of the palpable depression at this site. The dorsal ulnar aspect of the wrist can be injected through the interval between the distal ulna and the triquetrum and lunate bones (Fig. 3). The needle at this site is inserted between the extensor digitorum communis tendon of the ring finger and the extensor digiti minimi tendon at the ulnar aspect of this interval. The radial carpal area and the first carpometacarpal joints can be injected from the radial or lateral aspect of the wrist within the boundaries of the anatomic snuff box for pain apparently originating from this region of the wrist. The proximal border of the snuff box is formed by

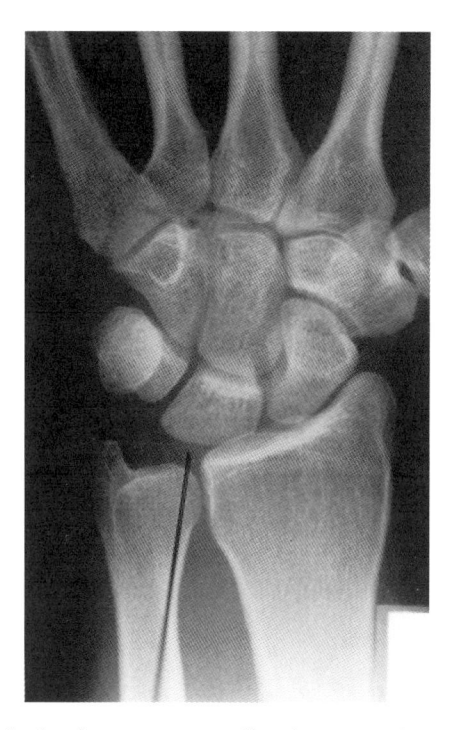

FIGURE 3. AP radiograph showing proper needle placement for wrist joint injection from dorsal ulnar approach. (From Obermiller JP, Lox DM: Peripheral joint injections. In Lennard TA (ed): Pain Procedures in Clinical Practice, 2nd ed. Philadelphia, Hanley & Belfus, 2000, pp 124–138, with permission.)

the radial styloid process, and the box extends distally to the thumb at the carpal base. To inject the radiocarpal joint through the snuff box, the needle should be inserted at the level of the joint just distal to the radius between the posterior dorsal extensor pollicis longus tendon and the anterior or volar border of the extensor pollicis brevis and abductor pollicis longus tendons. Care should be taken to avoid needling or intravascular injection into the radial artery that traverses the snuff box in this area; this can be avoided most easily by inserting the needle immediately proximal to the distal end of the radius.[20] The first carpometacarpal (CMC) joint is the articulation between the trapezium and the first metacarpal bone, and is located at the distal border of the anatomic snuff box. Needle insertion should be located just proximal to the palpable proximal end of the first metacarpal bone within the confines of the snuff box, avoiding proximal needle advancement toward the most common anatomic location of the radial artery.

Hand Interphalangeal Joints

The proximal and distal interphalangeal joints are affected mostly by arthritic processes and may benefit from intra-articular corticosteroid treatment. Smaller needles are required to enter these joints with use of a 25- or 27-gauge needle connected to a 2-ml or tuberculin syringe used to allow more precise control of the needle. These joints will accommodate only small amounts of injectate, usually less than 1–2 ml to avoid overdistention of the joint. Both the proximal and distal interphalangeal joints are best approached from the radial aspect with needle insertion at the level of the palpable interphalangeal joint line with needle placement in the superior half of the digit above the neurovascular bundle and lateral to the extensor mechanism (Fig. 4).

Hip Joint

Fluoroscopic guidance with the use of radiopaque contrast is necessary in the hip joint to confirm intra-articular needle placement. The joint may be accessed from

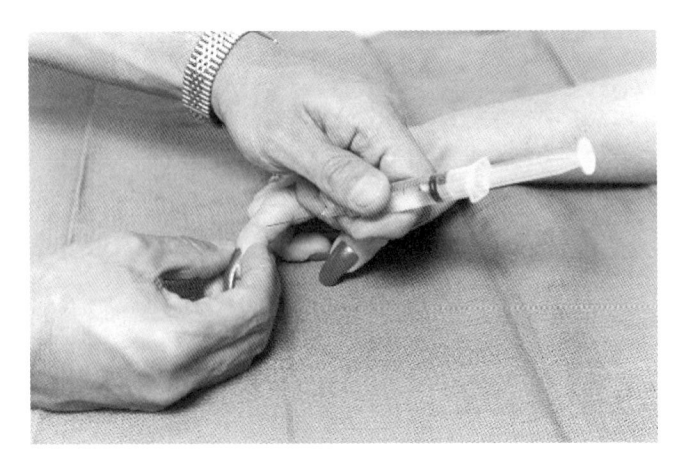

FIGURE 4. Needle placement into the interphalangeal joint. (From Obermiller JP, Lox DM: Peripheral joint injections. In Lennard TA (ed): Pain Procedures in Clinical Practice, 2nd ed. Philadelphia, Hanley & Belfus, 2000, pp 124–138, with permission.)

either an anterior or a lateral approach. The anterior approach places the needle in closer proximity to significant neurovascular structures. For the anterior approach, the patient is placed in the supine position, and the ipsilateral lower extremity is rotated externally. The needle is inserted at a point 2 cm directly inferior from the anterior superior iliac spine and 3 cm or about 3 fingerbreadths lateral to the palpated femoral artery pulse at a level in line with the superior margins of the greater trochanters. The needle is directed posteromedially at an angle of about 60° from the frontal plane aimed in the direction of the umbilicus, with needle advancement down to and through the tough hip capsular ligaments. From the lateral approach, the needle is inserted at the lateral hip just anterior or posterior to the greater trochanter and advanced in a medial and slightly cephalad direction. The needle passes through the iliotibial band and usually through the gluteus medius muscle before entering the thick iliofemoral ligament just superficial to the hip joint capsule.

Knee Joint

The knee joint is the most commonly aspirated and injected joint in the body. The knee joint is most easily accessed from either a medial or lateral approach with insertion of the needle between the patella and femur about midway between the superior and inferior pole of the patella. Mild manual pressure on the patella to push the patella toward the side of needle insertion can help open the joint space at the insertion site. The anterior approach into the knee joint is possible with insertion of the needle just inferior to the inferior patellar pole on either the lateral or medial side of the patellar tendon with the needle advanced parallel to the tibial plateau until the joint space is entered. The risk of injuring the articular cartilage or the infrapatellar fat pad is higher for this particular approach and is not recommended unless anatomic considerations preclude the use of needle insertion at the level of the midpatella, as described above.

PERINEURAL INJECTIONS

Perineural injections in the upper and lower extremity obviously pose the highest risk for potential direct nerve injury of all peripheral injection procedures. Thorough knowledge of the local anatomy including all major neurovascular structures is essential in performing any of these injections as safely as possible. Another important tool for many of these injections involves the use of a Teflon-coated needle, allowing localized electrical stimulation from the bare needle tip to help determine the exact location of the target nerve tissue. For safety considerations, it is also very important to inject only when there is no significant resistance to infiltration, or intraneural injection can occur, which has a greater risk of significant local nerve damage than does contacting the nerve with the tip of a small-gauge needle.[21] Needle advancement should be performed slowly and carefully particularly if electrical stimulation is not available, and typically patients will be able to report nerve-related paresthesias and pain just before damaging direct contact with nerve tissue occurs.

Radial Nerve Block at Humerus

The needle insertion point is located between the middle and distal third of the humerus on a line between the lateral epicondyle and posterolateral tip of the acromion process. The insertion site lies between the muscle bellies of the biceps brachii and the triceps and is typically located about 15 cm proximal to the tip of the olecranon. A 25-gauge needle can be used for the injection and advanced at this site until bone is contacted or, if using a nerve stimulator, until elbow flexion and wrist extension is elicited at a low level of electrical stimulation current. About 4–7 ml of anesthetic solution may be injected for neural blockade. Anesthetic injection at this site will usually affect all radial innervated muscles in the upper extremity except for the elbow extensors.

Ulnar Nerve at Elbow

The ulnar nerve can be blocked just above the elbow level as it courses medially between the triceps and brachialis muscle. For ulnar nerve blockade, a 25-gauge needle can be inserted at the interval between these two muscles approximately 5 cm directly superior to the medial epicondyle.[22] For some individuals, the ulnar nerve may be palpable at this level, allowing more detailed localization for the injection (Fig. 5). If the nerve is not palpable, the injectate can be placed just beneath the subcutaneous fat in a fan-like manner across the anatomic path of the nerve at this level. When a nerve stimulator is used, the needle tip will be adjacent to the nerve when wrist flexion and intrinsic hand muscles are activated, and then 5–8 ml of anesthetic solution can be injected after nerve localization is complete. The ulnar nerve may also be blocked within the ulnar groove closer to the elbow joint. The ulnar nerve can usually be carefully palpated at the level of the medial

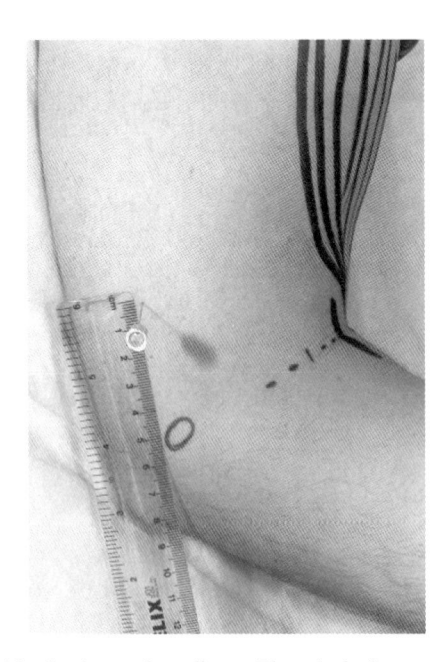

FIGURE 5. Ulnar nerve block above the elbow. The circle is over the medial epicondyle. (From Mauldin CC, Brooks DW: Arm, forearm, and hand blocks. In Lennard TA (ed): Pain Procedures in Clinical Practice, 2nd ed. Philadelphia, Hanley & Belfus, 2000, pp 96–107, with permission.)

epicondyle and with gentle manual pressure the ulnar nerve can be gently pushed toward the olecranon and a 25-gauge needle inserted carefully between the palpable nerve and the medial epicondyle. After the ulnar nerve is confined within the groove at this location, the total injection solution should be limited to less than 5 ml for nerve protection. Injection at this specific location should be used only for suspected compressive neuropathies at the ulnar groove and cubital tunnel.

Median Nerve at the Wrist

At the level of the carpal tunnel, the median nerve is enclosed within the ulnar bursa and surrounded by the forearm flexor tendons. The median nerve travels just beneath and between the flexor carpi radialis and palmaris longus tendons. The preferred injection site for the median nerve at the wrist is into the ulnar bursa just proximal to the carpal tunnel.[23] Several different injection techniques have been proposed for access to the median nerve at the wrist.[20] A $^5/_8$-inch-long needle is most easily controlled for this injection, and either the 25- or 27-gauge needle size is appropriate. Typically, the injection is performed just proximal to the distal wrist crease, with the needle angled at 30° from the proximal forearm and directed distally (Fig. 6). If no neuropathic symptoms are reported, a volume of 2 ml can be injected slowly. Active finger flexion and extension for 1–2 minutes by the patient after infiltration of steroid can help distribute the solution throughout the ulnar bursa. Following the injection, a gradual onset of numbness in a median nerve distribution is common with this procedure and typically is not associated with any significant pain and helps

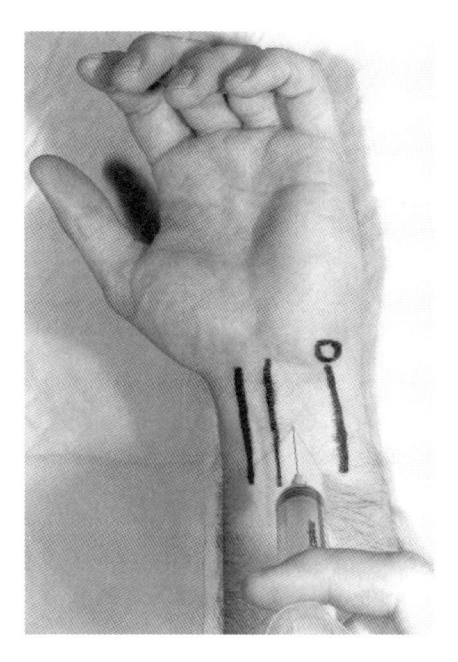

FIGURE 6. Ulnar bursal injection into carpal tunnel. Needle entry is just ulnar to the palmaris longus tendon. (From Mauldin CC, Brooks DW: Arm, forearm, and hand blocks. In Lennard TA (ed): Pain Procedures in Clinical Practice, 2nd ed. Philadelphia, Hanley & Belfus, 2000, pp 96–107, with permission.)

to confirm proper localization of the injection adjacent to the median nerve. Superficial hematomas can occur with this infection despite the best efforts of the physician to avoid subcutaneous veins. These typically are of no clinical concern, but patient reassurance is often extremely helpful after these events.

Lateral Femoral Cutaneous Nerve

The lateral femoral cutaneous nerve provides sensation to the anterior, lateral, and possibly, posterior aspect of the thigh and has a purely sensory nerve contribution from the L2 and L3 nerve roots. A lateral femoral cutaneous nerve block can be performed in suspected cases of neuropathic pain such as cases of nerve entrapment with meralgia paresthetica. The injection is performed with the patient in the supine position and the anterior pelvis exposed. The needle is placed perpendicular to the skin approximately 1 inch medial to the anterosuperior iliac spine and just inferior to the inguinal ligament and the needle is advanced into the soft tissue to a depth of about 2–3 cm. The exact depth of the nerve, however, may vary significantly depending on the patient's size. Once needle placement is believed to be satisfactory, 5–10 ml of injectate can be slowly injected after aspiration and, in some cases, paresthesias may be elicited soon after injection verifying correct needle placement.

Sciatic Nerve

The sciatic nerve is composed of the common peroneal and tibial nerves and receives nerve fibers from the L4–S3 nerve roots. The sciatic nerve exits the pelvis through the greater sciatic notch usually just inferior to the piriformis muscle and runs inferiorly through the posterior thigh. Sciatic nerve blocks can be used to assist casting of spastic ankle or knee flexion contractures and for diagnosis and treatment of suspected sciatic neuropathy such as following local trauma. The posterior approach to the sciatic nerve is most common. The sciatic nerve location can be identified by extending a line between the upper aspect of the greater trochanter over to the posterior superior iliac spine with the injection site 3-cm below the midpoint of this line (Fig. 7). An alternative method involves marking a line between the greater trochanter of the femur and a point about 2 cm below the sacral hiatus, with the midpoint of this line corresponding to the location of the sciatic nerve, which should correspond to approximately the same spot as determined by the first localization technique described earlier. A long needle up to 15 cm is typically required to reach the sciatic nerve, and when using a nerve stimulator, the needle should be slowly advanced until knee flexion contraction is noted.

Tibial Nerve at Knee

The tibial nerve block at the popliteal space can be used along or in conjunction with the common peroneal nerve block at the same location as described next for the treatment of complex regional pain syndromes involving the ankle and foot region. The patient is placed in the prone position, and the borders of the popliteal fossa are identified within a triangle having a base along the posterior knee crease and the semimembranosus muscle and biceps femoris muscle forming the medial and lateral borders of the triangle, respectively. A perpendicular line is

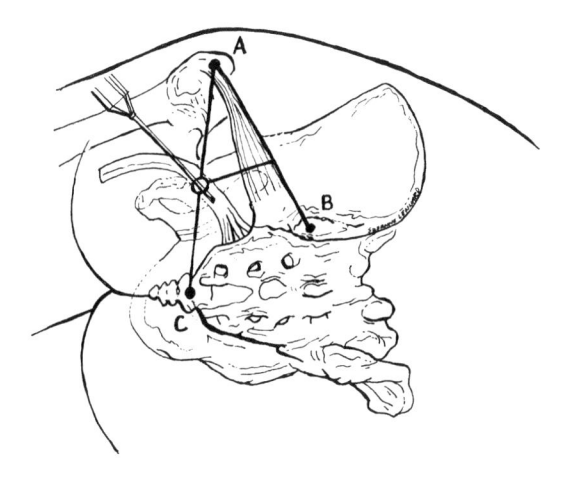

FIGURE 7. Landmarks for a sciatic nerve block. *A*, Greater trochanter of the femur; *B*, posterior superior iliac spine (PSIS); *C*, a point 2 cm below the sacral hiatus. (From Lennard TA, Shin DY: Proximal lower extremity blocks. In Lennard TA (ed): Pain Procedures in Clinical Practice, 2nd ed. Philadelphia, Hanley & Belfus, 2000, pp 108–116, with permission.)

extended from the midpoint of the base of the triangle up to the apex and the needle is inserted 6 cm proximal to the baseline and 1 cm lateral of the midline (Fig. 8). The needle is advanced to a depth of approximately 3 cm, or a needle stimulator can be used to provoke a plantar flexion muscle contraction (Fig. 9). Aspiration of the needle should be performed throughout needle advancement for identification of intravascular needle insertion into the large popliteal vessels as soon as possible. Relatively large volumes of anesthetic and corticosteroid solution can be injected at this location, although 10–12 ml should be adequate for treatment of pain conditions in most cases.

Common Peroneal Nerve

The common peroneal nerve can be blocked either at the popliteal space or adjacent to the fibular head. Needle insertion into the popliteal space would be most appropriate for all common peroneal nerve block conditions other than suspected compression neuropathy at the fibular head. In the popliteal fossa, the common peroneal nerve lies adjacent to the biceps femoris muscle and is located about 2–3 cm lateral to the tibial nerve. The needle can be inserted 5–6 cm superior to the posterior knee crease and just medial to the biceps femoris muscle. The needle should be advanced to a depth approximately midway between the skin and the underlying femur.

The common peroneal nerve can also be blocked as it travels adjacent to the fibular head. After identification of the fibular head, the common peroneal nerve can be localized as it crosses the lateral leg over the fibula 2–3 cm inferior to the fibular head. Using a nerve stimulator, contraction of the anterior and lateral leg compartment muscles should be observed at low current settings before injection. Usually less than 5 ml of injectate volume is recommended at this location to prevent postinjection pressure neuropathy.

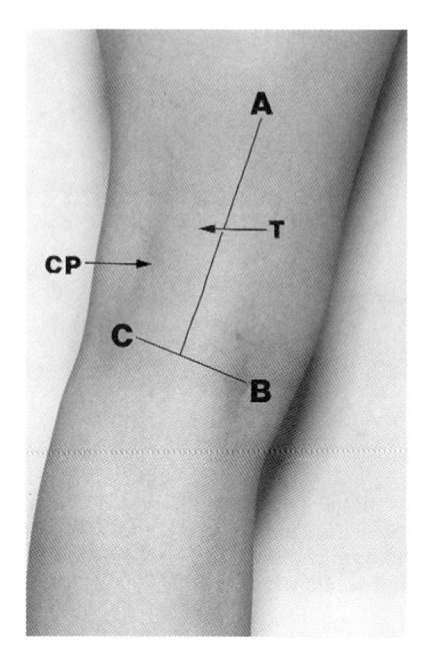

FIGURE 8. The borders of the popliteal fossa are outlined (ABC), as well as the surface location of the tibial nerve (T) and the common peroneal nerve (CP). (From Matthews D: Leg, foot, and ankle blocks. In Lennard TA (ed): Pain Procedures in Clinical Practice, 2nd ed. Philadelphia, Hanley & Belfus, 2000, pp 117–123, with permission.)

Posterior Tibial Nerve at Ankle

The evaluation of pain potentially originating from the posterior tibial nerve as it traverses the tarsal tunnel at the medial ankle can be helpful in the diagnosis and treatment of tarsal tunnel syndrome. A relatively easy approach to the posterior tibial nerve at this location first involves identification of the medial malleolus with the patient supine and the foot externally rotated. A needle is then inserted at the midpoint of a transverse line connecting the upper portion of the medial malleolus over to the medial edge of the Achilles tendon (Fig. 10). The needle is directed anterolaterally until the posterior surface of the tibia is contacted, and then the needle tip is withdrawn about 2 mm before starting infiltration of the injectate solution.

PERITENDINOUS AND BURSAL INJECTIONS

Corticosteroid injections adjacent to tendon sheaths and at tendon insertion sites, as well as bursal injections, are relatively common procedures used in the nonsurgical treatment of musculoskeletal pain conditions. Reports in the literature of potential tendon ruptures as a direct complication of repeated steroid injections seem to be associated with either multiple repeat injections at the same anatomic site or direct infiltration of steroid into the tendon substance, which is contraindicated.[24,25] The potential for postinjection tendon rupture is greatest in lower extremity weight-bearing regions, including the patellar and Achilles tendons, and many practitioners actually avoid the patellar tendon region for steroid injection

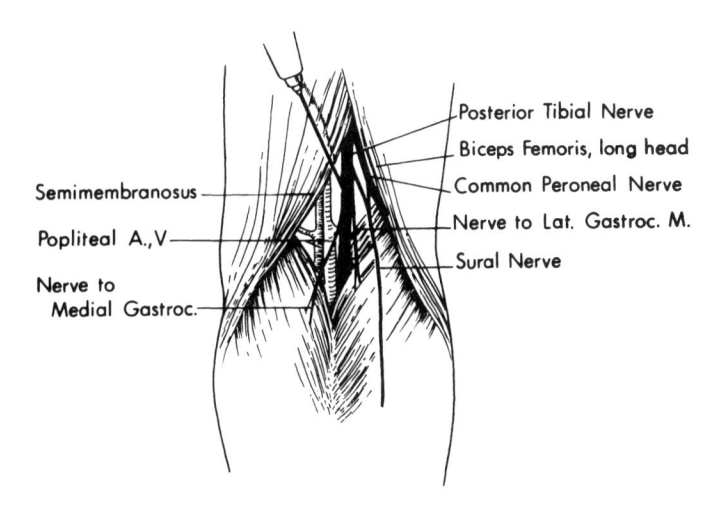

FIGURE 9. Needle is in position within the popliteal fossa to block the posterior tibial nerve. (From Matthews D: Leg, foot, and ankle blocks. In Lennard TA (ed): Pain Procedures in Clinical Practice, 2nd ed. Philadelphia, Hanley & Belfus, 2000, pp 117–123, with permission.)

for fear of possible rupture. It is a reasonable practice to restrict aggressive or vigorous weight-bearing activity for at least 48 hours after lower extremity peritendinous injection.

Subcromial Bursa and Rotator Cuff Tendons

The injection approach and procedure for subacromial bursitis is the same for suspected rotator cuff tendinitis because these two conditions often occur concurrently. A 25-gauge, 2-inch length needle is typically the most practical needle selection for this injection and may be inserted just inferior to the acromion process with an inferior, lateral, or posterior approach. Typically, the posterolateral approach provides easiest access and is most effective. The patient should place the arm in a dependent position, with the shoulder joint in the neutral position. The posterolateral angle of the acromion can be easily identified by palpation and the needle inserted just inferior to the acromion and advanced in an anteromedial direction at this location. Palpation of the skin and soft tissue surrounding the needle should be done during infiltration, and if any ballottement of these tissues is occurring, the needle tip location is too superficial and should be carefully advanced more deeply before reinjection. If the needle tip is safely within the subacromial space, then there should be absolutely no resistance to the injection. The total volume of approximately 4–6 ml is usually adequate for both diagnostic and therapeutic injections. This particular injection is often performed as strictly a diagnostic injection with only lidocaine or bupivacaine anesthetic in an attempt to confirm the subacromial space as the pain generator in patients with shoulder pain problems. Following anesthetic injection, a re-examination of the shoulder joint can be performed, and if the pain is originating from the subacromial tissues, then resisted rotator cuff activation and the shoulder impingement test typically become nonpainful.

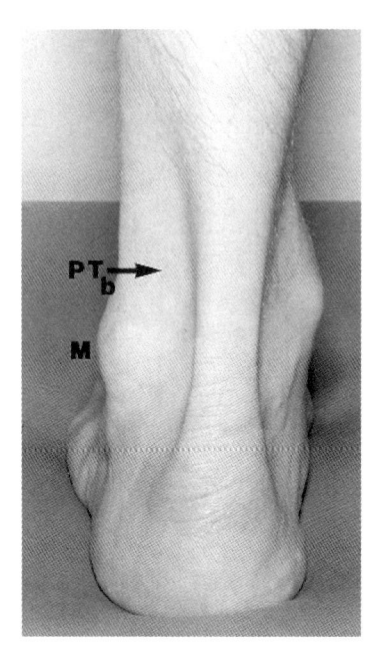

FIGURE 10. Posterior view of ankle indicating medial malleolus (M) and the block site region for the posterior tibial nerve (PTb) at the ankle. (From Matthews D: Leg, foot, and ankle blocks. In Lennard TA (ed): Pain Procedures in Clinical Practice, 2nd ed. Philadelphia, Hanley & Belfus, 2000, pp 117–123, with permission.)

Biceps Brachii Tendon

The presence of biceps brachii tendinitis is indicated by localized pain in the anterior glenohumeral region at the location of the proximal biceps long head tendon, which is often palpable at this location and is usually noted to have increased pain on firm resisted elbow flexion and forearm supination. Biceps tendon sheath injection can be performed with either a 25- or 27-gauge needle, with insertion just superficial to the palpable biceps tendon within the bicipital groove at the level of the greater tuberosity with the needle angled superiorly to reduce risk of direct tendon needling. The needle is then advanced slowly until reaching the region of the tendon sheath, and a mixture of anesthetic and corticosteroid solution injected to a total volume of about 2–4 ml (Fig. 11). The biceps tendon is often most easily palpable and accessible for injection with the glenohumeral joint placed in external rotation position.

Lateral Epicondyle

Lateral epicondylitis (tennis elbow tendinitis) is a common diagnosis encountered in the practice of occupational and sports medicine. Care should be taken so that accurate diagnosis is confirmed and that significant bony injury at the elbow is excluded before lateral epicondyle steroid injection. Typically, the site of maximum pain with this condition is at and just distal to the lateral epicondyle.[26] A 1- or 1^1/$_2$-inch, 25- or 27-gauge needle can be used for this injection. The needle

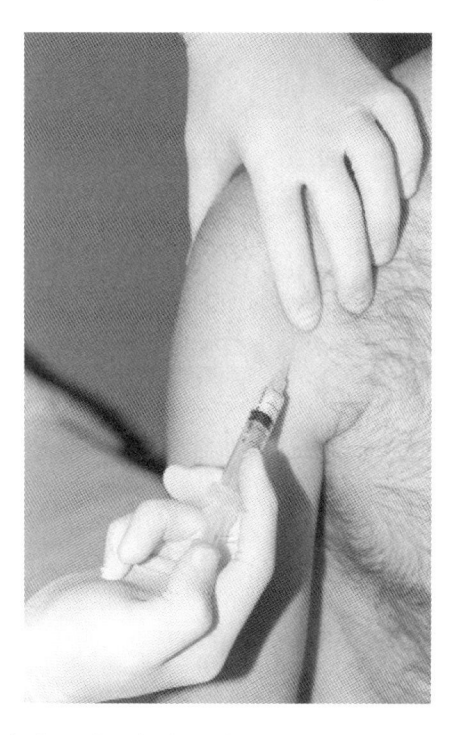

FIGURE 11. Injection technique for the long head biceps brachii tendon. (From Geiringer SR: Tendon sheath and insertion injections. In Lennard TA (ed): Pain Procedures in Clinical Practice, 2nd ed. Philadelphia, Hanley & Belfus, 2000, pp 147–152, with permission.)

is inserted 1–2 cm distal to the lateral epicondyle and angled superiorly, with infiltration of anesthetic and steroid solution along the tendon sheath during advancement of the needle tip superiorly to the lateral epicondyle. At least some tenting of the skin often results from this injection, particularly in slender individuals, and a total of 1.5–2 ml of solution is usually adequate. The lateral elbow area is a region more susceptible to visible skin depigmentation and fat atrophy, particularly after repeat injections, and care should be taken to avoid these potential complications.

Olecranon Bursa

After diagnosis of olecranon bursitis, any substantial bursal effusion should be aspirated following aseptic skin preparation and is most successfully performed using an 18-gauge needle. The needle may be started perpendicular to the skin at the posterior elbow in the region of maximum swelling with or without local skin anesthetic. Following aspiration or for milder cases of olecranon bursitis, intrabursal injection of corticosteroid solution can be performed with a maximum volume of injectate of 1–2 ml. Localized cellulitis infections at the posterior elbow are possible with olecranon bursitis conditions, particularly following aspiration or injection procedures, and should be excluded or treated appropriately prior to any initial or repeat injection at this location.

de Quervain's Tenosynovitis

de Quervain's tenosynovitis involves the abductor pollicis longus or the extensor pollicis brevis tendons at the radial wrist with focal tenderness in this region reported by the patient usually with pinch or key gripping maneuvers.[27] This injection may be performed with a 25- or 27-gauge $^1/_2$- or 1-inch needle inserted just proximal to the most painful portion of the tendons on palpation and the needle directed subcutaneously parallel with the course of the tendons until the needle is just superficial to the tendon sheath. Care should be taken to avoid penetration of these relatively superficial tendons with the needle tip. The needle should not be advanced beyond the distal radius to prevent advancing the needle into the anatomic snuff box in the region of the radial artery. One to two milliliters of total injectate volume is adequate for treatment.

Trigger Finger

Stenosing flexor tenosynovitis, or trigger finger, is more likely to have lasting response to corticosteroid injection than most other soft tissue conditions and can be curative. The most common site of tendon stenosis and triggering is the A-1 pulley with palpable tendon swelling and tenderness at the volar aspect of the metacarpal head of the involved digit. Severe stenosis is identified with visible and palpable triggering of the flexor tendon at this location. A 27-gauge, 1- to $1^1/_2$-inch needle can be used with a tuberculin syringe for best control during the procedure. The needle is inserted just proximal to the palpable tendon nodule and advanced through the skin until the syringe plunger can be depressed with no resistance to injection. When the appropriate needle position has been achieved, the needle tip should not move with passive flexion and extension of the finger. A total of 0.5 ml is usually adequate for treatment. Initial injection of local skin anesthetic is not recommended for this procedure, and the patient's hand should be firmly stabilized before needle insertion.

Greater Trochanter Bursa

Greater trochanteric bursitis is usually diagnosed with the patient having exquisite tenderness to gentle pressure and palpation directly at or just distal to the greater trochanter. For injection, the patient is placed in a side-lying position on the asymptomatic side. A 25-gauge, $2-3^1/_2$ inch needle is inserted directly over the greater trochanter perpendicular to the skin and advanced down to the bone. After withdrawing the needle 1–2 mm, a total volume of injectate of 6–8 ml can be infiltrated, usually with little resistance to injection.

Pes Anserine Bursa

The pes anserine bursa is located in the proximal medial tibia and surrounds the tendons of the gracilis, sartorius, and semitendinosus muscles. Directly beneath this bursa is the medial collateral ligament of the knee. Owing to the lack of any significant overlying soft tissue structures, this injection is relatively superficial and can be performed with a 1-inch needle. The site of maximal pes anserine bursa tenderness is palpated, and the needle is inserted perpendicular to the skin at this location and, after appropriate subcutaneous needle position, a total of 2–3 ml injected.

Intramuscular Injection

Myofascial trigger points are localized tender areas within various soft tissues but most commonly within muscle tissue. These tender points usually radiate pain into distant areas known as a *reference pain zone*. Myofascial trigger points may also involve the fascia and may be associated with a palpable taut fibrous band at the trigger point location. Dry needling of trigger points without infiltration of any anesthetic or corticosteroid solution has been shown to provide significant pain relief in some instances.[28] Trigger point injections are thought potentially to disrupt mechanically abnormal painful tissue in the fascia and muscle, resulting in significant pain relief. Use of local anesthetics, usually 1% lidocaine or 0.5% bupivacaine, can provide temporary diagnostic pain relief with long-term pain relief possibly resulting from repeated needling into the abnormal tissue. The most effective treatment of a myofascial trigger point occurs when a 22- or 25-gauge needle is inserted specifically into the most tender portion of the trigger point, with repetitive insertion and redirection of the needle within the entire abnormal painful area with as few skin penetrations as possible to treat the entire painful region.[28] The needling and infiltration should be extended over the entire length of the taut band. With each needle insertion into the muscle, a small amount of local anesthetic can be infiltrated to assist with immediate pain relief. Corticosteroids are not necessary for myofascial trigger point treatment, and repeated steroid injection may induce local myopathy. If corticosteroid is not used in a particular anatomic region, then there will be no concern if repeat trigger point injections are required in regard to any potential long-term steroid complications. Often, a more firm texture with increased resistance to needle advancement is palpable when the needle is penetrating the trigger point and taut fibrous band tissue, and needle advancement should be stopped when the needle tip is felt to have progressed completely through the firm trigger point tissue. Following myofascial trigger point injections, the patient should always be instructed in a thorough myofascial stretching and strengthening program with the trigger point injections acting as an adjunctive therapy for these conditions.

REFERENCES

1. Humar A, Ostromecki A, Direnfeld J, et al: Prospective randomized trial of 10% povidone-iodine versus 0.5% tincture of chlorhexidine as cutaneous antisepsis for prevention of central venous catheter infection. Clin Infect Dis 2000, Oct 31(4):1001–1007.
2. Mimoz O, Karim A, Mercata, et al: Chlorhexidine compared with povidone-iodine as skin preparation before blood culture. A randomized controlled trial. Ann Intern Med 131:834–837, 1999.
3. Sebben JE: Surgical antiseptics. J Am Acad Dermatol 9:759–765, 1983.
4. Plevak DJ, Linstromber JW, Danielson DR: Paresthesia vs nonparesthesia: The axillary block. ASA Abstracts, Anesthesiology 59, 1983.
5. Selander D: Paresthesias or no paresthesias? Nerve complications after neural blockades. Acta Anesthesiol Scand 23:173–174, 1988.
6. Selander D, Edshage S, Wolff T: Parethesiae or no parethesiae? Acta Anaesthesiol Scand 23:27–33, 1979.
7. Fauci AS, Dale DC, Balow JE: Glucocorticosteroid therapy: Mechanism of action and clinical considerations. Ann Intern Med 84:304–315, 1976.
8. Gallin JL, Goldstein IM, Snyderman R: Overview. In Gallein JI, Goldstein IM, Snyderman R (eds): Inflammation: Basic Principles in Clinical Correlates. New York, Raven, 1992, pp 1–4.

9. Fantone J: Basic concepts of inflammation. In Leadbetter WB, Buckwalter JA, Gordon SL (ed): Sports Induced Inflammation. Parkridge, IL, American Academy of Orthopedic Surgeons, 1990, pp 25–53.
10. Fauci AS, Dale DC: The effect of in vivo hycrocortisone on subpopulations of human lymphocytes. J Clin Invest 53:240–246, 1974.
11. Peters WP, Holland JF, Senn H, et al: Corticosteroid administration and localized leukocyte mobilization in man. N Engl J Med 286:342–345, 1972.
12. Goldfien A: Adrenocorticosteroids and adrenocortical antagonists. In Katzung BG (ed): Basic and Clinical Pharmacology, 2nd ed. Los Altos, CA, Lange Medical Publishers, 1984, pp 453–465.
13. Behrens TW, Goodwins JS: Oral corticosteroids. In Leadbetter WB, Buckwalter JA, Gordon SL (eds): Sports Induced Inflammation. Brockridge, IL, American Academy of Orthopedic Surgeons, 1990, pp 405–419.
14. Boumpas DT, Paliogianni F, Anastassiou ED, et al: Glucocorticosteroid action on the immune system: Molecular and cellular aspects. Clin Exp Rheumatol 9:413–423, 1991.
15. Crabtree GR, Gillis S, Smith KA, Munck A: Glucocorticoids and immune responses. Arthritis Rheum 22:1246–1256, 1979.
16. Lennard TA: Fundamentals of procedural care. In Lennard TA (ed): Physiatric Procedures in Clinical Practice. Philadelphia, Hanley & Belfus, Inc., 1995, pp 1–13.
17. Miceo WF, Rodreques RA, Amy E: Joint and soft tissue injections of the upper extremity. Physical Med and Rehabil Clin 6:823–840, 1995.
18. Bain LS, Balch HW, Weatherly JM, et al: Intra-articular triamcinolone hexacetonide: Double-blind comparison with methylprednisolone. Br J Clin Pract 26:559–561, 1972.
19. Woodward JL, Lennard TA: Anatomic principles for peripheral joint injections. Phys Med Rehabil State Art Rev 10:473–487, 1996.
20. Bridenbaugh LD: The upper extremity: Somatic blockade. In Cousins MJ, Bridenbaugh TO (eds): Neuro Blockade in Clinical Anesthesia and Management of Pain, 2nd ed. Philadelphia, J.B. Lippincott, 1988, pp. 387–417.
21. Lennard TA: Basic principles of neural blockade. In Lennard TA (ed): Pain Procedures in Clinical Practice, 2nd ed. Philadelphia, Hanley & Belfus, 2000, pp 33–39.
22. Mauldin CC, Brooks DW: Arm, forearm, and hand blocks. In Lennard TA (ed): Pain Procedures in Clinical Practice, 2nd ed. Philadelphia, Hanley & Belfus, 2000, pp 96–107.
23. Green DP: Diagnostic and therapeutic value of carpal tunnel injection. J Hand Surg 9A:850–854, 1984.
24. Tonkin MA, Stern SH: Spontaneous rupture of the flexor carpi radialis tendon. J Hand Surg 16B:72–74, 1991.
25. Halpern AA, Horowitz BG, Nagel DA: Tendon ruptures associated with corticosteroid therapy. West J Med 127:378–432, 1993.
26. Price R, Heinrich SI, Gibson T: Local injection treatment of tennis elbow. Hydrocortisone, triamcinolone and lignocaine compared. Br J Rheumatol 30:39–44, 1991.
27. Harvey FJ, Harvey PM, Horsley MW: De Quervain's disease: Surgical and nonsurgical treatment. J Hand Surg 15A:82–87, 1990.
28. Fisher A: Trigger point injection. In Lennard TA (ed): Pain Procedures in Clinical Practice, 2nd ed. Philadelphia, Hanley & Belfus, 2000, pp 153–161.

Chapter 18

Promoting Functional Independence through the Use of Assistive Devices and Durable Medical Equipment

Sarah Eggen-Thornhill, OTR, and Jennifer Fouché, OTR

This chapter reviews the tools commonly referred to as *assistive devices*. The purpose of these tools is to compensate for lost function and to make the job of living easier. This chapter is an introduction to assistive devices and durable medical equipment for health care professionals. It is not intended to be a comprehensive list because there are thousands of devices and custom-fabricated adaptations in use today. New devices and developments in assistive technology are developed on a daily basis.

This chapter includes devices and equipment that are designed to promote independence and increased functional outcomes. It does not include medical devices or equipment, such as splints, specialized mattresses, and mechanical lifts, used in health maintenance settings. This chapter focuses on the needs of the adult population and does not address the thousands of assistive devices and equipment in use with the pediatric population.

Many professionals working in health care can identify when a patient is having difficulty performing necessary self-care tasks or activities of daily living (ADLs), but occupational therapists are usually the ones who identify solutions to these problems. "Occupational Therapy Practitioners are uniquely qualified to provide, for individuals with disabilities, equipment that promotes the highest degree of independence in daily living."[1] "After assessing the ability and limitations of patients within their environments, the Occupational Therapist determines the types of assistive technology most effective for each individual. The equipment chosen may be commercially available, modified from existing products or custom fabricated."[1]

Occupational therapists are uniquely trained to analyze daily activities by breaking down the steps involved in ADLs. *Task analysis* is necessary to identify the specific subcomponents of functional skills, which need adaptation or remediation following disability. This profession is adept at teaching compensatory strategies until skills return, providing therapeutic interventions in skill redevelopment for function performance, and modifying tasks and environment for optimal independence.

A typical comprehensive evaluation includes an assessment of the physical, cognitive, psychological, and psychosocial aspects of disability. It is crucial to identify the origin of dysfunction before treatment.

Occupational therapists and others on the rehabilitation team use assistive devices and technology when functional remediation cannot be attained. When prescribing assistive devices, one must always consider whether or not the tool will increase or decrease function or hasten or prevent recovery.

Without proper assessment and correct identification of deficits, assistive devices have the potential to decrease overall health and well-being. A common example of this is decreased lower extremity strength and the need for reconditioning due to unnecessary scooter or wheelchair use when walking is an option. A second example is when patients rely on assistive devices for lower body self-care following a total knee replacement, which discourages active movement of the surgical knee. Dependence on a device to perform an ADL, even after the ability and/or strength has returned, is contraindicated.

This chapter provides a definition of each daily living skill area that should be addressed. Case studies and patient accounts are included to illustrate the use of the assistive devices. The device's function and the patient population that it benefits are briefly included in the tables.

SELF-CARE

The term *self-care* refers to the basic tasks each one of us performs daily to maintain cleanliness, health, and well-being. Often after disease, surgery, or injury, patients have difficulty performing these ADLs. These areas of function are often the most important for patients to perform independently (Table 1).

The following series of case studies and patient testimonials illuminate the impact of the assistive devices on self-care.

Modifying Basic Self-Care after Traumatic Brain Injury

Patient A suffered multiple injuries including a severe traumatic brain injury (TBI) following a motorcycle accident. His upper extremity (UE) function is limited to gross grasp only in the right hand, and he is able to use only his left UE as a gross stabilizer. This patient initially was dependent for all of his basic self-care, but when he was discharged, he was able to complete many tasks with set-up only (set-up constitutes having an aide or family member prepare the task items ahead of time). He was able to progress because of assistive devices, environmental modifications, and repetitive training of adaptive techniques for task completion. He uses an **electric toothbrush**, which is always available in its upright holder, with a large gripping base. The holder is **attached with Velcro to the side of the sink** to prevent it from falling because of his uncoordinated movements. Patient A lacks the grip strength to squeeze the pump-style toothpaste dispenser; therefore, the toothpaste is provided in a small medication cup, which is also attached to the side of the sink with Velcro. The patient can dip his toothbrush into the small toothpaste cup with his right hand. The patient was also taught to use his teeth to assist his right hand. For example, he was shown how to grab onto a washcloth with his teeth to drape the washcloth over his hand to wash his face. He was taught to use his left hand to stabilize items, such as his deodorant, while removing the cap with his right hand. His hairbrush handle was enlarged with a **built-up handle** and a **fabricated cuff** to allow the item to stay in his hand. Patient A uses an electric shaver because it is also easier to grip. The shaver base is also attached to the sink-side to prevent frequent unintentional dropping. This patient was taught to use the tip of the faucet to push the shaver on and off since he had lost the thumb function necessary to do so. Overall, with this set-up, the use of verbal cues, an **ADL checklist**, and

TABLE 1. ASSISTIVE DEVICES FOR SELF-CARE TASKS

ADL	Assistive Device or Equipment	Function/Patient Population
Self-feeding	Utensil with built-up handle	Provide better grip surface for patients with decreased hand strength, painful joints, etc.
	Cut-out cup (Fig. 1)	To prevent neck extension during swallowing for patients with limited neck movement who are unable to drink a full glass. Space for nose is cut out of cup.
	Rocker knife (Fig. 2)	To allow one-handed cutting for patients with decreased bilateral hand use
	Extended utensil	To compensate for inability to reach mouth secondary to limited ROM, weakness, etc.
	Swiveled utensil	To keep food level during transition to mouth when UE uncoordination is present
	Coated utensil	To protect teeth and lips during biting reflex, often used with neurologic impairments
	ADL checklist	To serve as a memory and sequencing cue for the patient who requires cognitive reminders to perform self-care tasks independently. The checklist is usually posted in the patient's bedroom/bathroom
	Universal cuff	To allow use of utensils (e.g., pencils, silverware, toothbrush, tools) for patients with limited grasp strength and movement of hand and wrist
	Weighted utensil	To decrease interfering muscle in coordination of UE and provide added sensory input to UE, for patients with neurological impairments
	Food clamp	It assists in reach and grasp of food to mouth when patient is unable to reach mouth or hold food
	Flexible utensil	To allow versatility in angle and position of handle for patients with decreased wrist/hand ROM, strength, etc.
	Mechanical feeding device	To provide assistance to patients for aspects of feeding they cannot perform independently due to limited UE function
Dressing	Velcro-adapted clothing	Provide access into/out of clothing by replacing buttons and zippers with hook-and-loop tape (Velcro). For patients limited by decreased strength, ROM, or restrictive medical devices, etc.
	Pant clip	To prevent clothing from dropping to the floor when the patient stands after toileting. It attaches to pants and shirt simultaneously. Used for patients with THP, hemiplegia, poor standing balance, etc.
	Button hook (Fig. 3)	To allow buttoning when fine motor coordination is decreased, joint protection needed, or limited by pain
	Long wall mirror	To provide visual feedback of entire body (after dressing or for positioning cue) for patients with decreased body awareness, neglect, etc.
	Clothing identifiers	To cue patient as to type, color, etc., of clothing. For patients with low vision. Identifiers are sewn onto clothing
	Panty hose aid	To provide donning assistance for patients who are limited by THP, pain, ROM, etc.
	Zipper hooks or ringed pulls for zippers	To allow zippering when fine motor strength or coordination is decreased, joint protection needed
	Sock aid (Fig. 4)	To allow donning socks when patient limited due to THP, back pain, decreased ROM, etc.

Continued on next page

Table 1. Assistive Devices for Self-Care Tasks (continued)

ADL	Assistive Device or Equipment	Function/Patient Population
	Extended shoe horn	To allow shoe donning when patient limited by THP, pain, decreased ROM, etc.
	Elastic shoelaces	To provide already tied shoes to patients with limited fine motor, THP, pain limitations, etc.
	Cuff and collar extenders	To allow collars and sleeves to remain buttoned during dressing/undressing for patients with amputation, painful joints, hemiplegia, etc.
	Shoelace adapters	To allow fastening with the use of 1-hand for patients with limited bilateral hand function
	Shoe remover	To allow shoe removal for those unable to flex due to THP, pain, ROM limitations, etc.
	Dressing stick	To allow an extended reach for dressing and accessing objects for patients with limited ROM, THP, SCI, etc.
	Leg lifter	To help patients lift leg using UE strength when LE strength is limited due to SCI, pain, joint replacement, etc.
	Reacher (Fig. 5)	To provide an extended grab to better access lower body and items out of reach for patients with COPD, SCI, THP, arthritis, poor dynamic standing balance, etc.
Toileting	Non-spill urinal	To help prevent urinal leakage during supine use in bed and with patients with decreased motor coordination, decreased sensation or poor body schema
	Toilet supports	To provide back support with stabilizing straps or feet supports for patients with poor sitting balance and high fall risk while toileting
	Urinary drainage bag holder	To provide a concealed holder for urine receptacle bag
	Bathroom tissue aid	To allow better access to peri-area for patients with limited ROM, decreased hand strength or obesity
	Incontinence-proof chair cover, mattress pad, and wheelchair cushion cover	To provide waterproof, easily washable surfaces for use with patients with incontinence
	3-in-1 Commode chairs (Fig. 6)	These chairs can be used as a bedside commode, as a tub bench, and over the toilet to raise the seat height for patients with neurological deficits, THP, etc.
	Long-handled digital bowel stimulators and suppository insertors	To allow rectal access for patients with limited ROM, strength, coordination, sensory loss
Hygiene/ Grooming	Suctioned denture/ finger nail-brush	To allow teeth/fingernail cleaning with one hand
	Long-handled hair washer	To compensate for impaired reach to hair with rubber-knobbed brush. For patients with limited ROM, limited hand strength, arthritis, etc.
	Long-handled comb and brush	To allow reach to hair for patients with limited ROM or strength
	U-cuffed toothbrushes, brushes	To facilitate hygiene for patients with limited grip strength, wrist ROM, etc.
	Suctioned nail clipper board	To provide assist with nail care for patients with limited hand function
	Individual dental floss sticks	To provide ability to floss one-handed or with limited bilateral hand function

Continued on next page

Table 1. Assistive Devices for Self-Care Tasks (continued)

ADL	Assistive Device or Equipment	Function/Patient Population
	Hands-free hair dryer holder	To dry hair with one hand. For patients with hemiplegia, amputation, etc.
	Long-handled nail clippers	To provide assistance with toenail clipping for patients with THP, obesity, pregnancy, etc.
	Modified toothpaste dispenser (pump style)	To provide toothpaste access for patients with decreased hand function, painful joints, etc.
Bathing	Long-handled and curved bath sponge and brush	To provide low back reach for patient with limited ROM, energy, strength, etc.
	Wheeled shower chair	To provide transport of patient from toilet into roll-in shower. Often used for patients who have difficulty performing multiple transfers
	Tub side rail (Fig. 7)	Clamps to tub side to provide support for tub transfers to patients with poor standing balance, high fall risk, etc.
	Inflatable bathing assist	Some are full tub-like bed baths that allow bed bathing; others provide transfer surface in tub that, upon deflation, bring patient to tub bottom. For patients with decreased functional mobility
	Wash mitt	Provides sensory re-education. Also encourages UE use for patients with limited hand function
	Foot brush and medication applicator	To allow access for proper foot cleaning and care for patients with limited ROM, THP, diabetes, etc.
	Soap-on-a-rope or bottled soap	To prevent falls in shower caused by slipping on dropped bar soap. For patients who may be unable to retrieve from tub floor
	Shampoo basin	To assist with shampooing at bed level for patients with decreased functional mobility
	Shower seat or tub bench	To allow safe showering for patients who are unable to stand safely, need assist with transfers to reduce fall risk, or need to practice energy conservation
	Commode chair	To provide free-standing toilet for patient who cannot access toilet due to functional mobility deficits
	Utensil holder with D-ring strap	Provides a snap in/out holder for items such as razors, typing sticks, brushes, etc., for patients with decreased grip strength, coordination, or sensation in hands
	Extended shower hose (Fig. 8)	To better wash body while seated. For patients with decreased ROM, strength, need for energy conservation and to better regulate water temperature for patients with sensory loss.
	Adapted towel with handles	To allow access to difficult to reach areas of the body for patients with decreased hand function or upper body ROM
	Bidet or sitz bath systems	To assist with peri-care for patients limited by decreased ROM, sensation, hand function, etc.
Meal preparation	Kitchen timer (tactile or regular)	To assist patient with poor memory, time sense, or vision to measure time
	Over-stove mirror	To provide visual feedback for safety while cooking for patients at wheelchair level. Mirror is mounted at an angle above stove top
	Adaptive handled cookware	Large handles provide ergonomic design and better bilateral weight distribution for patients with painful joints, decreased ROM, or UE injury
	Hand-held electric can opener	To allow can opening for patients with one nonfunctional UE or decreased strength
	Large print recipe book	To assist with recipe reading for patients with low vision

Continued on next page

TABLE 1. ASSISTIVE DEVICES FOR SELF-CARE TASKS (CONTINUED)

ADL	Assistive Device or Equipment	Function/Patient Population
	Adapted cutting board (Fig. 9)	To allow safe one-handed food preparation. Board offers clamps, food spikes, and edges to hold food in place
	Adapted angled knives	To allow safe one-handed cutting, adequate joint protection to prevent severe ulnar deviation, etc.
	Large-handled kitchen tools	To aid patients with decreased grip strength, painful joints, etc.
	Pan holder	To provide stabilization of panhandle while on stove top or during one-handed stirring for patients with decreased bilateral hand function or safety issues
	Suction bottle brush	To assist with one-handed dish washing
	Milk carton opener	To assist with one-handed opening
	Bowl holder	To assist the patient using one hand to cook to pour food from bowl to pan/dish
	Spread board	To hold food item (bread) for one-handed spreading
	Mounted jar or bottle opener	To assist jar opening for patients with painful joints, decreased strength
	Box top opener	To allow opening box one-handed for patients with decreased hand strength, painful joints, etc.
	Zip bag sealer	To assist with sealing zip top bags for patients with decreased pinch strength, painful joints, etc.
	Microwave dish gripper	To provide safe way to remove hot items from microwave without handling dish for patients with sensory problems, etc.
	Flame-retardant oven mitt and apron	To provide a protective barrier against heat contact, especially for patients with decreased sensation, etc.
Health management	Pill organizers (Fig. 10)	To help prevent mistakes in pill taking due to memory loss, confusion, or disorganization
	Braille pill organizer	To assist in self-medication for patients with low vision
	Electronic pillbox	To provide audio reminder for patients with low vision, poor memory, etc.
	Long-handled mirror	To help patients with amputations, SCI, diabetes, etc., inspect skin for hard to see or feel areas
	Wall-mounted insulin needle holder	Designed for one-handed IV medication and insulin users
	Syringe magnifier	To increase visibility of insulin needle holder for patients with low vision.
	Pill splitter and crusher	To increase ability to swallow pills for patients with dysphagia
	Vocalized glucose monitor	To provide auditory cues for glucose levels for patients with low vision
	Talking blood pressure monitor	To provide auditory feedback for BP levels to patients with low vision
	Audio thermometer	To provide auditory readout of temperature for patients with low vision
	Elbow pads	To protect elbows against pressure, accidental skin breakdown, etc.. for patients with fragile skin, sensory loss, immobility, or nerve compression
	Specialized wheelchair cushion	To provide adequate pressure relief and prevent skin breakdown for patients with sensory loss, prolonged sitting such as SCI, geriatrics, neurologic impairments, etc. *Therapy evaluation required due to the variety of alternatives specific to patient need*

Continued on next page

Promoting Functional Independence through the Use of Assistive Devices 267

TABLE 1. ASSISTIVE DEVICES FOR SELF-CARE TASKS (CONTINUED)

ADL	Assistive Device or Equipment	Function/Patient Population
	Medical alert tag	An emblem worn on a wrist or neck chain to communicate vital medical facts, a 24-hour hotline, and personal info. number so medical personnel can contact family members/caregivers on file
	Magnetic hearing aid battery dispenser	To provide access to battery for patients with decreased vision, fine motor, etc.
	Safety pill-bottle cap opener	To assist with opening safety bottles caps (e.g., pills, hazardous content bottles) for patients with decreased hand function

ROM = range of motion, UE = upper extremity, THP = total hip precaution, SCI = spinal cord injury, LE = lower extremity, COPD = chronic obstructive pulmonary disease, BP = blood pressure.

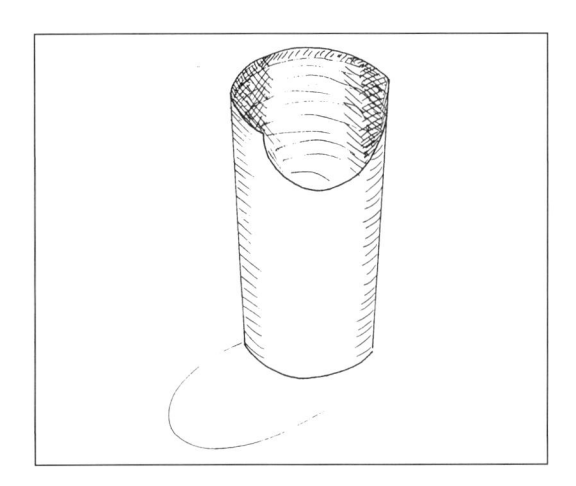

FIGURE 1. Cut-out cup.

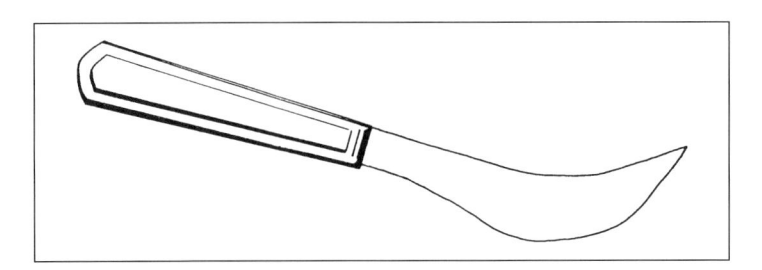

FIGURE 2. Rocker knife.

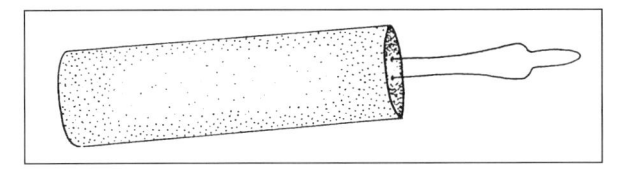

FIGURE 3. Button hook.

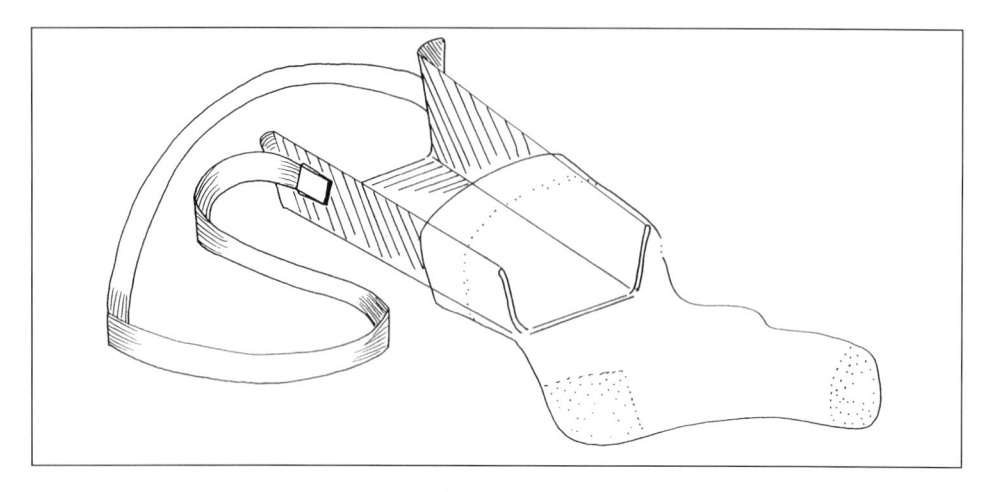

FIGURE 4. Sock-aid device.

the structure of a daily routine, this patient is physically able to perform all tasks and initiate and recall the sequence of the tasks.

Check-Off List for ADL Task Completion

Patient A initially needed constant cues to perform the most basic self-care tasks. His severe initiation, sequencing, and memory problems affected his ability to perform these familiar daily tasks. The patient was provided with a structured daily set of tasks and trained to check off each task on a checklist as he completed them. Without this list and the check-off method, this patient was unaware whether or not he had showered or changed his clothes, even if he had done so just minutes before. With this compensation method, he is able to look at the list and find whether the check is next to the task on today's date and perform any necessary tasks. The occupational therapist was able to grade the treatment and offer only supervision with an occasional reminder. The patient learned the routine and would look for the next step to be completed during his morning care activities. Prior to discharge this patient learned to apply the compensatory technique of the ADL checklist without staff assistance.

Wearing a Halo Vest

Patient B wears a halo vest following a cervical injury. Because of her decreased shoulder flexion and the size and awkwardness of the halo, she was unable to don

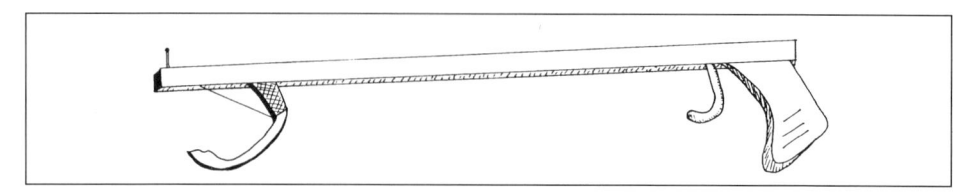

FIGURE 5. Reacher.

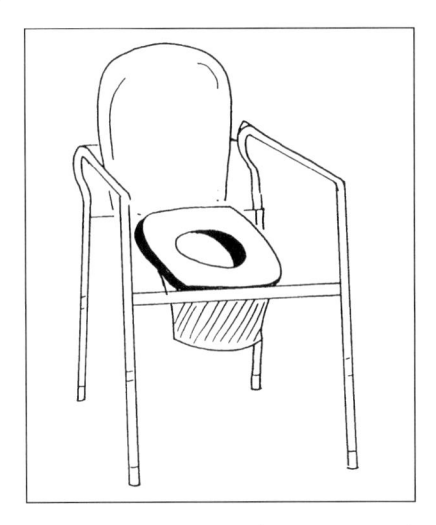

FIGURE 6. This commode also serves as a shower seat and a raised toilet seat.

her T-shirts. The occupational therapist modified several T-shirts with a vertical front separation and attached Velcro closures to the opening. With the use of a **dressing stick** to bring the shirt to her second arm, Patient B is able to don her shirts independently following the adaptation and training with the assistive device.

Neglect of the Left Side

Patient C, a stroke survivor, displayed severe left body neglect during all ADLs. The extent of the neglect became evident one day during dressing training. During

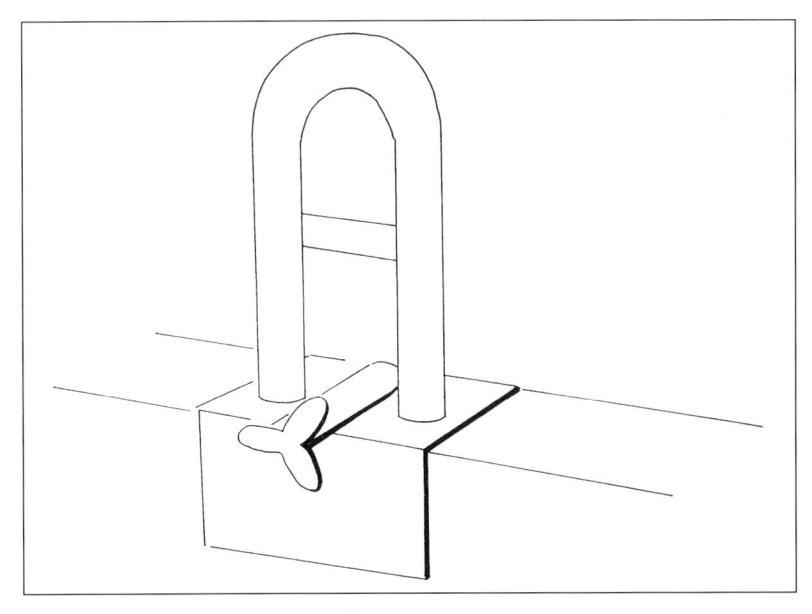

FIGURE 7. Bathtub grab bar.

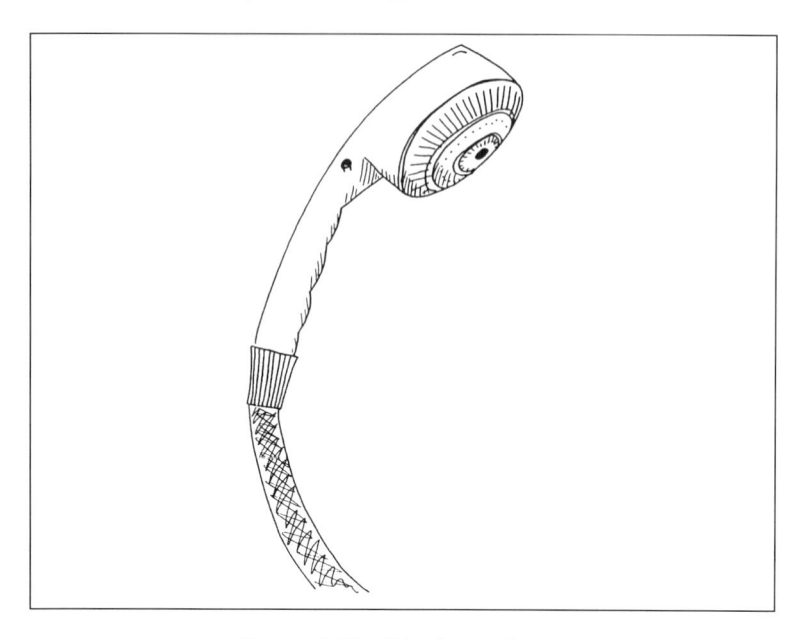

270 Promoting Functional Independence through the Use of Assistive Devices

FIGURE 8. Flexible shower hose.

her first week of sessions with the occupational therapist, she was able to use daily cues to attend to the left side of the body when donning all clothing and dressed without any physical assistance. At the end of the week, the therapist decided to schedule the therapy session after the patient had gotten dressed. However, the therapist failed to realize the extent to which the patient relied on her verbal cues to compensate for the left-sided neglect. This became evident to the therapist after meeting the patient in the hallway and finding the patient completely undressed on the left side while still fully dressed on the right side of her body. After further dressing training sessions, a comprehensive team approach to address the severe

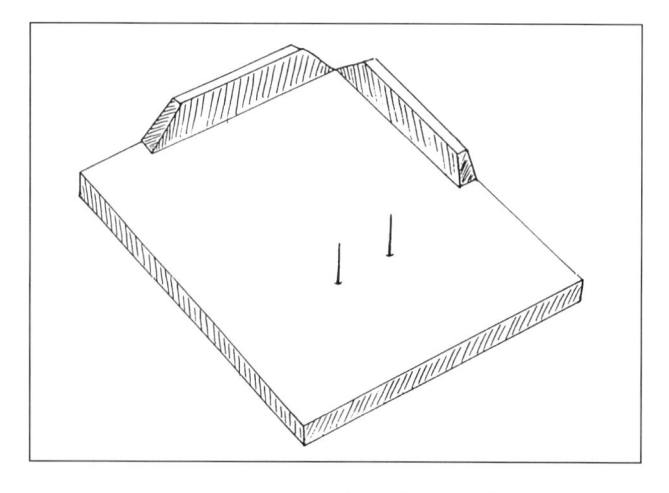

FIGURE 9. Adapted cutting board.

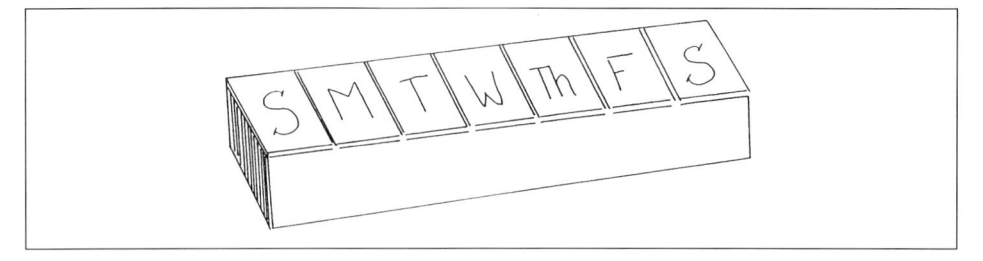

FIGURE 10. Pill organizer.

neglect, and teaching the compensatory technique of checking her body in a **long mirror** before leaving any dressing room, this patient was able to master this daily task without assistance.

Common Toileting Issues

Patients often find it difficult to bring up problems related to toileting. When the subject is discussed, it is often expressed as the most important ADL task to master. Problems can arise for a variety of reasons. Some patients lack the ability to reach the peri-area due to obesity or UE dysfunction. Other patients have a decreased ability to target or wipe effectively due to lack of proprioception or sensory loss in the hand. Poor trunk balance due to hemiparesis can greatly impair toileting skills. Limited pelvic tilt or flexibility combined with an impaired reach makes toileting independently and effectively almost impossible. It is important to distinguish the difference among the act of toileting, continence, and the actual toilet transfer. All three present different problems and therefore require separate treatments. All three problems are scored separately on the Functional Independence Measure (FIM).

Self-Care Issues after Stroke

Following a stroke, Patient D stated:

Since my stroke two months ago, I have had trouble doing the simplest things to take care of myself. It was a sad day when I got my **wheelchair**, but now I get out of the house and go places I want to go. I still have trouble using the toilet alone, feeding myself, getting dressed without help, and taking a shower like I used to. I always took these basic things for granted.

The gadgets I learned how to use while going through rehab, have made it possible for me to go home and not depend on my wife. I use a **tub bench** because I can't safely stand in the shower yet, and the grab bars help me get in and out without having to rely on my wife to help me. With the **toilet tissue aid** I was given, I can now wipe myself after using the toilet, and this means a lot to me. It still takes a long time to button my shirts, tie my shoes and ties, but with the different tools I was taught how to use, I can do this without getting so frustrated. With the special **eating equipment** that I have, I can use both hands and now feed myself. At first these tools made me feel handicapped, but I realize now how they allow me to do things alone, just in a different way.

Adaptations for Joint Pain

Patient E, a young single mother, suffered from severe pain in her hand joints due to arthritis. She is the primary caregiver for her two small children, and meal preparation is part of her ADLs. One of her main complaints to the occupational therapist was the inability to open jars and bottles. Consequently, she tended to use many premade foods to conserve her energy and reduce pain. She was issued a **jar and bottle opener**, which mounts under a kitchen cabinet, and she was instructed on joint protection techniques to apply to all ADLs. Patient E is now able to prepare meals without pain or frustration and with complete independence.

Medication Use after Traumatic Brain Injury

Seizures are a common sequela of TBI, so taking antiseizure medications routinely and on time becomes quite important. Patient F has severe short-term memory deficits, and for a time, could not recall when to take his medications even though written reminders were provided and he was using an organized **pillbox**. Fortunately, he was discharged to a large, supervised board and care setting from the inpatient rehabilitation unit, and his medications were administered to him. His only responsibility was to request his medications on time. This patient was issued a **pocket alarm** that was set to beep at the time he needed to take his medication. Despite this aid, the patient was unable to recall why his alarm was going off. The therapist provided a simple alteration by placing a sticker on the alarm that read, "go ask for your pill." He was able to learn where his medication was distributed and, with the alarm and written cue, was able to arrive on time independently.

Food and Figure-Ground Discrimination

The wife of a patient with Alzheimer's disease reported that her husband used to love mashed potatoes, but whenever she served them with dinner, Patient G would eat everything on his plate except the potatoes. The occupational therapist working with the family had assessed that the patient had poor figure-ground discrimination and suggested that his wife try serving the potatoes on a black or dark-colored plate instead of their usual white ones. From that point on, the patient was able to locate the potatoes successfully on his plate, and his quality of life increased through renewed his enjoyment of a favorite familiar food.

SAFETY AND HOME ACCESSIBILITY

This section highlights devices for personal safety and accessibility within the living environment (Table 2). Several case studies are included to illustrate the daily issues patients may face when it comes to their safety and their ability to access their homes.

Safety and Figure-Ground Discrimination

A patient with new-onset dementia was admitted to the hospital after falling several times at home. During his brief inpatient stay, Patient H did not fall. During a home safety visit, the occupational therapist found that his single-story home had one step dividing almost each room. The patient's wife pointed out where the falls

TABLE 2. ASSISTIVE DEVICES AND DURABLE MEDICAL EQUIPMENT FOR SAFETY AND HOME ACCESSIBILITY

AD/DME	Function/Patient Population
Door alarm	Alerts caregivers if patient wanders. For patients who require supervision for safety outside the home due to confusion and poor safety awareness
Seat and bed alarm	Lets caregiver know when patient is changing position or getting up. Used with patients who have a high fall risk and usually memory impairments/ confusion
Colored tape cues	Used on steps to cue patients with decreased depth perception or poor visual scanning or perceptual abilities. Applied to door jams, wheelchair brakes, tables, etc.
Butane gas match	Allows one-handed fire starting
Glow-in-the-dark safety marking tape	Allows taped items (e.g., exits, steps, table corners) to be seen in the dark for safety purposes. For patients with decreased visual discrimination and environmental awareness
Protective padding	Adheres to edges, corners. or overhead/under sink pipes to prevent injury
Audio monitors	Provides patient or caregiver communication when direct supervision is not possible
U-shaped handle on phone receiver	Allows persons without hand grasp to hold phone up to ear without assist
Long-armed phone receiver holder	Hands-free device that holds the receiver up for persons with UE dysfunction
Wheelchair ramp	Provides method of access to ingress/egress home or community for wheelchair user
Offset door hinges	Adds 2 inches to the width of doorway for extra wheelchair clearance
Grab bars and safety rails	Provides support to patients in a variety of areas throughout home to prevent falls and increase functional mobility
Furniture raisers and extenders	Increases height of bed, couch, or chair for safer and easier transfers. Increases height of tables/desks for wheelchair clearance
Transfer belt	Provides stabile assist for caregiver to move patient safely to/from surfaces
Dark-colored dishes	Provides figure-ground discrimination for patients lacking this perception to increase recognition of food items
Large-buttoned or modified phone (Fig. 11)	Provides accuracy with dialing to patients with low vision, poor hand coordination or sensation, or inability to recognize numbers
Visual ring indicator for phone calls	Provides visual signal of phone ringing for hearing impaired patients
Electronic environmental controls	Allow patient with limited physical movement to control their living environment such as temperature, lights, open doors, turn on stereo, call for emergency assistance, etc. using computer technology. *Home evaluation required to discern specific patient need*
Antiskid tape	Placed on indoor or outdoor surfaces (e.g., steps, decks, tub bottom) to provide nonslip surface to prevent falls
Transfer pole/bed handle	Assists with transfers and standing where grab bars are unable to be placed for unsteady patients who are a fall risk
Chair and bed alarm	Alerts caregiver that patient has changed his/her position. Used for fall prevention. Some also give patient a verbal cue (e.g., "sit down") or a visual cue (e.g., a stop sign)
Wireless alarm	Keeps track of patients at risk of wandering. The receiver for the alarm is attached to the patient and to the door that you do not want exited. The alarm is triggered when the patient goes past a certain point
Safety mat	Reduces injury if patient falls out of bed. To be placed on floor near bed. For patients with confusion, decreased mobility, high fall risk, etc.

Continued on next page

Table 2. Assistive Devices and Durable Medical Equipment for Safety and Home Accessibility (continued)

AD/DME	Function/Patient Population
Bed hoist	Allows patients with decreased strength to hoist themselves from supine to sitting up in bed. Used for patients with decreased strength, after surgical intervention, etc.
Seat lifter	Provides a spring-like device on seat to assist patients going from sit to stand more easily. Used for patients with decreased LE strength, higher fall risk with transfer, etc.
Door and faucet knob grips and extender	Provides better gripping surface to patients with painful joints, decreased grip strength, etc.
Light flashing/vibrating smoke alarm	Awakens or alerts hearing-impaired patients to fire alarm
Tactile adhesive dots	Assist with location of buttons on keyboards, telephone, calculators, etc. For patients with low vision
Portable location finder	Provides siren on portable device to locate car, apartment, house, etc. For patients with decreased memory, vision, pathfinding, etc.
Door viewer	Provides a wide-angle view of person on other side of the door to the patient at wheelchair level

AD = assistive device, DME = durable medical equipment, LE = lower extremity.

had occurred, and the sites were consistent with the step placement. Although grab bars were already in place near each step, the occupational therapist noted that when the patient ambulated alone, he did not remember to use the grab bars and seemed unaware of the steps altogether. Further evaluation revealed that there was not much visual distinction (i.e., difference in floor color) between rooms. Apparently, the patient's inability to negotiate the steps safely was caused by his lack of figure-ground discrimination, similar to Patient G's inability to distinguish mashed potatoes on a white plate. The occupational therapist suggested the application of **red vinyl tape** to each step. A follow-up phone call 1 month later reported that the patient had not fallen since the therapist's visit.

Sense of Smell

Patients with TBI often have a diminished sense of smell. Frequently, TBI patients are unaware of the deficit, and family members notice only decreased appetites or overuse of spices and condiments. The loss of the sense of smell can pose a safety risk, one that is often overlooked. It is imperative that the patient be able to recognize the deficit as a problem in order to teach compensations. Some recommended compensations are:

- Ensure that enough working **smoke alarms** are present in the living space
- Ventilate well when using chemicals or toxins
- Carefully check expiration dates on food
- Visually inspect foods prior to eating

Wheelchair Ramp

Often, patients and their families do not want to install a permanent **wheelchair ramp** into their home, claiming that it will decrease the value of the home. A good solution is to recommend a portable ramp (as long as there are no more than two

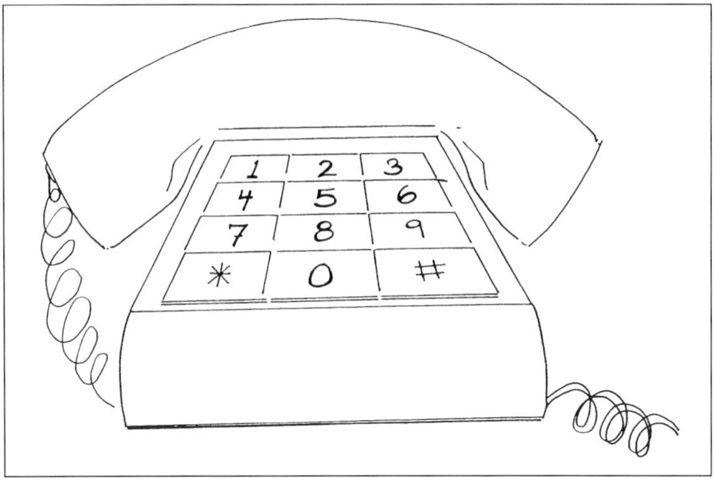

FIGURE 11. Large-numbered telephone.

steps to enter the home). A ramp is a necessary safety item that should be available in any household where there is a wheelchair user in residence. Other issues to consider with wheelchair accessibility are the door widths and the door jams. Hardware, known as **offset door hinges**, that will allow the door to open with the widest possible opening is commercially available. This can be particularly helpful in older homes where the doors are very narrow.

HOME MANAGEMENT SKILLS

Home management refers to the tasks needed to adequately maintain the living environment. Examples of these tasks are laundry, housekeeping, budgeting, gardening, and space organization (Table 3).

Telling Time

Many patients who are disoriented to time or have memory problems benefit from the routine reminder that **talking watches** provide them. ADLs such as taking medication, getting to appointments on time, and timing self-care routines are completed with more independence using these devices.

Typing Aids

Patient I was admitted to a hospital located far from his support system and family. He was unable to type because of abnormal muscle tone in his bilateral upper extremities. With the use of a **typing aid**, this patient was able to e-mail his loved ones daily, and his rehabilitation progress improved greatly.

Equipment Needed Following Spinal Cord Injury

Patient J has a spinal cord injury and uses a wheelchair to get around and take care of her home. Although she has movement in her arms, she is unable to grasp

TABLE 3. ASSISTIVE DEVICES AND DURABLE MEDICAL EQUIPMENT FOR HOME MANAGEMENT

AD/DME	Function/Patient Population
Long-handled dust pan	Allows use without bending for patients limited by pain, decreased ROM, THP, etc.
Angled stovetop mirror	Allows view of items cooking on stove top from wheelchair level
Hand-clip phone holder	Attaches to phone receiver and provides U-shaped handle for holding with limited hand function
Task checklists	Checklists that serve as reminders to cognitively impaired patients to perform household management activities
Electric iron guide	Allows safer ironing for patients with low vision or unilateral sensory loss, etc.
Rolling cart (Fig. 12)	Allows easier transport of objects for patients needing to conserve energy (reducing trips), using joint protection techniques, UE limitations, etc.
Modified lamp switches	Increases lamp use for patients with decreased fine motor ability
Key turner	Assists the patient with decreased fine motor, hand strength, wrist ROM, or pain
One-handed loop scissors	Allow cutting with one hand and decrease pressure on small joints
Slip-resistant matting	Provides nonslip surfaces under a plate or around pill bottle to increase grip, etc.
Talking watch/clock	Increases time awareness for patients with decreased memory, vision, etc.
Recording device	Provides memory cues or voice organizers to patients with low vision, decreased hand use, etc.
Long-handled dusters	Allows easier reach for cleaning from wheelchair level or for patients with decreased shoulder AROM
Grasping cuff	Assists with grabbing cleaning brushes, brooms, etc. For patients with limited grip strength
Various large-print and buttoned devices	Allows use of routine home devices for patients with low vision, decreased fine motor coordination, etc.
Modified keyboard	Allows computer use for patients with low vision, decreased fine motor coordination, decreased hand use, etc.
Check-writing/reading guides	Provide visual cues and guides for patients with visual scanning problems, poor coordination, etc.
Modified writing utensil	Some provide weight to increase coordination; others have built-up handle to increase grip; U-cuff for limited hand function; ball handle for limited fine motor coordination; splint type base for better use of pen, etc. Specific assessment required
Typing aid	Typing device that straps to hand to allow easier typing for patients with limited finger function
Walker bag and basket	Allow easier transport of items for ADLs and hand freedom to use walker properly

AD = assistive device, DME = durable medical equipment, ROM = range of motion, THP = total hip precaution, AROM = active range of motion, ADL = activity of daily living.

objects with her hands, and she has impaired sensation in both UEs. In order to cook safely and clean from her wheelchair, several assistive devices and modifications have been provided. Because she is unable to grasp appliance handles, **fabric loops** have been sewn and placed on the refrigerator and over door handles so that she can hook her arm through the loop to open the doors. An **angled stove-top mirror** was installed to facilitate safe cooking. **Universal cuffs** have been supplied so that she can use utensils with her limited grasp. Full oven mitts can be used to

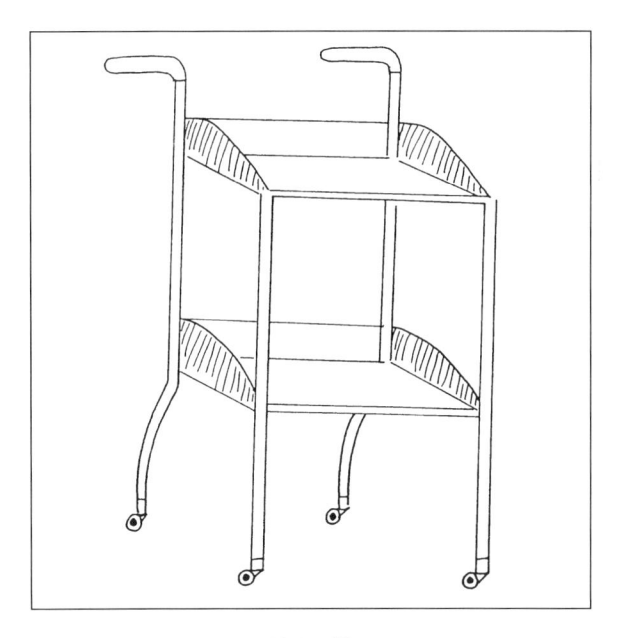

FIGURE 12. Rolling cart.

retrieve items from the oven because of her impaired sensation. Her pots are stabilized on the stove with **pan holders**. She uses a **special chopping block** that has suction cups on the bottom to hold it in place and edges to keep the food from sliding off the surface. It takes her more time to cook than it did before her injury, but she prefers to cook homemade food instead of eating out.

VOCATIONAL ACTIVITIES

Vocational activities refer to any aspect of a person's productivity that they consider work. There are thousands of job sites and types of work that allow modification or adaptation for a patient to return to a productive work role after a disabling injury or disease. There are also many ergonomic solutions for persons to remain injury free in jobs that require repetitive motion. Occupational therapists are trained in both custom modification of work sites and evaluation of job tasks to optimize productivity, while limiting possibility of injury.

Assistive technology devices include "any item, piece of equipment or product system whether acquired commercially off the shelf, modified, or customized that is used to increase or improve functional capabilities of individuals with disabilities" as defined by the Technical Assistance to the States Act in the United States.[5]

One-Handed Work Performance

Patient K works at a desk job that requires answering busy phones. Since his stroke, Patient K has only right UE function and, therefore, needs to have his right hand available to take messages. The **hands-free headphone set** allows him to multitask and complete his job effectively.

Ergonomic Modifications

Patient L suffers from a variety of strains and aches because of her office layout. The therapist suggested raising the monitor to eye-level and centering it in front of the keyboard. A **reverse tilted keyboard tray** was installed under the desk to reduce her wrist extension, which was contributing to her carpal tunnel syndrome. The patient's chair was raised to decrease hip flexion, and her armrests were raised to the appropriate height. After these few minor adjustments, the patient reported less pain and fatigue at the end of the day.

Hundreds of ergonomic modifications are available on the market today. Table 4 summarizes the most commonly used ergonomic equipment and devices.

LEISURE ACTIVITIES

Leisure activities are the activities one does that add fulfillment and enjoyment to life. Often times after a disabling event or disease, patients find it difficult to continue these activities and require adaptations to participate in them. Certified recreational therapists and occupational therapists train patients with assistive devices or custom adaptations either to explore alternative leisure options or to learn how to perform previously enjoyed activities in a new way (Table 5).

Golf

Many patients can no longer play the sports they love following a disease or accident. Golfing is a favorite to some. Patient M was having difficulty holding onto his golf clubs tightly enough to swing. He could stand tall and walk short distances, but he could not swing with confidence. The occupational therapist came up with a simple modification. A **fabric strap** was fastened with a grommet to his club handle so that the strap could wrap around his hand and attach to the club with Velcro. In addition, the handle of the club was **built-up** to make it easier to hold. The patient was so happy that he gladly participated in his therapy sessions, which consisted of actually playing golf to improve his balance and his walking.

Gardening

To many patients, gardening is a hobby that is soothing and energizing. Patient N is an elderly patient with Parkinson's disease. The goal of her therapy was to figure out ways to encourage movement and maintain strength so that the family and caregivers would be able to follow a home exercise program. However, she refused to participate in the usual therapy routine, citing lack of interest, and she sat in a wheelchair during most of the day, taking only a few assisted steps here and there. Because she had once loved to garden, she was presented with a **raised garden box** filled with new soil and some colorful flowers. Patient N responded immediately. The therapist noted that she began to reach, bend, lift, shovel, and even stand occasionally, all in the effort of tending her flowers. Not only was she exercising, but she had found a renewed interest that occupied her time during the day. Gardening modification such as this can easily be provided in either a home or institutional setting.

TABLE 4. ERGONOMIC MODIFICATIONS

ADL	AD/DME	Function/Patient Population
Sitting tasks	Specialized chair	Provides lumbar support or UE support or head/neck support during work tasks
	Custom-made ergonomic chair	Custom made to employees needs to reduce back, neck, shoulder, and muscle tension. It assists in proper positioning
	Footrest	Provides adequate support for feet during seated tasks to prevent back injury, leg discomfort
	Sit/stand frame	Provides a supported upright position for work tasks to limit leg strain
	Seat shock absorber	A foam or gel seat cushion placed in heavy machinery for operators to sit on and be protection by impact of full body vibration
Standing tasks	Standing mat	Provides cushioned standing surface that reduces fatigue and encourages LE circulation
Work supports	Spine supporter	Belts or supportive devices that assist patient to maintain good posture during work activity. Some have sensors in them and act as biofeedback devices to cue to stretch, change position
	Hands-free headset	Allows use of telephone or cellular phone while keeping a neutral head/neck position, to prevent repetitive strain.
	Phone amplifier	Assists with clarity of speech for persons with hearing loss
	Specialized gloves	Some are antivibratory for power tool use; others have gel pockets to protect against shock, pressure, or friction
	Elbow protectors	Provide support and shock absorption to prevent against or prevent further injury
	Knee protectors	Protect joint and soft tissue of knee from pressure while performing work tasks on knees
	Gel pads for elbows/knees	Limit pressure on joints against hard surfaces
	Built-up tool handle	Foam tubing slides over tool handles increasing grip circumference to protect joints, limit joint pain, decrease RSI, etc.
	Modified handle	Angles on tools (e.g., hammers) that have at least a 19° bend assist in the prevention of carpal tunnel syndrome, and better protect and position wrist
	Eye and ear protector	Safety glasses and ear plugs protect both ears and eyes from harmful objects, stimuli
	Ergonomic tool grip	Grip handles attached to straight tools, shovels, etc., to allow upright standing position with use, reducing the natural tendency to bend at waist
	Rolling ergonomic table	Work surface adjusts to limit neck, back, and eye strain for a variety of work tasks
Computer use	Specialized keyboard tray	Provides ergonomic typing position and mouse height for optimal use and limited potential for injury
	Keyboard tray for employee in wheelchair	Allows lateral adjustability and accommodates adjustment for wheelchair
	Split or fixed split keyboard	Allows proper wrist position (decreased ulnar deviation) when typing
	Armrest	Provides support for UEs while typing, to ensure proper position and prevent further injury
	Wrist support	Provides proper positioning of wrist and limits potential injury when using mouse, keyboard, 10-key machine, etc.
	Modified mouse	A variety of design solutions for optimal use and injury prevention. Will provide comfort and be more effective if fit properly to user (some range from extra small to extra large, measuring from tip of 3rd digit to distal wrist crease)

Continued on next page

TABLE 4. ERGONOMIC MODIFICATIONS (CONTINUED)

ADL	AD/DME	Function/Patient Population
	Hands-free mouse	Voice- or foot-operated mouse for patients with limited UE function
	Sip-and-puff operated mouse	An accurate mouse pointer that operates hands-free with sip-and-puff action. For patients with decreased UE function, quadriplegia, etc.
	Screen visors and filter	Decrease glare off screen for optimal vision of screen info
	Monitor positioner	Lifts monitor to eye level to increase proper position of head/neck for work tasks
	Mouthpiece and head pointer	Provide an alternative method of typing for patients with decreased UE function
	Voice-activated computer programs	Allow voice recognition for computer access for patients with limited hand function.
Workbench or tabletop tasks	Edge rest	Provides wrist rests and soft-edged work station to decrease pressure injury to wrists/forearms
	Adjustable work station	Adjustable for standing or sitting for patients that need to alternate between positions throughout the day

ADL = activity of daily living, AD = assistive device, DME = durable medical equipment, UE = upper extremity, LE = lower extremity, RSI = repetitive strain injury.

COMMUNITY FUNCTIONING

Community functioning refers to the instrumental activities of daily living (IADLs) that are performed in the community setting. Some IADL examples are shopping; banking; taking public transit; fulfilling social roles in clubs, churches, and committees; and participating in occupational roles (e.g., student, parent, employee, caregiver, and volunteer) (Table 6).

Power Scooter Use for Arthritis

One day Patient O phoned the occupational therapy clinic distraught. His multiple joint arthritis had progressed to the point that he was unable to use his manual wheelchair, even for short distances in his apartment. His meals were being provided two times a day, and he reported that the majority of his day was spent in his recliner because of his pain and immobility. The most crucial safety issue was that his apartment was on the second floor and he was unable to push his wheelchair to the elevator to exit his apartment. A home visit was arranged that week, and the patient was evaluated and trained in a **power scooter**. Patient O came to the clinic several weeks later and stated that his life was changed. He was now able to access his community again. He was no longer dependent on others and stated that he did not feel "like a prisoner in my own home anymore."

Using a Reacher

Many patients with total hip precautions (THP) use **reachers** to perform several ADLs such as lower body dressing, reaching laundry in and out of the washer and dryer, and retrieving objects dropped on the floor. Many patients use them to get objects overhead out of cupboards. This simple device has many uses and provides independence to many patients.

TABLE 5. ASSISTIVE DEVICES FOR LEISURE ACTIVITIES

ADL	AD/DME	Function/Patient Population
Computer use	(See Table 4)	
Writing	Note-size writing guide	Provides a guide for writing letters effectively for patients with some loss of visual or spatial functioning
	Built-up pens	Designed to decrease radial side pressure on small joints for patients with painful joints or decreased pinch strength
Woodworking	Vise grip	To be used with pliers, wrench, or clamp for patients with one functional UE
Bowling	Wheelchair bowling frame	Assists the patient seated in a wheelchair to bowl effectively
	Retractable bowling ball	Provides a retractable handle for ball for patients with decreased hand strength and function
Reading	Prism glasses	Allow effective reading for the patient who is supine in bed
	Book holders/stand	Provides support for book for patients with inability to hold own book while reading
	Cut newspaper	Newspapers are folded on the crease so patient with one functioning UE can handle one page at a time
	Multipurpose suction mouth wand	Assists with page turning, typing, etc. For patients with limited UE function
	Books on tape	Audiotape of books read aloud. For patients with low vision, difficulty recognizing words following a CVA, etc.
Card playing	Card holder	Assists patients with limited hand function
	Automatic card shuffler	Shuffles cards automatically (battery operated) without the need for hand function
Sewing	Knitting needle holder	Clamps to table side and assists with one-handed knitting
	Needle-threader	Assists with needle threading for patients with poor fine motor coordination or eyesight
	Loop scissors	For right- or left-handed use with limited grip strength
Stamp collecting	Illuminated magnifier	Assists patients with low vision to view stamps more easily
Gardening	Large-handled garden tools	Assist patients with painful joints, decreased grip strength, etc., to garden effectively
	Gardener seat and kneeler	Provides a seated surface to garden from and, when turned over, provides a cushioned kneeling surface
	Raised garden bed	Allows garden access from a seated or wheelchair position instead of kneeling
	Faucet and hose adapter	Converts twist controls to snap connections to increase access with limited hand function, painful joints, etc.
Television viewing	Large-buttoned, touch-sensitive remote control	Provides easier use for patients with low vision, decreased fine motor skills
	Closed captioning	Assists patients with decreased hearing to follow TV program
	TV screen enlarger	Could double the size of current TV screen for patients with visual loss
Music playing	Enlarged sheet music	Allows patients with low vision to read music notes
	One-handed sheet music	Music composed to be played one-handed by most functional UE, following an amputation, CVA, etc.
Playing board games	Enlarged or modified with braille	A variety of board games are available to be more effectively played by patients with low vision
Fishing	One-handed reel	Allows effective reeling with one functional UE
	Multipurpose fishing device	A two-piece graphite rod, holder, and casting device that clamps to left or right arm of wheelchair
Watching movies	Listening devices	Available at theaters upon request. These are worn to increase volume of film for patients with hearing loss

ADL = activity of daily living, AD = assistive device, DME = durable medical equipment, UE = upper extremity, CVA = cerebrovascular accident.

TABLE 6. Assistive Devices for Functioning in the Community

AD/DME	Function/Patient Population
Gas cap wrench	Eases gas cap opening for patients with painful joints, decreased hand function
Portable shopping cart	Light-weight handbag that folds into pulling shopping cart to provide assistance for patients needing one free hand to use a cane or hand rails
Talking and braille compass	Provides geographic direction to patients with low vision or poor directional sense
Cane rest	Provides a cane-rest (attached to cane) to free up both hands for ADL tasks
Key lever	Provides a lever to turn keys for patients with decreased pinch strength or painful joints
Ramp	Allows wheelchair access into buildings, over steep thresholds, within bilevel rooms
Car door opener	Assists patients with decreased hand function to open a variety of car doors more easily
Folding cane carrying case	Allows free hands during community activities without leaving cane behind
Reflective tape or flags	Tape adheres to mobility assistive devices or flag attaches to scooter or wheelchair to increase overall visibility at night or in parking lots
Adapted wallet	Provides separate sections for each type of coin or bills to allow more successful locating of items for patients with decreased memory, vision, etc.
Grocery store scooter	Provides accessibility and decreased risk of fatigue while shopping for patients with neurologic impairments, low endurance, pain, etc.
Wheelchair bag	Transports needed items while allowing hands to be free to perform tasks (e.g., hold grocery basket, clothing, etc.)
Reacher	Allows access to items in stores, businesses from wheelchair level
Seat swivel	A padded disk-type seat swivel that provides assistance to patients who have difficulty swinging legs into and out of cars
Memory book/day planner	Usually customized by therapy staff with patient to provide specific cognitive assistance for community functioning
Handbag hook	Attaches to the shoulder of a jacket or shirt so that a purse strap can hang from hook. For patients who have decreased shoulder musculature or a nonfunctioning UE

AD = assistive device, DME = durable medical equipment, ADL = activity of daily living, UE = upper extremity.

Vision Impairment

Patient P was no longer able to drive due to his impaired vision. Fortunately, he lived within walking distance of the local grocery store. After some training in community mobility, crossing streets carefully and using a **vision cane**, he was able to safely walk the streets again. He also found that carrying a **cellular phone** (with preprogrammed numbers) made him feel more secure. A **portable shopping cart** made it possible for him to continue shopping on his own. He went to the store two times a week and even started helping another neighbor with his shopping.

CUSTOM FABRICATED ADAPTATIONS AND MODIFICATIONS

Historically, many therapists and especially occupational therapists have been known for their creative use of materials and tools to assist patients with independence in performing their ADLs. With the use of fabrics, Velcro, a good sewing machine, thermoplastics, plastics, wood, metal, a band-saw, and a little ingenuity, therapists have created and modified just about anything that people use during their daily tasks. In today's world, many of these items have now been patented and are being mass produced. Therapists and doctors now only need to refer to catalogues to find most items that fits a need. Rarely do you see a therapist fabricate anything from scratch because of the time constraints of health care delivery and the limited budgets of facilities and insurance companies. Anything can be modified with the right tools and a little creativity. Sometimes the simplest modification can mean a whole new way of life for a patient.

CONCLUSION

The combined efforts of the health care team will ensure a holistic approach toward regaining functional independence for the patients being treated in our care. Assistive devices and durable medical equipment can greatly improve quality of life and independence in ADLs following a disabling incident, but they should be issued with great care. A comprehensive evaluation should preclude issuance of assistive devices and should always include the patient's goals and the life roles that are being impacted by disability.

REFERENCES

1. American Occupational Therapy Association: 1996.
2. Burnett PS: Independent Living Functioning with the Use of One Hand in a Two-handed World. Thorofare, NJ, Slack Inc., 1990.
3. Pedretti LW: Occupational Therapy: Practical Skills for Physical Dysfunction, 4th ed. St. Louis, Mosby, 1996.
4. Larkin M: When Someone You Love Has a Stroke: A National Stroke Association Book. Lynn Sonberg Book Associates, 1995.
5. Public Law 100-407 (Technical Assistance to the States Act in the United States).
6. Occupational Therapy Association of California.
7. Platt JV, Hahn R, Kessler S, McCarthy D: Daily Activities after Your Hip Surgery, revised edition. American Occupational Therapy Association, 1986.
8. Zoltan B, Siev E, Freishtat B: The Adult Stroke Patient, 2nd ed. Thorofare, NJ, Slack Inc., 1986.

Chapter 19
Mobility Aids

Kenneth D. Randall, MPT, GCS, ATC

The goal of any therapeutic intervention should include improved function and mobility. One of the major tasks rehabilitationists face daily is selecting the most appropriate mobility aid for accomplishing this goal. Mobility aids including wheelchairs, walkers, canes, and crutches are used by people of all ages with a variety of gait and movement disorders. These aids are especially helpful for persons with unsteady gait or those who are unable to bear weight due to recent injury or weakness. Primary indications for using mobility aids include (1) poor balance in standing, (2) inability to bear weight due to pain or structural damage, and (3) neuromuscular involvement including weakness of the lower extremities or trunk. Ambulatory assistive devices increase the user's base of support, creating a stable platform, which allows for safe ambulation, whereas wheelchairs allow those who are unable to ambulate to be mobile. The purpose of any of these assistive devices is to maximize functional independence and mobility. To accomplish this, physicians and physiatrists are often involved with prescribing these assistive devices. With the many styles and choices to be made today, this can be a difficult decision to make. Ultimately, the selection of an assistive device should depend on the cooperative effort of the physiatrist, physical therapist or athletic trainer, patient, and equipment supplier. This chapter describes the various types and models of assistive devices available and provides insight into how and when these devices should be prescribed. Additionally, we will cover safety considerations and techniques for properly instructing patients in the use of these devices.

DEFINITIONS

Ambulatory Assistive Device

Ambulation (gait) is defined as bipedal locomotion, or walking. An ambulatory assistive device is a hand-held aid used to help the user walk or stand safely. The most common ambulatory assistive devices are listed in Table 1.[1] Additionally, parallel bars are a form of ambulatory assistive device, commonly used in therapy clinics for those who need maximum stability.

Gait Stability

True stability necessitates that the center of gravity be well within the base of support. A larger base of support provides increased stability. Figure 1 shows how

TABLE 1. COMMON AMBULATORY ASSISTIVE DEVICES

Crutches	Canes	Walkers
Platform	Single point	Standard
Axillary	Quad cane	Front-wheeled
Lofstrand (forearm)	Hemicane	Four-wheeled
	Walker with seat	
	Surround walkers	

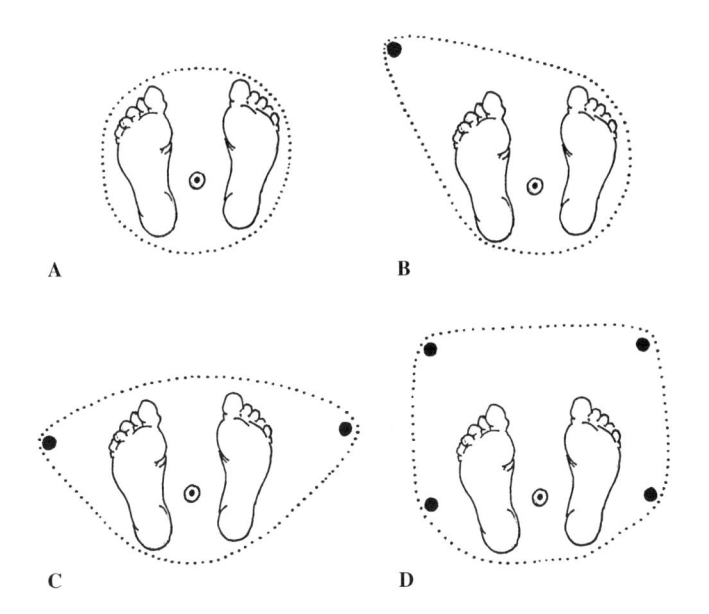

FIGURE 1. Base of support (*dotted line*) with two-legged stance (*A*) and its enlargement with use of a cane (*B*), crutches (*C*), and a walker (*D*). The bulls-eye represents the center of gravity forceline. (From Ogle A: Canes, crutches, walkers, and other ambulation aids. Phys Med Rehabil State Art Rev 14:485–492, 2000, with permission.)

the base of support is enlarged when an assistive device is used for improved balance.[1] Assistive devices increase the base of support, allowing a redistribution of weight within the base of support, and a larger area within which the center of gravity can shift without losing balance.[2] It is readily apparent that some devices provide more stability and support than others.

The primary assistive devices in order of most stable to least stable are:
Parallel bars
Walkers
Axillary crutches
Lofstrand (forearm) crutches
Two canes
One cane

Additionally, a referring physiatrist and therapist must consider the coordination required for the device. Some devices require more coordination than others. Assistive devices, beginning with those requiring the least coordination and progressing to those requiring the most coordination, are as follows:
Parallel bars
Standard walker
Wheeled walker
Cane
Lofstrand crutches (forearm)
Axillary crutches

TYPES OF AMBULATORY ASSISTIVE DEVICES
Canes

These lists demonstrate that, although crutches provide good stability, they may not be the device of choice for a patient who does not possess the coordination to use them properly and safely. Also, keep in mind that these are generalized lists and may not apply to all patients. Each patient has his or her own specific needs, and a therapist or referring physiatrist must ensure that the device chosen safely provides the patient with the greatest freedom of mobility.

As noted, the cane provides little stability compared with other devices; however, it is the most appropriate aid for those needing mild balance correction or a slight load reduction for joint protection. Several styles of single-point canes are available for patients. The standard cane is known as the J-line because of its shape.

Figure 2 shows the variety of single-point canes available. A common variation is the bent cane. This cane allows the force of weight bearing to be transmitted directly over the tip and into the ground. The grips on these canes come in a variety of textures and shapes to enhance control and comfort. A larger contoured grip is often better for patients with arthritic or coordination problems with their upper extremities and hands. A popular modification is the straight-handle cane, which provides the user with a comfortable platform on which to bear weight.

Figure 3 shows the two most common forms of four-point canes, known as quad canes. These canes typically come in two sizes: small base and large base. In the author's clinic, quad canes are most beneficial for those who have slower gait speeds and balance deficits such that a single-point cane does not provide enough support. As gait speed increases, the patient will not firmly plant the legs of the cane down together and the device can become a hindrance, either slowing the patient or causing him or her to trip over the cane itself. At this point, it is often

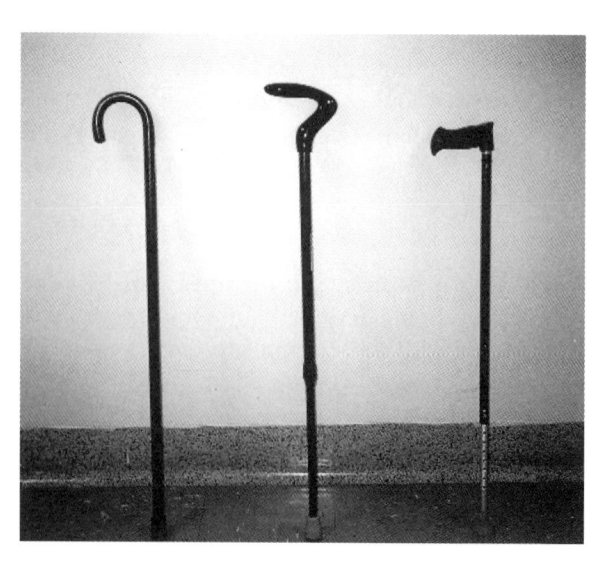

FIGURE 2. Single-point canes: J-line (*left*) and straight-handle variations (*middle* and *right*).

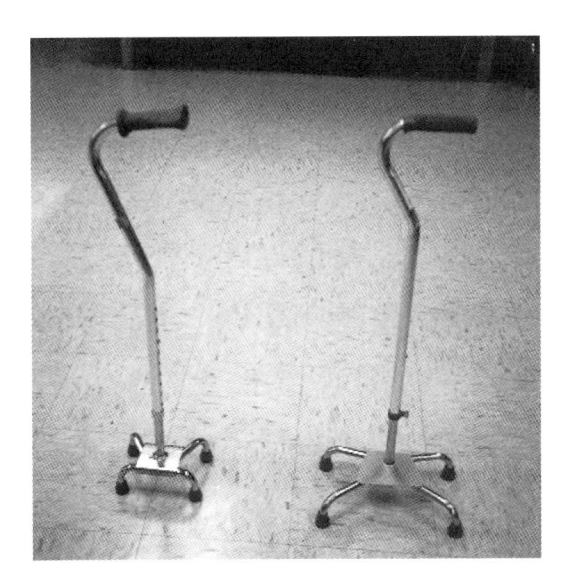

FIGURE 3. Four-point canes: small base quad cane (*left*) and large base quad cane (*right*).

helpful to progress the patient to a single-point cane. Quad canes are often used by patients who cannot use a walker secondary to upper extremity hemiparesis. For a patient recovering from a stroke, the quad cane is usually part of the progression of assistive devices used. The ideal gait progression for these patients is handrail, hemiwalker (discussed later in this chapter), quad cane, and single-point cane.

Unfortunately, many patients use canes that are faulty, are damaged, or are not set at the appropriate height. George and associates found this to be the case in up to 70% of the elderly population.[3] When issuing a cane or any assistive device, it should be inspected for safety and adjusted to fit the user properly. The elbow should be flexed 15–30° when standing upright.[4] This allows the triceps to provide the stability and force needed to bear weight through the arm most efficiently. In order to achieve 15–30° of elbow flexion, the cane should crest at the greater trochanter. Another popular way to measure cane height is by ensuring the cane handle is level with the crease of the wrist with the arm hanging freely at the side. A cane that is too short or tall may cause trunk leaning and will decrease the efficiency of the upper extremity muscles involved in stabilizing the cane.[5] This may result in further discomfort and increased energy expenditure.

Perhaps the most frequently asked question concerning canes is "which hand should I carry it in?" Ideally, the cane should be carried in the hand opposite that of the affected leg (the contralateral side). The placement of the cane on the side opposite the involved lower extremity allows the patient's weight to be shifted toward the stronger side by increasing the base of support on the stronger side. Figure 4 shows how the total force across a hip joint is reduced by almost two thirds when a cane is used to augment the hip abductor muscles and unload the hip joint.[1] Because of this principle, the loss of one pound can relieve the hip of three pounds of pressure. Placing a cane in the contralateral hand gives a large moment

288 Mobility Aids

Without cane

$F_1 \times d = F_2 \times d$
$F_1 \times 1 = 0.85\ BW \times 3$

Hip abductor force (F_1) = 2.55 BW

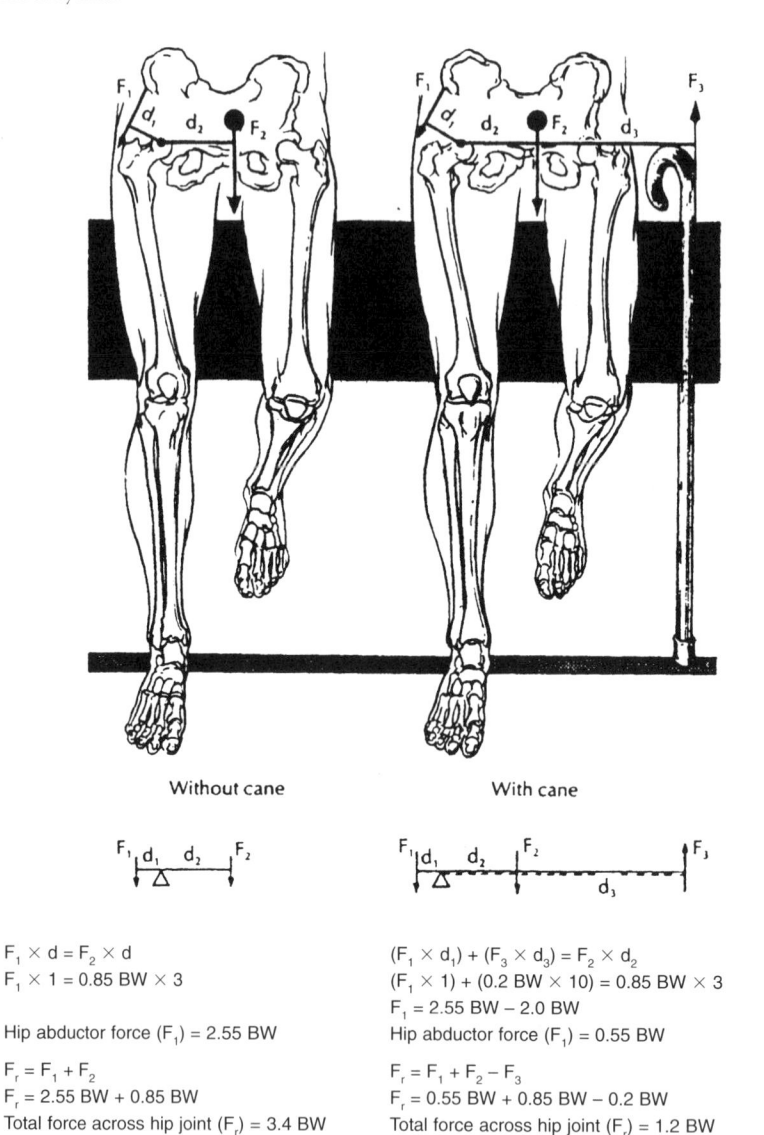

$F_r = F_1 + F_2$
$F_r = 2.55\ BW + 0.85\ BW$
Total force across hip joint (F_r) = 3.4 BW

With cane

$(F_1 \times d_1) + (F_3 \times d_3) = F_2 \times d_2$
$(F_1 \times 1) + (0.2\ BW \times 10) = 0.85\ BW \times 3$
$F_1 = 2.55\ BW - 2.0\ BW$
Hip abductor force (F_1) = 0.55 BW

$F_r = F_1 + F_2 - F_3$
$F_r = 0.55\ BW + 0.85\ BW - 0.2\ BW$
Total force across hip joint (F_r) = 1.2 BW

FIGURE 4. Why is a cane used in the hand *opposite* an affected hip? This figure shows that the total force across a hip joint is reduced by almost two-thirds when a cane is used to augment the hip abductor muscles and unload the hip joint. To simplify the calculations, the assumption is made that equilibrium exists; that is, the counterclockwise and clockwise moments of force must be equal. The moment of force (or torque) is the force (F) times the distance (d) that the force line is away from the axis of rotation. F_1 is the force of the hip abductors; F_2 is the force of gravity acting on the mass of the body, excluding the stance leg (F_2 = 0.85 × body weight [BW]); F_3 is the force that can be applied to a standard cane, about 0.2 BW; d_2 = 3 × d_1; d_3 = 10 × d_1. Implanted force transducers in hip prostheses have demonstrated forces of about 2.5 times body weight during one-leg support, empirically validating some of these calculations. (From Joyce BM, Kirby RL: Canes, crutches and walkers. AFP 43:535–542, 1991, with permission.)

arm between this and the hip joint, which complements the ipsilateral hip abductors and therefore reduces joint load.[6]

There are occasions when limitations such as upper extremity amputations or residual effects of stroke prevent the proper use of canes. In these instances, the cane can still be advantageous to the user for maintaining balance; however, the true benefit of a wider base of support is not accomplished. Interestingly, ipsilateral cane use has been shown to reduce the forces acting on the hip and the muscle activity around the knee.[7,8]

The recommended gait pattern for single cane use is to advance the cane with the involved lower extremity in a normal reciprocal gait pattern. For gait with use of two canes, several gait patterns can be used. The two-point alternating pattern is performed by advancing the left cane with the right leg, and the right cane with the left leg. This pattern maintains reciprocal motion and speed is ensured. In order to reduce the load on one lower extremity, the three-point gait pattern is recommended. The two canes are advanced with the affected lower extremity during swing phase, and they help reduce the load during swing phase of the opposite leg. The four-point pattern is beneficial for increased stability. The sequence for this pattern is left cane, right foot, right cane, left foot. At any given point in this pattern, three of the points are in contact with the ground.[2]

Crutches

The two most common forms of crutches are axillary and forearm. Axillary crutches are used when a patient requires significant reduction in weight bearing, but speed and mobility are still necessary. The various forms of crutches are shown in Figure 5. As mentioned earlier, axillary crutches require significant arm strength and good coordination overall. Some of the important anatomic functions for axillary crutch use include scapular depression to avoid glenohumeral elevation, shoulder adduction endurance to keep the crutch placed close to the chest wall, shoulder flexion and extension for proper forward and backward crutch placement, triceps strength for maintaining elbow extension during crutch weight bearing, and wrist positioning and grip strength for grasping the handpiece.[9]

In the author's experience, many elderly patients are not safe with crutches because of poor balance, poor coordination, and decreased upper extremity strength. It is crucial for the issuing therapist to allow the patient to experiment and try the assistive device before issuing it. Although this is important for all assistive devices, it is especially so for crutches. In general, axillary crutches are for patients who need temporary support to prevent weight bearing while an injury heals. Common uses include ankle sprains, fractures, and foot disorders.

For patients who require a more permanent form of mobility aid, forearm crutches are more appropriate. Forearm crutches, also known as Lofstrand or Canadian crutches, allow excellent mobility while substantially decreasing the weight-bearing load. Again, these crutches require significant coordination, and they may not be appropriate for those with strength or coordination limitations.

The gait patterns used for axillary crutches include the two-, three-, and four-point patterns. The best pattern for complete non–weight bearing is the two-point swing-through pattern. This pattern is performed by moving the crutches together

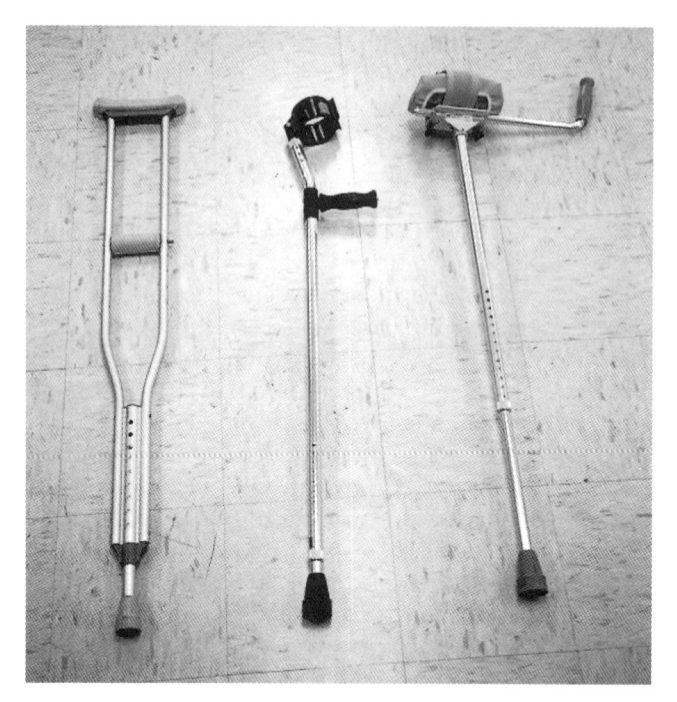

FIGURE 5. Crutches: axillary (*left*), forearm of Lofstran (*middle*), and platform (*right*).

and then advancing the uninvolved limb through, while keeping the involved limb elevated by knee and hip flexion.

A three-point pattern is used when one leg is involved and partial weight bearing is called for. The three-point pattern is performed by first advancing the crutches together, then stepping either to the crutch tips or past them with the involved limb, and finally having the uninvolved foot step forward. The four-point pattern is similar to the cane four-point pattern: right crutch, left foot, left crutch, right foot. This stable form of ambulation allows for maximum stability.

The fit of axillary crutches is important. With the patient in the standing position, the crutches are positioned so that the crutch tips rest on the floor approximately 6 inches away from the toes at a 45° angle. The therapist should be able to place two fingers between the axilla and the top of the crutch pad. The upper end of the axillary crutch should rest on the ribs 5 cm below the axillary fold. Patients should be instructed to bear weight through their arms and not to lean on the top of the crutches. Leaning on the axillary crossbar can lead to axillary artery thrombosis or nerve compression neuropathy of the radial nerve.[10,11]

The height of the handgrip should be adjusted as the height of a cane is. This will allow for 20–30° of elbow flexion when grasping the handgrip. When ambulating with axillary crutches, the lift is provided by the elbow extensors, shoulder depressors, and shoulder adductors. Forearm crutches are fitted in the same manner as axillary crutches with the exception of the cuff. The forearm cuff should be positioned as high as possible on the forearm without interfering with full elbow flexion. The cuff should be tight enough to stay on the arm but loose enough not to bind.

Walkers

Walkers are used to reduce weight bearing on one or both lower extremities and ensure balance. As stated, the walker is the device that provides the most stability. Walkers provide a wide base of support, improve lateral and anterior stability, and allow the upper extremities to transmit body weight to the floor.[12] Over the past three decades, walkers have changed dramatically. Persons needing walkers today can choose from a wide variety of styles, functions, colors, and models. There are walkers with wheels, seats, baskets, and even hand-breaks. Whether the need for a walker is permanent or temporary, a walker should be chosen after actual trials, which take into account living situation, personal needs, and abilities. Walker size is also important. Most walkers are height adjustable, but the width and depth vary with style. The height of the walker should be adjusted, as that of the cane, to yield a bend in the elbow of approximately 20–30°.

The most common standard walker has an aluminum rigid frame with four legs that are adjustable in height. Most of these walkers fold for ease of transport in vehicles. When folded, these walkers can be used as walking aids on stairs, although it is advisable for patients to use a handrail and avoid carrying the walker on stairs, if possible. Walkers are most useful for patients with balance difficulties. Although walkers have their limitations, they are the most stable platform for patients in need of fall prevention. Some disadvantages of walkers include decreased speed, poor patient posture, and danger on stairs. A standard walker and hemiwalker are shown in Figure 6.

The hemiwalker is an excellent assistive device for patients recovering from stroke or those limited to the use of one upper extremity. It provides outstanding stability compared with quad and single-point canes. It is, however, more bulky and sometimes difficult to maneuver. As mentioned, the hemiwalker is typically the first mobile assistive device used by patients in their poststroke gait rehabilitation.

Walkers can be divided into two groups: those that have three points of contact with the floor and those with four points of contact. In the author's experience, the

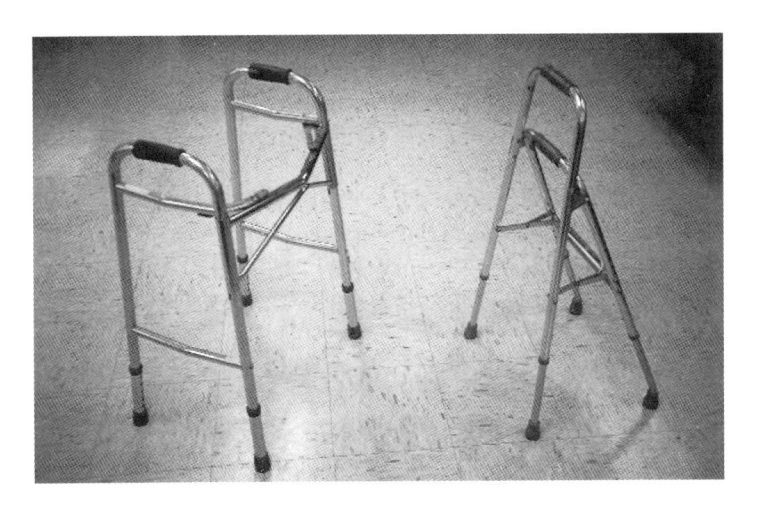

FIGURE 6. Standard walker (*left*) and hemiwalker (*right*).

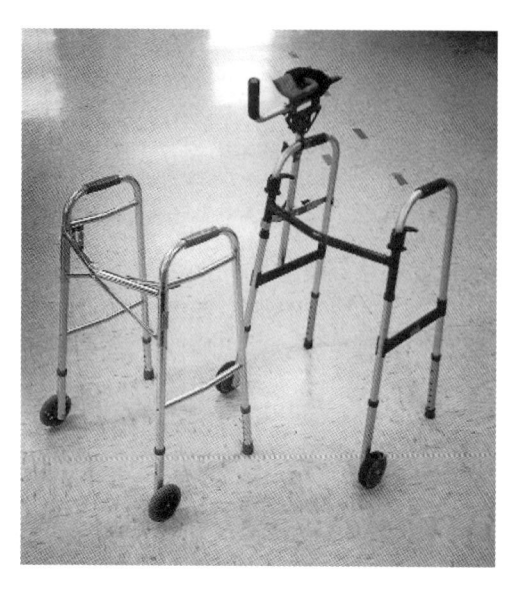

FIGURE 7. Standard front-wheeled walker (*left*) and a variation with a platform handle (*right*).

four-point walker with two wheels on the front is the most widely use in extended care and rehabilitation facilities. This walker affords the patient good stability while allowing him or her to progress without the interruption of picking up the walker each step (Fig. 7). The rear legs of this walker usually have rubber or plastic tips, which can provide good traction or glide, depending on the floor surface. The rubber tips provide excellent traction on tile flooring, which helps prevent falls for those who are not able to control a more mobile all-wheeled walker.[13]

By attaching tennis balls to the rear legs of the walker, patients are able to glide the walker in the facility more easily and more quietly (Fig. 8). Additionally, this inexpensive technique protects the floor from scrapes, which sometimes occur with the hard plastic tips.

Another popular modification in the author's extended care facility has been the use of walker pouches (Fig. 9). These handy attachments allow the user to bring items with them while freeing the hands for control of the walker.

In the past decade, all-wheeled walkers have become popular. These walkers, sometimes called rollators, come in three- and four-wheeled models, and usually have some form of braking system, either hand-activated or weight-bearing activated. The four-wheeled walkers often have a seat and carry basket (Fig. 10). This type of walker allows for better mobility on outdoor surfaces such as asphalt. The hand-activated brakes on these walkers are critical for the control and ability of the walker to support the user. In the author's clinic at a Veterans Affairs hospital in California, the feedback has been overwhelmingly positive on the benefits of these new walkers.

Several recent studies also indicate the value and functionality of these walkers. Bohannon looked at several groups of studies comparing standard two-wheeled walkers to these new all-wheeled walkers. He noted that the wheeled walkers were associated with faster speeds and cadences, lower energy demands, and more

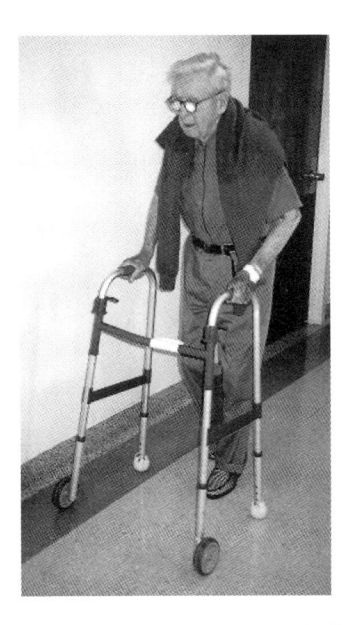

FIGURE 8. Front-wheeled walker fit with tennis balls on the rear legs.

normal-appearing gait. Additionally, patients preferred the rolling walkers.[14] Another study comparing performance of the four-wheeled rollator with a front-wheeled walker, found that healthy subjects, 21–65 years of age, ambulated faster and farther on smooth sidewalk, uneven asphalt, and rough, uneven grass when using the rollator.[15] Mahoney and colleagues found that elderly patients using the rollator had increased stride length and decreased obstacle course times and that they subjectively preferred the rollator over standard front-wheeled walkers.[16]

Results from a questionnaire administered to over 200 veterans has shown that they appreciate several aspects of the four-wheeled walker with seat:

1. It improved control on rough terrain.
2. It allows them to ambulate at a more normal pace.
3. It provides them with a convenient place to rest at any time.
4. They feel more control with the use of hand-brakes.
5. They like the image of themselves with this more modern sleek walker.

Energy Demand

Ambulating with an assistive device has proven to create an increased metabolic demand. Holder and colleagues compared heart rate, blood pressure, perceived exertion, and oxygen cost of non–weight-bearing ambulation using standard walker, axillary crutches, and a wheeled walker.[17] They found that use of any assistive device resulted in an increase in metabolic and cardiovascular responses compared with unassisted ambulation. The subjects in this study were young female physical therapists. Additionally, Holder and associates found that subjects using axillary crutches had the least oxygen costs during non–weight-bearing ambulation compared with using walkers or canes.

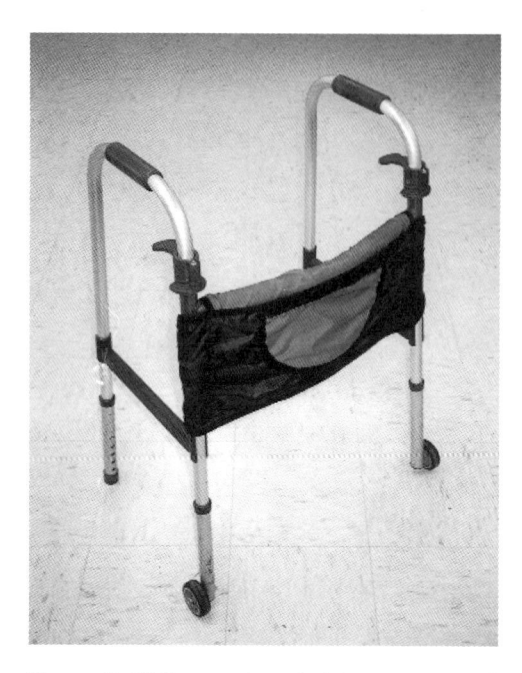

FIGURE 9. Walker equipped with a carry pouch.

A later study used elderly subjects ages 50 to 74. In this study, Foley and coworkers found that ambulation with a standard walker required 212% more oxygen per meter than unassisted ambulation and 104% more oxygen than ambulation with a wheeled walker.[115] They concluded that it may be better to prescribe a wheeled walker for patients with impaired cardiorespiratory systems. This is true in the author's clinic. The front-wheeled walker is much less taxing on the elderly patients in that they do not have to lift it with every step—they simply glide it on the floor.

A number of variables are responsible for the increase in energy demand found when using an assistive device. They include changes in speed of ambulation; prevention of normal arm swing, which may disrupt normal gait biomechanics; and an increased metabolic demand imposed on the upper extremities.[18] The effects of gait speed and energy demand have been studied. Interestingly metabolic demand can be increased by walking more slowly.[19] Because using an assistive device often slows the user, we can assume that this is one reason for the increased energy demand.

In another relevant study, Nielsen and colleagues found that individuals with either normal or pathologic gait appear to self-select the most efficient ambulation speed.[20]

This author has found that individual patients vary extremely in regard to energy demand and fatigue with various assistive devices. For example, an elderly man may walk over 200 feet with a pick-up walker. This same patient may fatigue by 25 feet when trying to use a cane, owing to his tenuous balance, fear of falling, and need to slow and steady himself continuously. Additionally, patients with respiratory disease may be able to ambulate further with the use of a wheeled walker versus no assistive device.

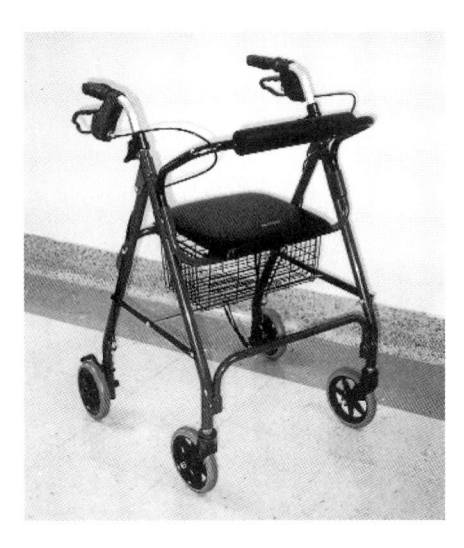

FIGURE 10. Four-wheeled walker with seat.

Many dynamics and factors are at play when attempting to select the correct assistive device for patients. Having patients try various assistive devices under the supervision of a therapist is the best way to choose the most safe and functional device.

Wheelchairs

For patients who lack the ability to ambulate safely or effectively, a wheelchair is the logical assistive device to select. Often, patients who can ambulate for only short distances because of decreased endurance use a combination of ambulatory assistive devices and a wheelchair to maximize their functional mobility. Wheelchairs come in a variety of styles and functions including powered chairs, scooters, reclining chairs, and basic manual chairs. The focus here is on a "standard" wheelchair, and some of the more common varieties of wheelchairs are briefly examined.

The standard wheelchair found in most clinics is made of a collapsible metal frame with a vinyl seat and armrests. The rear wheels are large with narrow, hard rubber or inflatable tires. The front wheels, called casters, rotate to allow for easy turning mobility. A standard wheelchair weighs 35–45 pounds and comes equipped with hand brakes and footrests (Fig. 11). The hand brakes lock the rear wheels to allow the user to transfer safely to and from the chair. The foot rests can either fold up or swing away to allow for safe transfers. Some wheelchairs come with removable or swing-away armrests that allow for a more debilitated patient to slide transfer to or from the chair (Fig. 12).

Popular modifications to these wheelchairs include reclining backrest and elevating legrest (Fig. 13). Another common modification is the one-arm drive. The one-arm drive allows patients with use of only one upper extremity to propel themselves safely in a wheelchair. This is accomplished by adding a rim to the wheel on the patient's functional side, which drives the opposite wheel via an axle.[21] Other possible modifications include:

296   Mobility Aids

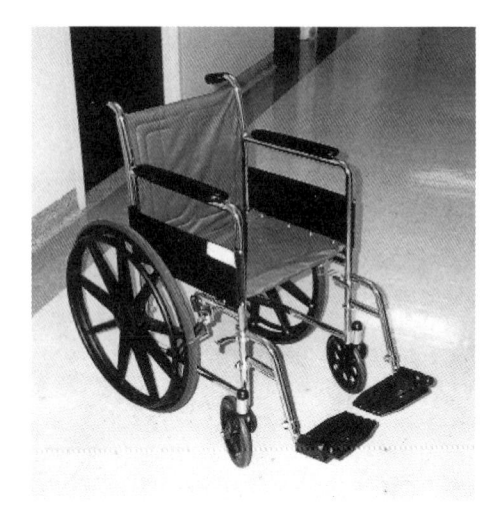

FIGURE 11. A standard wheelchair with hand brakes and footrests.

1. **Heel loops**. These loops on the rear of the footplate prevent the feet from sliding rearward off the plate.
2. **Brake lever extensions**. The extension allows a patient who may be unable to reach the normal brake lever to safely set the brakes independently.
3. **Antitipping extensions**. These project from the rear of the frame and prevent the chair from tipping over backward (Fig. 14).

Patients lacking the strength or coordination to propel a wheelchair often benefit from a motorized scooter or wheelchair (Fig 15). Powered chairs are normally controlled by means of a toggle switch, although some have specialized controls such as a mouthstick, which can be used by quadriplegic patients. Although pow-

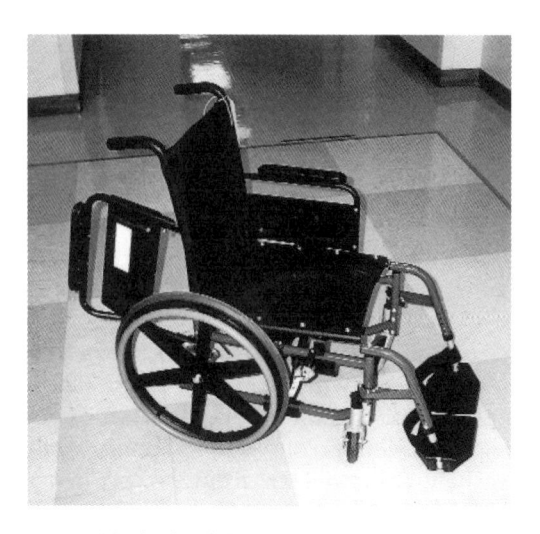

FIGURE 12. A wheelchair with swing-away armrests.

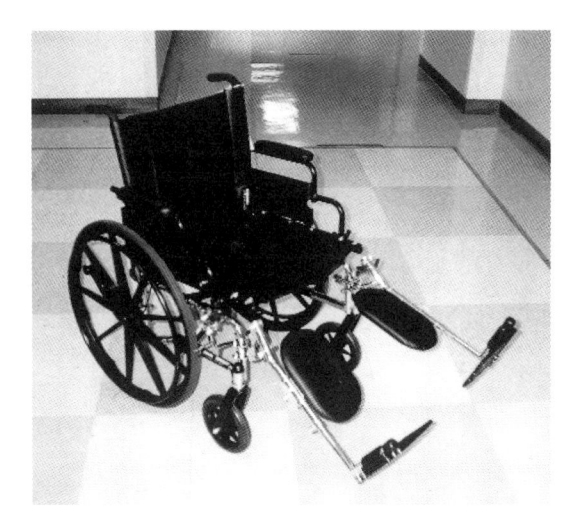

FIGURE 13. A wheelchair with elevating legrests.

ered chairs and scooters are heavy and difficult to transport, they allow a patient to regain independence in community mobility. Recently, a powered chair that can extend the user to a standing position has been developed.

Wheelchair Prescription

Knowing what type of wheelchair to order and selecting appropriate accessories can be difficult. The main considerations in choosing a wheelchair are:
1. Measurement of the wheelchair and parts to facilitate good posture, comfort and mobility
2. Easy storage and transport
3. Ability to provide a close approach for transfers to bed, toilet, or car
4. Ability of the patient to be independent and safe with self-propulsion and functional activities from the chair
5. Ease of mobility in the home

Wheelchair Size

Seat Depth. The seat depth should be 2–3 inches less than the distance to the patient's popliteal crease. This allows enough support for the thigh while not interfering with the popliteal area.

Seat Width. The seat width should be 2 inches wider than the patient's hips. Allowing 1 inch on each side of the hips leaves enough room for the greater trochanters.[22]

Seat Height. Seat height should allow for comfort and proper alignment of the hips and knees. Foot pedal adjustment should allow for a 1-inch space between the thigh and the seat edge. It is important that the footrest not be too high in order to maximize even weight distribution through the thigh and buttocks area. Foot pedals should be at least 2 inches from the ground to prevent contact on ramps or uneven terrain. Seat height can also be adjusted by use of cushions. Cushions come in a variety of materials and sizes.

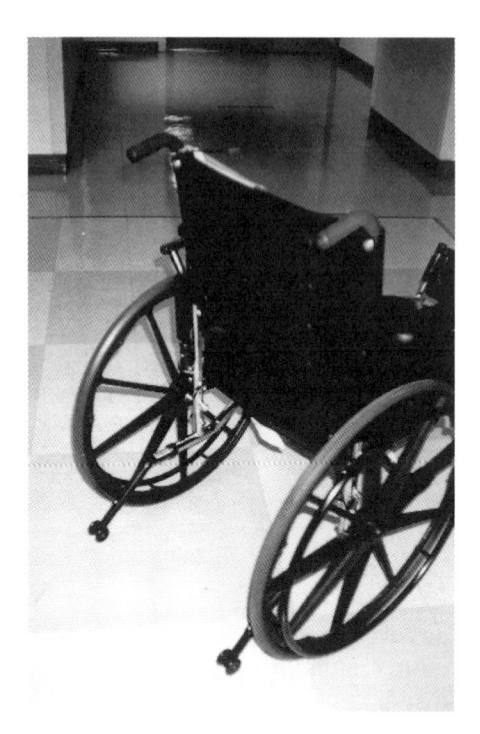

FIGURE 14. A wheelchair with antitipping extensions.

Consideration should also be given to the distance between the armrest and the flexed elbow. The elbows should rest comfortably without causing elevation of the scapulae or slouching posture.

Back Height. The seat back should be 3–4 inches below the axilla to allow for free arm movement. Exceptions to this include reclining chairs and chairs for those who lack trunk and head stability.

Wheelchair Mobility. Independent mobility in a wheelchair requires strength and endurance in the shoulder muscle groups. In a wheelchair user, ground reaction forces are no longer available for transmission in performing trunk and upper extremity activities.[23] Shoulder stabilizers, previously involved with the shoulder girdle, now become prime movers. This increases the vulnerability of the pectoralis major, supraspinatus, and other muscles to fatigue and possibly injury.[24] Therefore, it is important to have wheelchair patients perform a strengthening and endurance program. When starting patients in wheelchair propulsion, a gradual progression should be followed: smooth level ground, rough ground, inclines, and finally curbs.

CONCLUSION

In helping patients regain maximum levels of function, physiatrists and therapists are called on to prescribe and issue mobility aids. Unfortunately, many patients receive little or no professional advice in acquiring an assistive device. The patient's abilities and functional requirements should be correctly matched with the appropriate mobility device. As our elderly population grows, this becomes

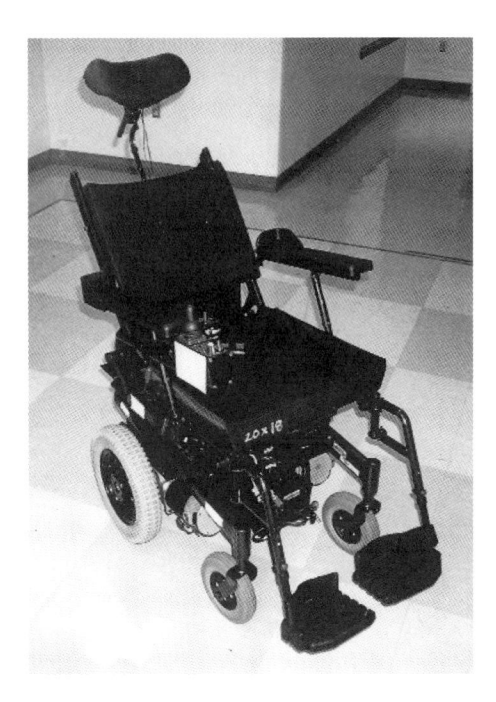

FIGURE 15. A powered wheelchair with controllable reclining feature and a toggle control.

increasingly important. Falls and decreased mobility are a major concern for the elderly. Statistics on falls and resulting injuries are alarming. The incidence of falls in the community-dwelling elderly is 25% at age 70 and 35% after age 75.[25] Although death is a less frequent consequence of falling, complications caused by falls are the leading cause of death from injury in men and women older than age 65.[26] Given the risk and associated emotional and monetary costs, falls are of significant concern and should be aggressively prevented. The correct use of appropriate assistive devices is one of the best preventive measures.

Consideration should also be given to patient preference. The use of an assistive device can sometimes be perceived negatively by patients, especially the elderly. Therapists encounter this often with patients who refuse to use a particular device because of the image of frailty and dependence it portrays. Today, therapists have more options to present patients as they work toward the common goal of improved gait safety and mobility. With new products and technology available, as well as increased emphasis on cost-effectiveness, the evaluation and treatment of gait disorders will continue to evolve.[27]

REFERENCES

1. Joyce BM, Kirby RL: Canes, crutches and walkers. AFP 43:535–542, 1991.
2. Minor MD, Minor SD: Patient Care Skills, 2nd ed. Norwalk, Appleton & Lange, 1990, p 223.
3. George J, Binns VE, Clayden AD, et al: Aids and adaptations for the elderly at home: Underprovided, underused, and undermaintained. Br Med J 296:1365–1366, 1988.
4. Hartigan C, Morgan RF, Hunter FP Jr, et al: Ergonomics of support cane handles. J Burn Care Rehabil 8:150–154, 1987.

5. Sainsbury R, Mulley GP: Walking sticks used by the elderly. Br Med J 284:1751, 1982.
6. Blount M: Don't throw away the cane. J Bone Joint Surg 38A:695–708, 1956.
7. Edwards BG: Contralateral and ipsilateral cane usage by patients with total knee or hip replacement. Arch Phys Med Rehabil 67:734–740, 1986.
8. Vargo MM, Robinson LR, Nicholas JJ. Contralateral vs ipsilateral cane use. Effects on muscles crossing the knee joint. Am J Phys Med Rehabil 71:170–176, 1992.
9. Shankar K, et al: Anatomic considerations: Therapeutic and exercise mobility aids. Phys Med Rehabil State Art Rev 10:580–581, 1996.
10. Brooks AL, Fowler SB: Axillary artery thrombosis after prolonged use of crutches. J Bone Joint Surg 46A:863–864, 1964.
11. Rudin LN, Levine L: Bilateral compression of radial nerve (crutch paralysis). Phys Ther Rev 31:229-231, 1951.
12. O'Sullivan SB, Schmitz TJ: Physical Rehabilitation: Assessment and Treatment, 2nd ed. Philadelphia, FA Davis, 1988, pp 293–306.
13. Nabizadeh SA, Hardee TB, Towler MA, et al. Technical considerations in the selection and performance of walkers. J Burn Care Rehabil 14:182–188, 1993.
14. Bohannon RW: Gait performance with wheeled and standard walkers. Percept Mot Skills 85:1185–1186, 1997.
15. Cornerly H, Garcia J, Pereda A: Comparing ambulation with a rollator walker and a two wheeled rolling walker [abstract]. Phys Ther 77:S72, 1997.
16. Mahoney J, Eudardy R, Carnes M: A comparison of two-wheeled walker and a three-wheeled walker in a geriatric population. J Am Geriatr Soc Mar 40:208–212, 1992.
17. Holder CG, Haskvitz EM, Weltman A: The effects of assistive devices on the oxygen cost, cardiovascular stress, and perception of nonweightbearing ambulation. J Orthop Sports Phys Ther 18:537–542, 1993.
18. Foley MP, Prax B, Crowell R, Boone T: Effects of assistive devices on cardiorespiratory demands in older adults. Phys Ther 76:1313–1319, 1996.
19. Blessey RL, Hislop HJ, Waters RL, Antonelli D: Metabolic energy cost of unrestrained walking. Phys Ther 56:1019–1024, 1976.
20. Nielsen DH, Shurr DG, Golden JC, et al: Comparison of energy cost and gait efficiency during ambulation in below-knee amputees using different prosthetic feet: A preliminary report. J Prosthet Orthot 1:23-30, 1988.
21. Lawton EB: Activities of Daily Living for Physical Rehabilitation. New York, McGraw-Hill, 1963, p 265.
22. Trombly CA, Scott AD: Occupational Therapy for Physical Dysfunction. Baltimore, Williams & Wilkins, 1977, p 385.
23. Sherman MO: Anatomic Considerations in the Prescription of Therapeutic Exercises and Mobility Aids. Phys Med Rehabil State Art Rev 10:581, 1996.
24. Mulroy SJ, Gronley JK, Newsam CJ, Perry J: Electromyographic activity of shoulder muscles during wheelchair propulsion by paraplegic persons. Arch Phys Med Rehabil 77:187–193, 1996.
25. Campbell AJ, Reinken J, Allan BC, et al: Falls in old age: A study of frequency and clinical factors. Age Aging 10:264–270, 1981.
26. Sattin RW: Falls among older persons: A public health perspective. Annu Rev Public Health 13:489–508, 1992.
27. Alexander NB: Gait disorders in older adults. J Am Geriatr Soc 44:434–451, 1996.

Index

Entries in **boldface** type signify complete chapters.

Acne vulgaris, ultraviolet therapy, 84
Acromioclavicular joint
    intra-articular injections, 246
    mobilization, 191
Acupuncture, **227–226**
    acupoints
        characteristics, 227–228
        Chengshan, 231
        Hegu, 229–230
        Huantiao, 231
        Sanyanglo, 231
        Taichong, 230
        Tiaokou, 231
        Tiaoshan, 231
        Weichung, 231
        Yanglingquan, 231
        Yaotiew, 231
        Zusani, 230
    auricular acupuncture, 235–236
    electrical. *See* Electrical acupuncture
    functional magnetic resonance imaging, 234–235
    historical background, 5–6, 227
    indications
        analgesia, 232–233
        musculoskeletal disorders, 229–232
        osteoarthritis, 232
        phantom limb pain, 233
        spinal cord injury, 234
        stroke therapy, 233–234
    massage, 157
    neuromodulation, 228–229
    scalp acupuncture, 235
    sensations on needling, 228
Ai chi. *See* Aquatic therapy
Ambulatory assistive devices, **284–299**
    cane, 286–287, 289
    crutches, 289–290
    definition, 284
    energy demand in use, 293–295
    falls in elderly, 299
    gait stability, 284–286
    indications, 284
    types, 284
    walker, 291–293
    wheelchair
        designs, 295–297
        prescription, 297
        size, 297–298

Analgesia
    acupuncture, 232–233
    magnet therapy, 90
    superficial heat therapy, 8
Anesthetic injection
    nerve characteristics, 240–241
    perineural injection
        common peroneal nerve, 253
        lateral femoral cutaneous nerve, 252
        median nerve at wrist, 251–252
        posterior tibial nerve at ankle, 254
        radial nerve block at humerus, 249–250
        safety, 249
        sciatic nerve, 252
        tibial nerve at knee, 252–253
        ulnar nerve at elbow, 250–251
    site of injection, 241
    structure of anesthetics, 241–242
    types and features of anesthetics, 240
Angina, transcutaneous electrical nerve stimulation, 111
Ankle, joint mobilization, 189
Aquatic therapy, **55–73**
    ai chi, 69
    Bad Ragaz ring method, 66–67
    Burdenko method, 69
    contraindications and precautions, 62–64
    exercise therapy
        equipment, 62
        exercise types, 61
        goals, 60
        indications, 59–60
        progression, 60–61
    Halliwick method, principles of instruction, 67–68
    historical background, 55
    immersion physiology
        circulatory system effects, 58
        conditioning effects, 59
        musculoskeletal system effects, 59
        pulmonary system effects, 58–59
    pool selection and maintenance, 64–65
    water properties. *See* Water
    Watsu, 65–66
Aromatherapy, with massage therapy, 151
Assistive devices, **261–283**. *See also* Ambulatory assistive devices
    assessment of patients, 261–262
    community functioning devices

assistive devices (continued)
  power scooter, 280
  reacher, 280
  table of devices, 281–282
  vision impairment, 282
 custom fabricated adaptations and modifications, 282–283
 home management devices
  clocks, 275
  spinal cord injury, 275–277
  table of devices, 276
  typing aids, 275
 leisure activity devices
  gardening, 278
  golf, 278
 safety and home accessibility devices
  figure-ground discrimination, 272, 274
  smell sensation, 274
  table of devices, 273–274
  wheelchair ramp, 274–275
 self-care tasks and devices
  bathing, 265
  check-off list for task completion, 268
  definition, 262
  dressing, 263–264
  feeding, 263
  figure-ground discrimination of food, 272
  halo vest, 268–269
  health management, 266–267, 272
  hygiene and grooming, 264–265
  joint pain, 272
  meal preparation, 265–266
  spinal cord injury, 268–269
  stroke, 269–271
  toileting, 264, 271
  traumatic brain injury, 262, 268, 272
 vocational activity devices
  ergonomic modifications, 278–280
  one-handed performance, 277
ASTM. *See* Augmented soft tissue mobilization
Athletic taping
 application difficulties and tips for taping, 202–204
 historical background, 194
 tape types, 194, 195–196
 uses, 194–195
Augmented soft tissue mobilization (ASTM), overview, 148
Auricular acupuncture, overview, 235–236

Bad Ragaz ring method. *See* Aquatic therapy
Bathing, assistive devices, 265
Beam nonuniformity ratio, ultrasound, 20
Biceps brachii tendon, corticosteroid injection, 256

Biofeedback, **209–226**
 conroversies, 224
 contraindications, 223
 definition, 209–210
 historical background, 4, 209, 211
 indications
  general rehabilitation, 222
  myofascial pain, 221
  overview, 223
  urinary incontinence, 222–223
 insurance reimbursement, 224
 modalities
  electroencephalography, 212
  electromyography, 211–212, 214, 221–223
  heart rate, 213
  respiration, 213–214
  skin conductance, 212
  temperature, 213
 prescription, 225
 protocol establishment, 214–215
 psychophysiology overview, 210–211
 resources, 225
 training courses
  relaxation-based training, 215–219
  surface electromyography biofeedback, 220–221
Bulimia, massage therapy, 149
Buoyancy, water, 56
Burdenko method. *See* Aquatic therapy

Cane. *See* Ambulatory assistive devices
Chipped ice bag, cryotherapy, 51
Chronic obstructive pulmonary disease (COPD), exercise prescription, 133
Codetron, overview, 113–114
Common peroneal nerve, perineural injection block, 253
Contraction, muscle
 concentric, 129
 eccentric, 129
 isokinetic, 129
 isometric, 128
 isotonic, 128–129
 plyometric, 129
Contrast bath
 contraindications and precautions, 72
 indications, 72
 procedures, 72–73
COPD. *See* Chronic obstructive pulmonary disease
Corticosteroid injection
 bursal injection
  greater trochanter bursitis, 258
  olecranon bursitis, 257
  pes anserine bursa, 258
  subacromial bursitis, 255
 mechanism of action, 242–243

peritendinous injection
  biceps brachii tendon, 256
  de Quervain's tenosynovitis, 258
  lateral epicondyle, 256–257
  rotator cuff tendon, 255
  safety, 254–255
  trigger finger, 258
trigger point injections, 259
types of steroids, 242
Crutches. *See* Ambulatory assistive devices
Cryotherapy, **47–53**
  administration
    chipped ice bag, 51
    gel ice pack, 50–51
    ice massage, 51
    iced bath immersion, 52
    iced towels, 51–52
    vapocoolant spray, 47, 49, 52–53
  conduction, 47
  contraindications, 49
  historical background, 47
  indications, 48–49
  insurance reimbursement, 53
  mechanisms of action, 47–48
  range of motion effects, 49–50

Deep heat, **18–34**. *See also* Microwave diathermy; Short-wave diathermy; Ultrasound
  diathermy overview, 2–3, 18
  historical background, 2–3
Density, water, 56
de Quervain's tenosynovitis, corticosteroid injection, 258
Diabetes
  exercise prescription, 133–134
  neuropathy, magnet therapy, 93
Diathermy. *See* Microwave diathermy; Short-wave diathermy
Drag, water, 57
Dressing, assistive devices, 263–264
Duty cycle, ultrasound, 19

EEG. *See* Electroencephalography
Effective radiating area, ultrasound, 20
Elbow
  intra-articular injections, 246–247
  joint mobilization, 188
Electrical acupuncture
  outcomes analysis, 112
  percutaneous electrical nerve stimulation, 112–113
Electroencephalography (EEG), biofeedback, 212
Electromyography (EMG), biofeedback, 211–212, 214, 220–223
Electrotherapy, **98–115**. *See also* Codetron; Electrical acupuncture; H-wave; Inferential current therapy; Neuromuscular stimulation; Transcutaneous electrical nerve stimulation
  historical background, 98
  interpulse interval, 99–100
  outcomes analysis with visual analog scale, 98–99
  pulse duration, 99–100
  pulse parameters, 100–101
  specifications for different modalities, 101
EMG. *See* Electromyography
Ergonomic modifications, assistive devices, 278–280
Exercise. *See* Therapeutic exercise

Feeding, assistive devices, 263
Flow, water, 57
Fluidotherapy, superficial heat therapy, 15–16
Fluoromethane. *See* Vapocoolant spray
fMRI. *See* Functional magnetic resonance imaging
Forearm, joint mobilization, 189
Fracture, magnet therapy, 94–95
Functional magnetic resonance imaging (fMRI), acupuncture studies, 234–235

Gardening, assistive devices, 278
Gel ice pack, cryotherapy, 50–51
Gel pack, superficial heat therapy, 16
General rehabilitation, biofeedback, 222
Glenohumeral joint, intra-articular injections, 245–246
Golf, assistive devices, 278
Greater trochanter bursitis, corticosteroid injection, 258
Grooming, assistive devices, 264–265

Halliwick method. *See* Aquatic therapy
Halo vest, assistive devices, 268–269
Heart rate, biofeedback, 213
Heating pad, superficial heat therapy, 16
Heat therapy. *See* Deep heat; Superficial heat
Heat transfer
  conduction, 7
  convection, 8
  conversion, 8
Hip
  intra-articular injections, 248–249
  joint mobilization, 189
Historical background, physical modalities, **1–6**
Hot pack, superficial heat therapy, 11–12
Hubbard tanks. *See* Hydrotherapy
H-wave, overview, 113
Hydrocortisone, phonophoresis, 43–44
Hydrostatic pressure, water, 56–57
Hydrotherapy, **55–73**
  contraindications and precautions, 70–71

Hydrotherapy (continued)
    contrast bath
        contraindications and precautions, 72
        indications, 72
        procedures, 72–73
    disinfection of tanks, 71
    duration, 70
    entries, 70
    historical background, 55, 73
    Hubbard tanks, 70
    immersion physiology
        circulatory system effects, 58
        conditioning effects, 59
        musculoskeletal system effects, 59
        pulmonary system effects, 58–59
    pulsed lavage
        advantages, 71–72
        contraindications and precautions, 72
        overview, 71
    sitz bath, 73
    temperature, 70
    water properties. *See* Water
    whirlpool baths, 70
    wound healing, 69
Hygiene, assistive devices, 264–265
Hyperemia, superficial heat therapy, 9

Inferential current therapy, overview, 114
Infrared lamp, superficial heat therapy, 12–14
Injection techniques, **239–260**
    anesthetic injection
        nerve characteristics, 240–241
        site of injection, 241
        structure of anesthetics, 241–242
        types and features of anesthetics, 240
    bursal injection
        greater trochanter bursitis, 258
        olecranon bursitis, 257
        pes anserine bursa, 258
        subacromial bursitis, 255
    corticosteroid injection
        mechanism of action, 242–243
        trigger point injections, 259
        types of steroids, 242
    intra-articular injections
        acromioclavicular joint, 246
        contraindications, 244
        elbow joint, 246–247
        glenohumeral joint, 245–246
        hand interphalangeal joint, 248
        hip joint, 248–249
        knee joint, 249
        technique, 244
        temporomandibular joint, 244–245
        wrist joint, 247–248
    nerve block, 240

Injection techniques (continued)
    perineural injection
        common peroneal nerve, 253
        lateral femoral cutaneous nerve, 252
        median nerve at wrist, 251–252
        posterior tibial nerve at ankle, 254
        radial nerve block at humerus, 249–250
        safety, 249
        sciatic nerve, 252
        tibial nerve at knee, 252–253
        ulnar nerve at elbow, 250–251
    peripheral injection, 243–244
    peritendinous injection
        biceps brachii tendon, 256
        de Quervain's tenosynovitis, 258
        lateral epicondyle, 256–257
        rotator cuff tendon, 255
        safety, 254–255
        trigger finger, 258
    soft tissue injection, 240
    technique
        needle insertion, 239
        patient positioning and relaxation, 239
        skin preparation, 239
Insurance. *See* Reimbursement
Intensity, ultrasound, 19–21
Interphalangeal joint, intra-articular injections, 248
Interstitial cystitis, transcutaneous electrical nerve stimulation, 110
Iontophoresis, **37–44**
    application principles, 40
    factors affecting iontophoretic transport
        continuous versus pulsed current, 39
        current strength, 38
        electro-osmotic transport, 39
        ionic strength, 38
        pH of vehicle, 38
        physiologic factors, 39
        solute concentration, 38
    historical background, 37
    indications, 39–40, 42
    instrumentation, 40–41
    ions and polarity, 40
    mechanism of action, 37–38
    principles, 37

Joint mobilization, **177–192**
    articulary movement, Maitland's grading system, 183–184
    case study, 185–187
    compression, 180
    contraindiations, 183
    definition, 177
    direction of treatment, 181, 182
    dysfunction philosophy, 177–178

Joint mobilization (continued)
  examination, 184–185
  exercise prescription, 192
  historical background, 177, 192
  immobilization effects on joint
    bone, 179
    cartilage, 178
    joint capsule, 178
    ligaments and tendons, 178–179
    muscle, 179
    synovium, 178
  indications, 183
  manipulation comparison, 177
  movement classification for joints, 179
  planes of motion, 180
  positions of joint, 180
  specific joint positions
    acromioclavicular joint, 191
    ankle, 189
    elbow, 188
    fingers, 188
    forearm, 189
    hip, 189
    knee, 189
    scapulothoracic joint, 190–191
    shoulder girdle, 190
    sternoclavicular joint, 191–192
    thumb, 188
    wrist, 188
  technique
    communication with patient, 181
    direction of treatment, 182
    mobilization, 182
    Mulligan techniques, 182–183
    patient positioning, 181
    slack uptake, 182
    stabilization, 182
    testing, 182
    therapist positioning, 181–182
  traction stages, 179–180

Kinesio taping
  application difficulties and tips for taping, 202–204
  historical background, 198–199, 204
  tape properties, 201–202
  uses, 194, 199–200
Knee
  intra-articular injections, 249
  joint mobilization, 189

Lactic acid, accumulation in blood, 121–122
Laser therapy, **77–85**
  historical background, 84
  indications, 84–85
  laser types, 84

Lateral epicondyle, corticosteroid injection, 256–257
Lateral femoral cutaneous nerve, perineural injection block, 252
Low back pain
  magnet therapy, 94
  spinal traction contraindication, 164
  transcutaneous electrical nerve stimulation, 108–109
Lymphdema, massage therapy, 149

Magnet therapy, **87–96**
  clinical uses
    diabetic neuropathy, 93
    fracture, 94–95
    indications, 95
    literature review, 91–95
    localized musculoskeletal pain, 91
    low back pain, 94
    migraine, 91, 93
    multiple sclerosis, 90, 91
    nerve regeneration, 90
    neurogenic bowel, 93
    osteoarthritis, 94
    pain reduction, 90
    postpolio pain, 93–94
    sleep, 93
    wound and ulcer healing, 95
  contraindications, 95
  delivery systems
    commercial products, 89–90
    permanent static magnet therapy, 89
    pulsed electromagnetic field therapy, 89
  historical background, 4–5, 87
  mechanisms, 87–88
  physics
    fields and measurement, 88–89
    poles, 88
    right hand rule, 88
  transcranial magnetic stimulation, 96
Massage, **143–158**
  contraindications, 157–158
  definition, 143
  historical background, 3, 143–144, 158
  hospitalized patient benefits, 149
  ice massage, 51
  mechanism of action, 144–145
  studies
    abdominal massage, 147
    aromatherapy, 151
    atopic dermatitis, 149
    augmented soft tissue mobilization, 148
    bulimia, 149
    caregivers, 150
    chair massage, 151
    infants, 145–146

Massage (continued)
  lymphdema, 149
  pain treatment, 146
  pregnancy, 147–148
  pulmonary and critical care patients, 146–147
  rheumatoid arthritis, 150
  smoking cessation studies, 148–149
  spasticity, 149
  sports massage, 149
  wounds and burns, 150
  types
    acupuncture, 157
    classic Western massage, 152–153
    connective tissue massage, 156
    cross-fiber friction massage, 154–155
    manual lymph drainage, 155–156
    myofascial release, 153
    reflexology, 157
    Rolfing, 153–154
    selection of technique, 151–152
    shiatsu, 157
Meal preparation, assistive devices, 265–266
Median nerve, perineural injection block at wrist, 251–252
Microwave diathermy (MWD)
  contraindications, 33–34
  historical background, 31
  indications, 33
  instrumentation, 33
  overview, 18, 30–31
Migraine, magnet therapy, 91, 93
Mobility aid. *See* Ambulatory assistive devices
MS. *See* Multiple sclerosis
Multiple sclerosis (MS), magnet therapy, 90, 91
MWD. *See* Microwave diathermy
Myofascial pain, biofeedback, 221

Neonatal jaundice, ultraviolet therapy, 84
Neurogenic bowel, magnet therapy, 93
Neuromuscular stimulation
  combination therapy, 103
  contraindications and precautions, 102
  electrical parameters, 102
  indications, 101, 102, 103
  muscle fiber recruitment, 101–102
Neuropathic pain, transcutaneous electrical nerve stimulation, 110–111
Nitric oxide (NO), exercise response, 125
NO. *See* Nitric oxide

Obesity, exercise prescription, 135
Olecranon bursitis, corticosteroid injection, 257
Osteoarthritis
  acupuncture, 232
  Codetron treatment, 113–114
  magnet therapy, 94

Pain control. *See* Analgesia
Paraffin bath
  superficial heat therapy, 14–15
Parkinson's disease (PD), exercise prescription, 134
PD. *See* Parkinson's disease
PENS. *See* Percutaneous electrical nerve stimulation
Percutaneous electrical nerve stimulation (PENS), overview, 112–113
Peripheral vascular disease (PVD), exercise prescription, 134
Pes anserine bursa, corticosteroid injection, 258
Phantom limb pain, acupuncture, 233
Phonophoresis, **37–44**
  applications, 42–43, 44
  contraindications, 43
  definition, 42
  equipment, 43
  historical background, 42
  hydrocortisone delivery, 43–44
  mechanism of action, 42
  piezoelectric effect, 42
Piezoelectric effect
  phonophoresis, 42
  ultrasound, 21
Posterior tibial nerve, perineural injection block at ankle, 254
Postoperative pain, transcutaneous electrical nerve stimulation, 108, 111
Postpolio pain, magnet therapy, 93–94
Power scooter, assistive devices, 280
Psoriasis, ultraviolet therapy, 83–84
Pulsed lavage
  advantages, 71–72
  contraindications and precautions, 72
  overview, 71
PVD. *See* Peripheral vascular disease

Radial nerve, perineural injection block at humerus, 249–250
Range of motion (ROM)
  cryotherapy effects, 49–50
  definition, 121
  exercises, 127–128
  superficial heat therapy with exercises, 9–10
Reacher, assistive devices, 280
Reflexology, overview, 157
Reflex sympathetic dystrophy (RSD), contrast bath, 1
Reimbursement
  biofeedback, 224
  cryotherapy, 53
  therapeutic exercise, 137–138
Relaxation-based training, biofeedback, 215–219
Respiration, biofeedback, 213–214

Rheumatoid arthritis
    exercise prescription, 135
    massage therapy, 150
    superficial heat, 1, 2
Rigid proprioceptive taping
    application difficulties and tips for taping, 202–204
    historical background, 196–197, 204
    tape types, 194, 198
    uses, 194, 197–198
ROM. *See* Range of motion
Rotator cuff tendon, corticosteroid injection, 255
RSD. *See* Reflex sympathetic dystrophy

Scalp acupuncture, overview, 235
Scapulothoracic joint, mobilization, 190–191
Sciatic nerve, perineural injection block, 252
Shiatsu, overview, 157
Short-wave diathermy (SWD)
    capacitive versus inductive applications, 32
    contraindications, 33–34
    historical background, 31
    indications, 33
    instrumentation, 32–33
    overview, 18, 30–31
Sitz bath. *See* Hydrotherapy
Skin conductance, biofeedback, 212
Sleep, magnet therapy, 93
Smoking cessation, massage studies, 148–149
Spasticity
    massage therapy, 149
    superficial heat therapy, 8–9
Specific gravity, water, 56
Specific heat capacity, water, 57
Spinal cord injury
    acupuncture, 234
    assistive devices, 268–269, 275–277
Spinal traction, **161–174**
    contraindications and precautions, 163–164, 173
    controversies, 170–172
    definition, 161
    historical background, 3–4, 161–162
    indications, 162–163
    literature review, 172–173
    methodology
        autotraction, 169
        cervical traction, 168–169
        continuous traction, 165–166
        gravity tration, 166
        home traction, 169–170
        inversion traction, 166
        lumbar traction on table, 167–168
        manual traction, 164–165, 174
        motorized traction, 166–167
        positional traction, 165

Spinal traction (continued)
        prone pelvic traction, 168
    safety, 163
    soft tissue stretching, 174
Sternoclavicular joint, mobilization, 191–192
Stroke
    acupuncture therapy, 233–234
    assistive devices, 269–271
Subacromial bursitis, corticosteroid injection, 255
Superficial heat, **7–17**
    adjunct therapy, 7, 16–17
    contraindications, 10–11
    delivery
        fluidotherapy, 15–16
        gel pack, 16
        heating pad, 16
        hot pack, 11–12
        infrared lamp, 12–14
        paraffin bath, 14–15
    heat transfer
        conduction, 7
        convection, 8
        conversion, 8
    historical background, 1–2, 7
    indications
        analgesia, 8
        hyperemia, 9
        range of motion and stretching, 9–10
        spasticity, 8–9
    temperature range, 11
Supportive taping. *See* Rigid proprioceptive taping
SWD. *See* Short-wave diathermy

Taping, **194–205**. *See* Athletic taping; Kinesio taping; Rigid proprioceptive taping
Temperature, biofeedback, 213
Temporomandibular joint, intra-articular injections, 244–245
TENS. *See* Transcutaneous electrical nerve stimulation
Therapeutic exercise, **121–138**
    aquatic exercise. *See* Aquatic therapy
    endurance training, 131
    energy production during exercise, 121
    flexibility training and stretching, 127
    historical background, 4
    lactic acid accumulation in blood, 121–122
    muscle contractions
        concentric, 129
        eccentric, 129
        isokinetic, 129
        isometric, 128
        isotonic, 128–129
        plyometric, 129

Therapeutic exercise (continued)
  physiologic response
    cardiovascular system, 123–124
    endocrine response, 126
    gastrointestinal system, 123
    hematologic response, 126
    muscle, 122
    nervous system, 122–123
    psychological response, 126
    pulmonary system, 124
    renal system, 124–125
    reproductive system, 125
    vascular response, 125
  prescription
    cardiac patients, 132
    children, 136
    chronic obstructive pulmonary disease, 133
    diabetes, 133–134
    elderly, 135–136
    frequency, 131–132
    mode, 132
    musculoskeletal conditions, 135
    neurologic disorders, 134
    obesity, 135
    perceived exertion, 131
    peripheral vascular disease, 134
    psychiatric patients, 134
    target heart rate, 131
  range of motion exercises, 127–128
  reimbursement, 137–138
  strength training
    open-chain versus closed-chain exercises, 129
    protocols, 129–130
Tibial nerve, perineural injection block at knee, 252–253
TMS. *See* Transcranial magnetic stimulation
Toileting, assistive devices, 264, 271
Traction. *See* Spinal traction
Transcranial magnetic stimulation (TMS), overview, 96
Transcutaneous electrical nerve stimulation (TENS)
  contraindications, 107
  costs, 115
  indications
    angina, 111
    gastroenterology, 112
    interstitial cystitis, 110
    low back pain, 108–109
    neuropathic pain, 110–111
    obstetrics and gynecology, 109–110
    pediatrics, 111
    postoperative pain, 108, 111
  physiology of action, 103–107

TENS (continued)
  stimulation parameters
    frequency, 104, 106, 107
    intensity, 106–107
Traumatic brain injury, assistive devices, 262, 268, 272
Trigger finger, corticosteroid injection, 258

Ulnar nerve, perineural injection block at elbow, 250–251
Ultrasound. *See also* Phonophoresis
  absorption, 19
  attenuation, 19
  beam nonuniformity ratio, 20
  continuous versus pulsed waves, 19
  contraindications, 24–25
  controversies, 30
  definition, 19
  depth of penetration, 30
  duty cycle, 19
  effective radiating area, 20
  healing facilitation studies, 25–27
  indications, 23–24
  intensity, 19–21
  joint contracture treatment, 27
  medical applications, 18
  nonthermal effects, 2, 23
  overview of deep heating, 2, 18
  piezoelectric effect, 21
  scattering, 19
  sonication frequency, 19
  techniques and parmeters for delivery, 27–30
  thermal effects, 2, 22–23
  variables, 21
Ultraviolet therapy, **77–85**
  application tetchniques, 80–81
  beneficial effects, 80
  classification of light, 79
  dosing parameters, 81–82
  equipment, 82
  exposure types, 81–82
  historical background, 77
  indications
    acne vulgaris, 84
    neonatal jaundice, 84
    overview, 83
    psoriasis, 83–84
  monitoring of dose, 81
  photobiologic effects, 79
  physics, 77–79
  precautions, 82–83
Urinary incontinence, biofeedback, 222–223

Vapocoolant spray, cryotherapy, 47, 49, 52–53

Walker. *See* Ambulatory assistive devices

Water
   buoyancy, 56
   density, 56
   drag, 57
   flow, 57
   hydrostatic pressure, 56–57
   specific gravity, 56
   specific heat capacity, 57
Watsu. *See* Aquatic therapy

Wheelchair
   designs, 295–297
   prescription, 297
   size, 297–298
Wheelchair ramp, assistive devices, 274–275
Whirlpool bath. *See* Hydrotherapy
Wrist
   intra-articular injections, 247–248
   joint mobilization, 188